Principles and Techniques of Patient Care

Principles and Techniques of Patient Care

Second Edition

Frank M. Pierson, M.A., P.T.

Assistant Professor Emeritus
The Ohio State University
Columbus, Ohio

W.B. SAUNDERS COMPANY
A Division of Harcourt Brace & Company
Philadelphia ■ London ■ Toronto ■ Montreal ■ Sydney ■ Tokyo

W.B. SAUNDERS COMPANY
A Division of Harcourt Brace & Company

The Curtis Center
Independence Square West
Philadelphia, Pennsylvania 19106

Library of Congress Cataloging-in-Publication Data

Pierson, Frank M.

Principles and techniques of patient care / Frank M. Pierson.—
2nd ed.

   p.   cm.

Includes bibliographical references and index.

ISBN 0–7216–7524–7

1. Physical therapy—Technique.   I. Title.
    [DNLM: 1. Physical Therapy—methods.   2. Patient Care Planning.
    WB 460 P624p 1999]

RM700.P545 1999   615.8'2—dc21

DNLM/DLC   98–5492

Principles and Techniques of Patient Care   ISBN 0–7216–7524–7

Printed in the United States of America

Last digit is the print number: 9   8   7   6   5   4   3   2

The decision of W.B. Saunders Company to request the development of a second edition of this book and the level of acceptance of the first edition by many students, faculty, and practitioners has been very gratifying. During the past three years several suggestions and comments about ways to improve the book have been received and reviewed carefully. Although not all the recommendations were incorporated into this edition, many of them have been used to increase the amount of material in it and to make the book easier for faculty and students to use.

The first chapter was revised to include more information about communicating with a person with a disability and about the process of informed consent. Greater emphasis was placed on the development of functional goals (outcomes) and the use of goal statements in the documentation of patient care. Also, the relationship of goals and functional outcomes has been tied more closely to the treatment planning process.

The chapter on "Vital Signs" was repositioned toward the beginning of the book to emphasize the importance of evaluating a patient prior to initiating treatment or physical activity. Information about and some techniques used to measure a person's body composition were added to this chapter.

Photographs of types of special equipment used for patients in an intensive care unit, including ventilation and intravenous infusion equipment and patient monitors, appear in Chapter 9. Supplemental information about selected reference laboratory values is also provided in this chapter.

More information about the management of nonsurgical wounds, particularly of pressure ulcers, including preventive measures, has been added to Chapter 10. This chapter also contains information about the use of an intermittent compression unit and the measurement and application of graduated compression garments for the upper and lower extremities. The material related to the general use of bandages, previously contained in this chapter, has been relocated to Chapter 11, which seems a more appropriate location.

A new chapter containing information about the Americans with Disabilities Act was developed to assist the reader to become aware of the more significant aspects of the act.

Overall, readers will notice a greater use of procedure outlines, boxes, and tables and the addition of directional arrows on many photographs to enhance their understanding and comprehension of many techniques or activities. Finally, new photographs appear in several chapters, and some previous photographs have been replaced to clarify or better depict specific procedures, equipment, or activities.

It is hoped that the additions and revisions presented in this edition will add to the value of the book as a teaching and learning tool for all readers.

Acknowledgments

Many persons, organizations, facilities, and institutions provided assistance and support in the development of this edition. My appreciation and gratitude are extended to the following:

Cynthia (Cindy) Pomeroy, for her time and efforts to prepare a print copy of the new material and revisions contained in this edition.

Peg Waltner, Developmental Editor, for her encouragement, constructive suggestions, and editorial recommendations.

Jenny Torbett, senior medical photographer, and Theron Ellinger, medical photographer, for their photographic skills and the quality of their photographs.

Those who served as subjects or who participated in the photographs: Larry Mengelkoch; John and Sarah Chidley; Kenneth Sims; S.L. Bellas, RN; Rae Ann Anderson, PT; Brenda Applegate, PT; Bobbi Lou Bates, PT; Diane Barrick, PT; Laura Collins; Ashley Hartlaub; Ashley Dye; Peter Cameruca; Chandler Daily; Megan Newsome; Ashley Bennett; Theron Ellinger; and Victor Davis.

Ronald Scott, JD, PT; Professional Education Systems, Eau Claire, WI; and KCI, San Antonio, TX, for granting permission to include information or photographs that originated from them.

The several reviewers of the additions and revisions of this edition, whose suggestions and comments were very helpful.

The Surgical Intensive Care Unit, Ohio State University Hospitals, Columbus, Ohio; The Easter Seal Society of Central Ohio; and the Physical Therapy Division and the Bio-Medical Communications Services, School of Allied Medical Professions, The Ohio State University, for providing access to facilities and equipment.

ADA-Ohio, Columbus, OH; Meacham and Apel Architects, Inc., Dublin, OH; the Central Ohio Transit Authority, Columbus, OH; and the President's Committee on Employment of People with Disabilities, Washington, DC, for material and access to transportation vehicles associated with the Americans with Disabilities Act.

Christa Fratantoro, Editorial Assistant; Andrew M. Allen, Editor-in-Chief; Frank Polizzano, Production Manager; and the other staff and departments of W.B. Saunders Company for their excellent support and assistance during the development of this edition.

Contents

Introduction to Patient Care Activities

OBJECTIVES

After studying this chapter, the reader will be able to:

1 Describe a process for the general evaluation of a patient.

2 List the four components of a problem-oriented status note.

3 Identify information that would be classified as "subjective" and information that would be classified as "objective."

4 Describe how subjective and objective information could be obtained through an evaluation.

5 Identify the major components or categories of the evaluation process.

6 Discuss the importance of evaluating each patient before establishing a treatment program.

7 Describe the major components or categories of the program planning process.

8 List five barriers to communications and describe how you would overcome them.

9 Describe five guidelines to use to communicate with a person with a disability.

10 Describe the major components or categories of a written home program.

■■■ **K E Y T E R M S**

Caregiver: The person who is treating or working with the patient; examples are the therapist, therapist assistant, aide, or family member.

Communication: The exchange of information through verbal or nonverbal means.

Documentation: Written or printed matter conveying authoritative information, records, or evidence.

Electrodiagnosis: The use of an electrical current to assist with the diagnosis of a patient's condition.

Goniometry: The measurement of the range of motion of a joint of the body.

Kinesthesia: The sense by which position, weight, and movement are perceived.

Orthosis: An orthopedic appliance used to support, align, prevent, or correct deformities or to replace the function of parts of the body; a brace or splint is an example of an orthosis.

Outcome measure: A quantifiable or objective means to determine the effectiveness of treatment or performance that is usually expressed with the use of functional terms.

Problem-oriented medical record (POMR): A system developed to organize a medical record that uses a common list of patient problems as its base.

Proprioception: Perception mediated by proprioceptors or proprioceptive testing; sensation and awareness about the movements and position of body parts or the body.

Prosthesis: The artificial replacement of an absent body part; an artificial limb is an example of a prosthesis.

Radiograph: An image or a record produced on exposed or processed film through radiography.

SOAP: An acronym whose letters identify each section of a patient's status note: S, subjective; O, objective; A, assessment; P, plan.

Stereognosis: The ability to recognize the form (shape) of an object by touch.

Two-point discrimination: The ability to recognize or differentiate two blunt points when they are simultaneously applied to the skin.

INTRODUCTION

This book has been prepared to assist persons responsible for and involved with patient care in providing safe and effective care. The term *caregiver,* rather than therapist, nurse, health care practitioner, therapist assistant, technologist, technician, aide, or family member, will be used to designate the person who is treating or working with the patient or client. It is recognized the term client is sometimes more appropriate to describe a person who receives treatment. Furthermore, the term consumer may be used to describe the receiver of care. However, for consistency, the term patient is used throughout this text to describe the person who receives treatment. Similarly, the term intervention may be used rather than the term treatment, but for consistency, the term treatment is used in this text. The procedures and techniques contained in the text were selected because they can be applied or adapted for use for a variety of patients to assist them to fulfill their functional needs or goals. The knowledgeable and experienced practitioner will realize there are alternative techniques or procedures that provide safe and effective ways to perform many of the patient activities described in the text. However, it was necessary to select and describe a limited number of activities and procedures.

It is anticipated and expected that the health care practitioner or caregiver will modify or adjust any technique or procedure to benefit the patient or better suit a specific situation or environment. The safety of the patient and the persons involved with his/her care must be maintained at all times. The patient should be encouraged to perform to his/her maximal ability whenever his/her active involvement is desired.

The caregiver will need to guide, direct, and instruct each patient. For many patients a brief demonstration of an activity or the use of equipment by the caregiver or another patient will enable him/her to understand his/her role better. Verbal, nonverbal, and written communication between the caregiver and the patient and his/her family members will be necessary. The purpose of each activity, its expected outcome, and the method of performance should be explained to the patient.

No activity should be attempted unless sufficient personnel and equipment are available to accomplish the task safely. All persons who assist with the patient's care must be trained and competent; the equipment must function properly and be safe and stable; and the patient must be evaluated to determine his/her capacity to assist with or perform a particular activity.

Patient evaluation, communication between the caregiver and the patient, and patient safety are required to promote quality patient care. Lack of attention to any one of these areas will usually adversely affect the quality of care the patient receives.

INTERPROFESSIONAL COLLABORATION

A team of caregivers from different professions who review a patient's condition, determine his/her problems amenable to treatment, discuss potential treatment solutions, and make decisions to resolve his/her problems is used by many organizations. This interprofessional collaboration approach is particularly useful for the patient with complex medical, social, economic, or other problems. To be successful, interprofessional collaboration requires the team members to meet collectively and periodically to problem solve and reach decisions about management of the patient. Collaboration, coordination, and communication are the important factors used by the team to assist the patient to effectively fulfill his/her goals or needs. The interprofessional team members must be competent professionals who are willing to function interdependently to maximally benefit the patient. Team members must be prepared to recognize and accept the value of other members' professional knowledge, skills, and expertise; work through role conflicts that may develop due to overlapping roles of the members; understand the basic components of each member's profession; be able to communicate effectively with each other; and participate in leadership. The interprofessional team approach must be patient centered, rather than profession centered, so team members must be able to provide advice, counsel, and recommendations based on each member's knowledge and expertise that will lead to the best outcome for the patient. Group members need to be adept in the application of group process skills; therefore, it is recommended a portion of their formal education be devoted to an introduction to and practice of techniques, skills, and activities associated with group interaction. Furthermore, the opportunity to collaborate with students from various professional programs (i.e., medicine, social work, nursing, law, theology, allied health professions) to discuss and resolve complex case study patient scenarios would be beneficial in preparation for future interprofessional team collaboration. Table 1–1 presents rationales for the support of and opposition to the use of interprofessional collaboration from the perspective of the patient and the participating professional.

ORIENTATION

Before providing any form of treatment, including an evaluation, the caregiver must initially orient the patient. This orientation consists of a personal in-

Table 1–1 INTERPROFESSIONAL COLLABORATION	
Rationale for Client/Patient	**Rationale Against Client/Patient**
1. Comprehensive approach	1. Process may overwhelm the patient
2. Reduction in duplication or fragmentation of professional services and activities	2. May not produce better quality care
3. Team is better able to address complex problems	3. May not result in best decisions due to professional role conflicts
4. Team decision making is better due to input from different professionals	4. Apt to be more costly (time, money, effort)
5. Results in interventions for complex problems that exceed what an individual could accomplish	5. May reduce the one-on-one relationship between the patient and individual professionals
Rationale for Professional	**Rationale Against Professional**
1. Opportunity for members to better understand the skills, expertise, and roles of other professionals	1. May have personal and professional identity reduced; may lose professional autonomy
2. Opportunity for members to become more aware of and effective in own professional role and application of professional expertise and knowledge	2. Reduces personal decision making
3. Enhances ability and provides opportunity to network and refer to other professionals	3. Takes time away from other patients; is time-consuming process
4. Broadens interaction with other professionals; leads to professional development	4. Causes separation from professionals, peers, and colleagues
	5. Interprofessional collaboration may not be a value of the profession; professional becomes reluctant to participate

troduction; informing the patient of the treatment goals, expected outcome, and potential risks; interviewing the patient (as part of the evaluation) to obtain information; instructing the patient regarding his/her participation; and initiation of the treatment or evaluation.

In a treatment setting, the caregiver should greet and identify the patient, state his/her own name clearly, and indicate his/her professional or technical status. The patient should be informed why he/she has been referred to the service unit, the type of treatment he/she will receive, and any potentially serious risks or adverse effects associated with the proposed treatment. At this time the patient should have the opportunity to ask questions, obtain additional information, and agree to or decline treatment. During the interview the caregiver should confirm the patient's name and diagnosis and then progress to the remainder of the evaluation. After the patient interview and evalua-

---

P R O C E D U R E   1 – 1
Orientation of the Patient

1. Introduce yourself by name <u>and</u> title or professional designation.
2. Verify or confirm patient information you have received such as his/her name, diagnosis, purpose of treatment, and referral source.
3. Interview the patient to obtain relevant information about him/her as part of the evaluation process.
4. Perform additional evaluation activities to establish the patient's capabilities, condition, problems, needs, and goals.
5. Inform the patient of the treatment plan and techniques selected to fulfill outcome goals; include information about potential risks or adverse effects associated with the treatment.
6. Encourage the patient to ask questions to obtain information to enable him/her to consent to or decline treatment.
7. Request that the patient sign an informed consent document or record his/her verbal consent in the medical record.

---

tion, the caregiver should instruct the patient more specifically about the treatment and the patient's role or expected level of performance. The last step in the process is the initiation of the treatment session. During subsequent treatment sessions, several of the steps can be eliminated or modified as the patient becomes more familiar with the treatment process. However, the caregiver should always discuss each treatment activity with the patient and instruct or guide his/her performance (Procedure 1–1).

INFORMED CONSENT

Before the initial treatment of a patient, the caregiver has the responsibility to inform the person about the proposed treatment, some of the alternative treatments available, and associated primary, known risks. The patient then has the right to consent to or reject the proposed treatment. This is the process of informed consent.

To ensure the patient is properly informed, the caregiver must provide sufficient information about the proposed treatment and alternative treatment, appropriate for the person's condition, to permit him/her to arrive at an intelligent and knowledgeable decision. The patient must be able to understand the information, so it must be presented with the use of terms and in a language he/she can comprehend. A translator or an interpreter may be required for persons who do not speak or comprehend English.

Known or potential primary risks associated with the treatment should be explained, and he/she should have an opportunity to ask questions, and receive responses to them, about any aspect of the proposed treatment. The caregiver should provide responses that are within his/her level of knowledge, training, and competence and based on expected or anticipated results or outcomes. The caregiver should not state or imply that certain results or outcomes will occur, and he/she should not offer any indication to guarantee that specific results or outcomes will be attained.

If the patient has not reached the legal age of consent or has been judged to be mentally confused or incompetent to participate in the informed consent decision-making process, it probably will be necessary to obtain consent from a legally qualified surrogate, such as a parent, guardian, family member, or court-appointed advocate.

The caregiver should document that he/she applied the process of informed consent in accordance with pre-established, written policies and procedures of the service unit or agency with which the caregiver is associated (i.e., hospital department, school system, home health agency, outpatient facility, skilled nursing facility, or subacute care facility). In some situations, it may be prudent to have the patient, or his/her surrogate, sign a document to indicate he/she has been informed of the proposed treatment and consent to the treatment is authorized. The caregiver will need to use his/her judgment and follow the recommendations of the facility or agency, risk manager, or legal counsel to

BOX 1–1

Elements of the Informed Consent Process

Description of the patient's condition, diagnosis, or evaluative data and information

Description or outline of the proposed, recommended treatment plan, techniques, or procedures

Primary, known, anticipated, or potential risks; complications; and precautions associated with the proposed treatment

Expected prognosis or outcome of the proposed treatment without a stated or implied guarantee of results (i.e., decrease or absence of pain, specific functional improvement, specific flexibility or strength gain)

Alternative forms of treatment appropriate for the person's condition with potential risks, complications, and precautions and the expected prognosis of the alternative treatment

Questions from the patient and responses from the caregiver that are thorough and honest; if you are unsure of or do not know the response to a question, indicate that to the patient but attempt to locate the information or refer the patient to a qualified resource (i.e., nurse, physician, social worker, pharmacist)

Explain the potential or possible consequence of no treatment if the patient refuses or rejects treatment

Document you provided the patient with the opportunity for informed consent before initiation of treatment and his/her decision to consent to or refuse treatment

PRINCIPLES OF DOCUMENTATION

The *documentation* of patient care is an important component of the written record maintained for each patient. Documentation is performed by physicians, nurses, therapists, social workers, and many other persons involved with providing patient care. Lawrence Weed developed the concept of the *problem-oriented medical record (POMR)* in the 1960s. This system has been accepted for use by many health care facilities throughout the United States, some of which have developed their own variations. This system is based on a list of patient problems, a database, and a series of status (progress) notes designated as the "initial," "interim," and "discharge" notes. When all departments or service units of a given facility use the POMR approach to record keeping, a higher quality of patient care may be anticipated, better communication between and among the caregivers is more likely to occur, and better decisions about the patient's treatment can be made. Information about the patient and his/her plan of care is contained in the status notes, which are written in the following format: subjective, objective, assessment, and plan information, or *SOAP.*

POMR DESCRIPTION

The POMR has four phases: formation of a database (current and past information about the patient); development of a specific, current problem list (problems to be treated by various practitioners); identification of a specific treatment plan (developed by each caregiver); and assessment of the effectiveness of the treatment plans. When the POMR system is used, each practitioner relates his/her evaluation, treatment planning, and treatment decision making to the patient's database and problem list.

The SOAP notes should contain important, relevant information about the patient; they should indicate and clearly reflect the patient's condition and subsequent changes in his/her condition; and they should be written periodically and frequently so information is reported promptly and regularly. The method used to gather the information and the development of the assessment and planning phases are described in the section related to the evaluation process. The relationship of the SOAP notes to the decision-making process and the purposes of documentations are described in several articles and textbooks. Excellent resources for information about the POMR and SOAP notes are listed in the Bibliography.

Some suggestions of ways to improve the quality and meaningfulness of documentation are listed in Box 1–2.

determine whether each patient should be required to sign an informed consent authorization for treatment. If signed documents are not used, policies and procedures of the facility or agency must be specific and clearly indicate the process each caregiver is to use when discussing informed consent decisions with the patient. Failure by the caregiver to fully inform a patient about the proposed treatment before the initiation of treatment and obtain his/her consent to receive treatment can, in some situations, constitute professional negligence. Informed consent is a right to which each patient is entitled; therefore, the caregiver has the obligation to inform the patient of the proposed treatment, its alternatives, and its foreseeable risks before initiation of treatment (Box 1–1).

BOX 1–2

Ways to Improve Documentation

1. Avoid general statements and provide specific, clarifying information. Instead of stating "The patient is uncooperative," state in what manner he/she is uncooperative: "Patient refused to perform active assistive exercise."

2. Use objective statements. Instead of stating "Patient ambulates," state "Patient ambulates 25 feet in 1 minute using bilateral axillary crutches on a level surface, with assistance, using a three-point pattern for three repetitions, with a 5-minute rest period between ambulations." Functional *outcome* measure statements will more accurately describe the patient's condition and assist with obtaining reimbursement for the services provided.

3. Be complete with your statements; record the significant or important information about the patient's condition, progress, or response to treatment. Remember: If an activity is not documented, it may be considered as not having occurred. If an unusual activity or procedure is used, document why it was selected and used. Unusual incidents and the action taken after the incident should be recorded. An objective description of the patient's condition or reaction after the incident should be recorded. An incident report should be filed with the risk manager or similar individual, but there is no need to document that it was prepared and filed.

4. Provide continuity with your status (i.e., progress) notes; be certain to indicate why or how you reached a particular decision about the care or treatment you provided, particularly if it deviated from the usual, acceptable care or treatment. Programs or treatment plans designed for the patient to follow at home should be well documented and should include precautions. Your documentation should indicate how you determined (or the steps taken to ensure) that the patient or family member understood and could comply with the instructions.

5. Identify that you informed the patient of the treatment he/she was to receive and its potential risks or hazards; that this information was understood by the patient; and that he/she consented to the treatment. If a consent form was used by the service unit, a copy signed by the patient should be in the medical record.

6. Be prompt and timely with your entries and be certain your writing is legible, including your signature and professional or staff designation; be certain the information is accurate and there is consistency between entries; investigate and clarify contradictory information. For example, is it the right hip or the left hip that requires treatment?

7. Use abbreviations that have been standardized or accepted and approved by the facility or the profession.

8. Be certain there are no empty or open lines between entries and that there are no open spaces within the notes; use the format approved by the human information systems department or used by the facility or profession.

9. Outline the major elements of the notes in your mind or on paper before you enter it in the record to avoid having to make a correction or a change in the notes. Avoid omissions, such as the date of initial or subsequent treatments, a change in treatment, or a discharge summary.

10. Properly countersign the entries of other persons according to state statutes and facility requirements; read the entry before countersigning it. In many cases it will be prudent to review the proposed entry before it is placed in the record to be certain it is accurate and complete.

ENTRY CORRECTIONS

Occasionally it may be necessary to correct an entry. Careful and proper correction of an entry will help to avoid accusations of tampering, changing the entry for self-serving reasons or intent, or capricious alteration of the medical record, especially if litigation is involved or being considered. Standard procedures should be followed when correcting a note:

1. Draw a single line through the inaccurate information, but be certain the material remains legible.
2. Date and initial the correction, and add a note in the margin stating why the correction was necessary.
3. Enter the corrected statement in the chronologic sequence of the record, and be certain it is clear which entry the correction replaces.

In some situations it may be beneficial to have the corrected statement witnessed by a colleague. Avoid alterations that create the appearance of tampering (e.g., erasing or writing over a word or phrase to improve legibility). Never attempt to obliterate material in the record by using a felt marker, correction fluid, a typewriter overstrike, or an eraser. Improper alteration of an entry can create many problems for the practitioner if the entry is questioned or used as evidence during litigation. The practitioner's credibility, honesty, and intent will be challenged, which may lead to charges of incompetence, negligent behavior, or poor judgment. Many errors of judgment are not negligent acts, but any attempt to hide them can create serious problems for the practitioner. Never enter a note or sign an entry for someone else, and do not ask someone else to perform such acts for you. During litigation or when questions arise about the patient's care, the medical record is the primary source of information about the care a patient received and his/her response to treatment; therefore, accurate, timely, and proper documentation is important. Failure to maintain proper documentation and records can delay or cause denial of reimbursement, lead to dismissal or disciplinary action against the practitioner, affect the accreditation status of the facility, weaken the defense of the defendant during litigation, or cause improper or poor quality treatment to be delivered. A basic principle to follow is this: maintain the record so if all the persons who were originally treating a patient were to disappear suddenly, the next group of practitioners could immediately continue to provide the best quality treatment by using only the information from the record.

Documentation is becoming more and more important as a means to assess or measure the quality of care received by the patient so the caregiver or facility will be more likely to receive payment from a third-party payer (e.g., Medicare or an insurance company).

When a caregiver documents the treatment he/she has provided or supervised, it is necessary to indicate the functional outcome or outcomes attained by the patient. Through the use of objective and measurable terms, language, or data, the documentation must report the extent of change in the patient's condition that resulted from the treatment. The results of initial and repeated muscle strength tests, *goniometric* measurements, and vital signs data are examples of objective, measurable information. However, it is also necessary to provide objective information that indicates the patient's ability or capacity to perform functional activities that are related to his/her activities in the home, workplace, and community and during recreation. Strength and range-of-motion data could be linked to the person's functional ability to perform dressing, feeding, and personal hygiene tasks at home; reaching, lifting, and carrying objects or use of office equipment at work; transfer and mobility activities in the community; and various sport or recreational activities. The reader is encouraged to propose other examples that would associate treatment techniques with functional outcomes. The caregiver should be certain the functional outcomes relate directly to the pre-established treatment goals or outcome measures stated in the treatment plan.

Persons who review claims and make reimbursement- and treatment-related decisions have focused on indicators of functional outcomes of treatment contained in the caregiver's documentation. This process can be expected to continue; therefore, the caregiver must be aware of the need to provide accurate, current function-oriented documentation. In addition, the use of function-oriented, objective, and measurable data in the documentation process will result in the greatest likelihood of obtaining a favorable reimbursement response to submitted claims and gaining approval to continue treatment from the third party payer. Furthermore, it seems reasonable to anticipate that a patient will have more motivation to accomplish a functional goal or task that is meaningful to him/her than to strive to attain a given strength or range-of-motion value. In addition, well-organized, accurate, relevant, and prompt documentation improves communication among the persons providing care.

PRINCIPLES OF TREATMENT PLANNING

Before the initial treatment of a patient, the caregiver must establish an organized, preplanned treatment approach and process. A four-step process can be used: (1) evaluate the patient, (2) develop a treatment program, (3) implement the program and re-evaluate the program frequently, and (4) terminate the program.

Information about the evaluation phase is presented in the next section of this chapter; however, it is important to understand the evaluation establishes a baseline of data and information to measure the patient's progress and response to treatment. The evaluation assists in establishing a functional diagnosis for the patient, setting outcome goals, and developing the treatment plan and program. Goals of treatment should be established cooperatively by the patient and caregiver once the patient has been informed of the various approaches available or possible for his/her care. These goals are usually designated as interim, or short-term, and terminal, or long-term, goals. Short-term goals are usually a specific component or lead-in activity for a long-term goal. An example of a short-term goal is the patient will be able to perform a sitting push-up in a wheelchair 10 times in 1 minute within 2 weeks. This would be a lead-in goal for the long-term goal of the patient being able to perform an independent sitting transfer from his/her bed to a wheelchair within 2 minutes and then return to the bed in 2 minutes within 4 weeks. These goals must be stated in objective, measurable terms and should indicate who will perform the activity, by what means the goal will be accomplished, the need for equipment or assistance, the time frame in which to accomplish the goal, and the functional outcome expected. Goals can and should be revised or modified depending on the patient's performance and progress. Finally, goals should be realistic and attainable for each patient.

The treatment plan and program developed by the caregiver should contain treatment procedures, techniques, and activities that will have the greatest effectiveness to fulfill the previously established goals and outcome measures. The sequence and frequency of the program must be determined, as well as the need for equipment and level of assistance required by the patient. Consideration should be given at this time to planning for the termination of treatment. Due to the cost-containment requirements of most third party payers, many patients will receive only a few treatment sessions from a qualified caregiver; therefore, the caregiver must begin planning a program for extended treatment activities after the patient's formal treatment program is terminated. Equipment needs, financial assistance, family education and training, referral procedures, and follow-up or extended care may need to be considered as alternate treatment plans are developed.

Implementation of the procedures, techniques, and activities selected by the caregiver should be performed using the sequence and frequency determined previously. The caregiver must frequently and consistently re-evaluate and measure the patient's progress and response to treatment. The extent to which the patient fulfills the short- and long-term goals and accomplishes the functional outcomes must be measured and documented. It is not sufficient, for example, to document a patient's active range of motion of shoulder flexion has increased from 90 to 120 degrees. Reporting a functional outcome, such as the independent application and removal of clothing over the head, should be a component of the documentation. The caregiver must be prepared to continue, revise, or modify the treatment plan or the individual components of the treatment program based on the patient's progress and response to the treatment. During this phase, greater attention will need to be given to the plan and program for extended treatment if it is determined extended treatment will be necessary. Education and training of the patient and a family member should be provided, as well as the opportunity to practice activities to be performed at home.

When the treatment program is to be terminated, the caregiver should evaluate and measure the patient's functional outcomes and compare them with the expected outcomes, and the extended treatment program should be reviewed and finalized. The written or printed program should be given to the patient or family member, and a copy should be placed in the medical record or maintained in a separate file.

A summary of the patient's condition and the functional outcomes and goals he/she has accomplished, future treatment plans, and any re-evaluation or follow-up care appointments should be documented in the medical record.

Additional information about the treatment planning process (Procedure 1–2) can be found in several of the resources listed in the Bibliography.

PRINCIPLES OF PATIENT EVALUATION

Patient evaluation guidelines are given in Box 1–3. In addition to these, the evaluation should consider the patient's emotional response to his/her condition, family unit interactions and the support system available to the patient, potential for improvement or regression of the patient's condition, and goals or expectations the patient has for the treatment program. The patient should be informed of the findings or results of the evaluation, and he/she should be consulted about and assist with the development of the goals for treatment.

The material in Box 1–3 is intended as a guide to the general areas that should be considered for an evaluation before initiation of treatment. Not all of the activities will be necessary or appropriate for every pa-

PROCEDURE 1 – 2
Treatment Planning Process

1. Patient evaluation
   a. Determine his/her present condition, including functional abilities and limitations
   b. Establish a functional diagnosis and outcome goals
   c. Gather data and information to use to develop a treatment plan and program
   d. Gather data and information for documentation

2. Develop treatment program
   a. Based on outcome goals related to function
   b. Determine and select appropriate treatment activities, techniques, procedures, and equipment
   c. Determine the sequence and frequency of the treatment methods
   d. Initiate planning for extended treatment, after formal treatment is terminated, as necessary
   e. Prepare and document the treatment plan and program

3. Implement treatment program
   a. Techniques, activities, and procedures performed or applied according to the predetermined sequence and frequency and the equipment used
   b. Patient's response to treatment is evaluated frequently and consistently; progress toward accomplishment of functional outcomes is determined
   c. The program is revised or modified depending on patient progress or response to treatment
   d. Planning for termination of treatment is intensified; patient/family member receives instruction, if necessary, for extended treatment program
   e. Patient's progress or performance is documented and linked to functional outcomes

4. Termination of treatment
   a. Patient's condition and functional abilities are assessed; the need for extended treatment is determined
   b. Patient/family member practices activities for additional treatment program as necessary
   c. Written extended treatment program (home program) is prepared and given to patient/family member
   d. Patient's condition and functional outcome abilities are documented; the date for re-evaluation or follow-up care is established and documented

tient, and selection of the most appropriate tests or procedures is the responsibility of the practitioner. In many instances a specific evaluation will be required to obtain the information or data necessary to develop the best treatment program for the patient. Remember that frequent re-evaluation of the patient is an important part of the evaluation and treatment process; without re-evaluation, the patient's response to treat-

ment or his/her change in function or achievement of the treatment goals or objectives cannot be identified. This information is necessary to maintain the most beneficial treatment plan and to enhance quality care.

The patient assessment or evaluation is used to identify the problems to be overcome, abilities of the patient, and patient's needs and goals. The development of a treatment program should include estab-

BOX 1-3

Guidelines for Patient Evaluation

Subjective Information

Subjective information can be obtained through interviews with the patient, family members, friends, or other practitioners and by reading the medical record. Effective listening skills and interview techniques by the evaluator are necessary to obtain the most beneficial information. The following information should be elicited:

1. Patient's concept of his/her primary complaint or problem.
2. Patient's description of the progression or regression of his/her condition (e.g., better, worse, or unchanged) over a period of time.
3. General health of the patient.
4. Any previous history of any similar condition, complaint, or problem.
5. Patient's description of the primary cause of his/her condition, complaint, or problem.
6. The patient's description of the results of any previous treatment for a similar condition, complaint, or problem.
7. The patient's occupation, lifestyle, recreational activities, social interactions, goals, needs, and values.

Objective Information

Objective information can be obtained with observation, palpation, and specific tests.

 I. Observe the patient's
  A. General appearance, body build, or configuration and any deformities or absence of any body part.
  B. Posture as he/she stands, sits, and walks.
  C. Skin condition and its appearance (i.e., color, lesions, or scars).
  D. Locomotion or mobility activities: these could include ambulation; use of a wheelchair; functional abilities, such as reaching, bending, or a change in position; and his/her level of performance (i.e., dependent, semidependent, or independent).
  E. Use of assistive devices, ambulation aids, *orthoses*, *prostheses*, bandages, slings, or casts.
  F. Balance and stability while he/she sits, stands, and ambulates.
  G. Coordination and motor control in his/her extremities and total body.
 II. Palpate the patient's
  A. Skin and subcutaneous tissue to determine its texture, temperature, flexibility, and pain response.
  B. Muscles, tendons, and ligaments for their tone, pain response, bulk, composition, strength, and stability/laxity.
  C. Joints to determine any swelling, change in shape, tenderness, amount of joint space, and pain response.
  D. Skeletal components, such as bone surfaces, bone ends, and specific landmarks.
  E. Arterial pulses to establish their rate, force, presence/absence, and rhythm.
III. Assess the patient's
  A. Muscle strength by performing a muscle test either manually or mechanically.
  B. Joint motion, both active and passive, by performing goniometric measurements.

BOX 1–3

Guidelines for Patient Evaluation—*Continued*

Objective Information—*Continued*

   C. Sensory mechanisms, including
      1. Protective reactions to pain, temperature, and touch.
      2. Discriminative reactions to pressure, *kinesthesia, proprioception*, response to textures, *stereognosis*, and *two-point discrimination*.
      3. Reflexes, including those related to stretch, posture, and "righting," or equilibrium.
      4. Automatic reactions, such as synergies or other movement patterns.
 IV. Assess functional activities and abilities, including
      A. Ambulation, by observing the patient's gait pattern and any gait deviations.
      B. The patient's ability to transfer and to change position.
      C. The patient's ability to perform personal care and hygiene.
      D. The patient's mental status and cognitive abilities.
      E. The patient's ability to apply, remove, and use assistive devices.
      F. The patient's communication abilities.
      G. The patient's mobility, other than ambulation.
  V. Evaluate cardiopulmonary function by
      A. Measuring the patient's vital signs, including the heart rate, respiration rate, and blood pressure at rest and during and after activity.
      B. Reviewing the results of exertion tests or electrocardiographic data.
 VI. Consider special tests, such as
      A. *Radiography*.
      B. Laboratory tests.
      C. *Electrodiagnosis*.
      D. Biopsy.
      E. Tests performed by other practitioners, such as speech, hearing, sensory integration, and psychological tests

lishing objective and measurable goals, which are usually related to functional tasks or abilities and are identified as outcome measures. Implementation of the treatment program requires the application of specific techniques, procedures, or activities that have been selected to accomplish the pre-established objectives and goals. Finally, re-evaluation of the patient is necessary to determine his/her response to treatment; identify the need to modify, alter, or revise the treatment program; and measure the extent to which treatment objectives and goals have been accomplished (Box 1–4).

The caregiver must be vigilant and consciously re-evaluate the patient frequently to provide quality care. Failure to adjust or revise the treatment program, based on the patient's response to the current program, will delay the patient's recovery of or limit the extent of his/her recovery of functional independence.

To summarize the evaluation process, remember that it is necessary to include evaluation as a primary component of the treatment planning and implementation process, to provide a solid base for all patient care.

PATIENT/FAMILY EDUCATION

Currently the public is exhibiting a greater interest in and desire to become better informed about medical/health care in general and about the specific medical/health care that individuals receive. Patients and family members expect to be consulted and informed about the care they receive. Questions related to the need for, efficacy of, and expected results or outcome of treatment are routinely asked by patients and family members. The practitioner must be prepared to provide appropriate and accurate responses without expressing or implying a guarantee or promise that a specific outcome or result will be achieved. The patient must be informed, with language and terminology he/she can understand, about the treatment he/she is to receive so he/she can make an informed decision about its value and safety.

The caregiver has the responsibility to educate the patient and family about the treatment program and activities, but he/she must respect patient confi-

---

BOX 1–4

Principles of Patient Evaluation

1. Establish a baseline of the patient's condition and functional status.
2. Provide data and information to develop the treatment plan and program.
3. Provide data and information to measure the patient's progress and response to treatment.
4. Provide data and information to determine need to revise or modify current treatment plan and program.
5. Provide data and information to determine need to revise or modify goals or functional outcomes.
6. Measure the patient's attainment of goals or functional outcomes.
7. Provide data and information to be used by others.
8. Perform before initial treatment and frequently and consistently as treatment continues.

---

he/she is required to provide. The patient and family member should practice the specific activities included in the home program while the caregiver observes and corrects improper performance. The home program should be printed or written and given to the patient for future reference. A copy is maintained with the patient's medical record or documentation materials at the treatment facility.

Instructions should include an outline of the exercises or activities to be performed, frequency of performance of the program, number of repetitions for each exercise, precautions or contraindications for each exercise, required equipment or supplies, specific instructions and diagrams to guide and direct the patient, therapist's name and telephone number so he/she can be contacted, and information regarding any scheduled re-evaluation or reappointment sessions (Procedure 1–3).

Frequently, the caregiver is the primary liaison between the patient and his/her family and other practitioners; therefore, the caregiver has the responsibility to educate all persons involved about the treatment program and its anticipated or projected outcomes. Information about the health care delivery system may need to be provided to assist the patient or family

dentiality and have the patient's permission before sharing information with the family. Goals of treatment should be established cooperatively by the patient and caregiver once the patient has been informed of the various possibilities for his/her care. These goals should be stated in objective, measurable terms, which should include a time frame, how or by what means the goals will be accomplished, the need for equipment or assistive aids, and an indication of the expected functional outcome.

Interim, or short-term, goals and terminal, or long-term, goals must be developed and agreed on. After the goals have been established, the therapist can provide an overview or explanation of the types of techniques or procedures that will be used to accomplish the goals. The effectiveness of the treatment program is measured by the accomplishment of the goals by the patient. Goals can be revised when it is apparent the goal was an under- or overestimate of the patient's ability or progress (Box 1–5).

Another component of patient and family education is instruction for a home program. Many patients will require assistance from others to perform exercises and other activities in the environment of a home, health club, school, or other nonmedical facility. The home program should be performed by the patient before termination of his/her treatment, with a family member present and under the direction of the caregiver. The family member must be instructed about his/her responsibilities and level of assistance

---

BOX 1–5

Goal Statements

1. General concepts
   a. Objective terms are used.
   b. Measurable outcomes are stated.
   c. Realistic, attainable outcomes are identified.
   d. Statements are oriented to the person involved, performance expected, time frame anticipated, functional outcome expected, and equipment or assistive aids needed.
2. Short-term (interim) goals
   a. Preparatory component of long-term goal
   b. Lead-in activity for long-term goal
   c. Sequential activities that produce cumulative effect
   d. Support and promote functional outcome
3. Long-term (terminal) goal
   a. Evolves from short-term goals
   b. Maximal performance or outcome is expected.
   c. Functional outcome is a necessary component.
   d. May be revised or modified based on the patient's progress and performance

---

PROCEDURE 1 – 3
Home Program Components

1. Determine the need or value for the patient to continue treatment after the formal activity treatment concludes.
2. Determine the environment and assistance available: home (family member), health club (health care practitioner), school (friend), or other.
3. Prepare the program before termination of the scheduled treatment sessions.
4. Instruct and supervise the patient and his/her assistant as they practice the program activities before termination of scheduled treatment sessions.
5. Provide a written (typed or printed) program with specific instructions and individualized for each patient:
   a. Outline and describe the activities, exercises, and positions to be used; provide diagrams as necessary.
   b. State goals and expected results, as necessary.
   c. Provide objective indicators of performance (i.e., repetitions, distance, time) and the frequency and duration of the program.
   d. Provide indicators of successful completion, fulfillment, or accomplishment of goals, functional outcomes, or activities.
   e. List equipment and supplies that will be needed.
   f. Indicate precautions or contraindications associated with the exercises or activities.
   g. Provide the date, time, and location of scheduled re-evaluation or re-appointment.
   h. Provide the caregiver's name, telephone number, and address.
6. Document the preparation and assignment of the home program and maintain a copy in the medical record or patient's file.

---

member to contact a particular agency or to obtain available benefits.

Education can be performed through direct contact between the patient and family members and the caregiver, printed materials, slides or videotapes, and demonstrations by other patients. The specific instructional methods selected should coincide with the social, economic, mental, and physical factors manifested by or available to the patient and his/her family members.

COMMUNICATION

Communication between and among persons is a primary function of life. For a therapist or other caregiver, communication with patients, family members, other practitioners, and coworkers is a necessity. The caregiver should recognize that different forms of communication, such as verbal, nonverbal, and listening, may be required depending on the purpose or situation related to the communication. Various barriers to communication should be recognized and avoided whenever possible. Patient–caregiver rapport can be established quickly through the use of effective communication or delayed by the lack of it. The information presented in this chapter is designed to provide guidelines or reminders for the caregiver and should not be considered all-encompassing or complete.

Instructions and information can be presented to the patient verbally, nonverbally, and with various audiovisual methods. Verbal communication is the most prevalent style used. When you communicate verbally, terms and concepts should be presented in language the listener understands. Lay language is the most satisfactory for most patients and family members. For example, use "bend" rather than "flex"; "turn" or "twist" rather than "rotate"; and "straighten" rather than "extend" when instructing the patient or family. Directions should guide the patient to perform or act and should be brief and concise. Functional terms or phrases such as "push," "stand," "sit," "turn toward me," and "reach to the left" are more effective than nonfunctional terms such as "Now, the first thing I want you to do is . . ." or "The next thing I want you to do is. . . ." However, it is necessary to provide some transitional terms and phrases, such as "Push with your hands on the armrests," "Straighten your hips and knees," or "Move your right crutch and left leg forward." The patient should be given time to process the message he/she receives, and this time will vary from person to person.

The tone, volume, and inflection of your voice can detract from or add to your message. You can either stimulate or calm a patient with your voice and behavior. For example, consider the mixed message you may give to a patient if you scowl or grimace while telling the patient that he/she performed well. When you desire to encourage or stimulate a patient to act quickly, use a louder than normal volume and a sharper tone to your voice as you say, "Stand up, now!" and simultaneously clap your hands. For the nervous or apprehensive patient you can use a lower than normal volume and a softer tone as you talk with him/her. It may also help assure the patient if you sit next to him/her or rest a hand on his/her shoulder while you talk with him/her. Think of other examples how the volume, tone, and inflection of your voice, along with your nonverbal cues, can add to or detract from your message.

Observation of the patient's reaction to the message will help you to determine whether he/she understands it, has questions, or is puzzled by it. Maintaining eye contact between yourself and the patient allows both persons to relate to nonverbal cues and maintain better interaction. For example, when you are working with a patient's foot and ankle and he/she is supine or sitting, be certain to look at the patient's face, rather than at the patient's foot, as you give your instructions.

It will be helpful to provide an overview or a description of the total activity and its components before giving specific instructions or directions. The specific responsibilities or activities expected of the patient can be presented and emphasized later. Many caregivers find it helpful to have the patient repeat the instructions to determine his/her ability to comprehend and retain the information and to estimate his/her preparedness to perform. It is not sufficient to ask, "Do you understand what you are to do?" or "Do you understand the instructions?" because most patients will respond affirmatively even when they do not understand. Listen for the appropriate sequence and completeness of the repeated instructions. You may request the patient to demonstrate certain activities,

Table 1–2 FORMS OF NONVERBAL COMMUNICATION	
Form	**Examples**
Appearance	Dress, grooming, cleanliness
Body movements	Abrupt, slow, threatening, caring
Body positions	Sitting, standing, walking
Facial expressions	Smiling, frowning, grimacing
Gestures	Using hands and arms to guide or direct
Pantomime	Demonstrating the activity
Posture	Erect, slouched
Touch	Therapeutic, caring, directive, guiding
Spontaneous response to stress	Blushing, perspiring, trembling

such as prepositioning an extremity or his/her body or performing wheelchair tasks such as locking or unlocking the wheels, swinging away the front rigging, or positioning other equipment. These activities, when performed properly, will assist the caregiver to assess the patient's level of comprehension and readiness to function.

Nonverbal communication (NVC) makes up the majority of human communication and may be even more effective than verbal communication. Nonverbal communication is done through facial expressions, posture, gestures, body movements, or changes in body responses. Some forms of NVC are planned, whereas other forms are spontaneous, uncontrollable, or involuntary (Table 1–2). Most of us have been in embarrassing or stressful situations and have sensed a change in the color of our skin or noticed an increase in perspiration. These are examples of spontaneous, uncontrolled, or involuntary NVC. Facial expressions tend to be spontaneous, but at times they are planned for a specific effect. A frown or smile will indicate a negative or positive response to a patient's performance. When we use specific hand gestures or pantomime or demonstrate activities, we are using planned NVC. The skilled caregiver will know when and how to best use these various forms of NVC.

The caregiver should also observe the patient to identify his/her NVC. Often, more information and a more accurate estimation of the patient's response or reaction to instructions can be obtained through his/her NVC.

The use of touch by the caregiver is another form of NVC that can add to the communication process. A brief hug, a hand squeeze, or a pat on the back can convey a message to a patient, and to other persons as well, that cannot be sent as effectively verbally. However, touch must be used in a therapeutic, caring way, and the caregiver must avoid any suggestion of sexual implications. Examples of improper and unacceptable forms of touch include patting, slapping, or stroking a patient's buttocks; squeezing the thigh; or stroking various body parts, except during a therapeutic massage or exercise activity. You must demonstrate care when you grasp, handle, or touch the patient, especially during massage and exercise when sensitive body areas are touched. The perineum and buttocks of all patients and the breasts of women and sometimes men should be draped as described in Chapter 3. When it is therapeutically necessary to massage, grasp, hold, or touch a potentially sensitive area, it may be prudent to state the reason the area is being touched or handled. In some situations, it may be wise to have another person observe or assist as you perform a particular treatment to protect yourself and to demonstrate your concern for the patient. Because touch may be construed to have a sexual implication by any patient, regardless of how careful the caregiver has been, any indication of impropriety must be avoided.

Written communication should follow guidelines similar to those listed for verbal communication. It should be brief, concise, and specific and should use language the reader will be most likely to understand. The guidelines previously given for the development of home programs are applicable here. Typed or printed instructions are more easily read than handwritten ones. Diagrams, drawings, or photographs are extremely useful to show specific positions or the sequence of movements. Films, videotapes, and slides are other forms of communication that can be useful to educate or instruct a patient or his/her family.

The use of consistent language and the manner in which verbal or written instructions or directions are given to a patient by the various persons involved with the patient's care should enhance the patient's level of understanding and capacity to learn. This concept is particularly important when complex activities are being taught and when a patient's mental capacities have been altered. Repetition and practice of activities that require motor control or coordination usually will enhance the patient's skill and ensure a safer performance. A complex activity should be performed consistently in the same or a very similar manner, regardless of the person assisting or guiding the patient (Box 1–6).

There are many barriers that can adversely affect verbal and nonverbal communication between a caregiver and his/her patients. A noisy treatment area, an excessive distance between the two persons, distractions in the treatment area, the language used by the caregiver (i.e., technical language instead of lay language), the position of furniture or equipment and of the persons who are communicating, the time available to communicate, and the individual values or biases of each person are some examples of deterrents and potential barriers to verbal and nonverbal communication. The astute caregiver will be aware of and able to identify these factors and avoid, eliminate, or

BOX 1–6

Barriers to Effective Communication

Distance between the sender and receiver; excessive distance decreases effectiveness.

Noise and environmental confusion interfere with and may distort the message.

Inability of the receiver to comprehend the message

Inability of the receiver to interpret or understand technical, medical, and professional terms, language, or abbreviations

Inadequate feedback occurs between the receiver and sender.

Complex messages are difficult to interpret and comprehend.

Sender and receiver may interpret the message differently; therefore, feedback from the receiver is important.

Cultural, gender, or age differences between the sender and receiver may affect the interpretation or comprehension of the message.

Illegible writing affects the accuracy and comprehension of the message.

reduce them. This awareness and the subsequent action to overcome these conditions or factors are important keys to effective communication (Box 1–6).

Being an attentive listener is another communication skill the caregiver should develop. Evaluating the patient's tone of voice; observing the nonverbal cues provided by him/her; listening for the main theme of the message; focusing on the content of the message, rather than on the way the message is communicated; and providing verbal feedback to clarify understanding of the message are examples of being an attentive listener. This aspect of communication may be overlooked or slighted by the caregiver, and the result may be a loss of information.

COMMUNICATING WITH A PERSON WITH A DISABILITY

Caregivers must become aware of their responsibility to communicate appropriately with a person with a disability. You should first and foremost maintain the person's self-esteem by considering the person first in your words and thoughts. The person's disability should be described accurately, if it needs to be included in the message, but it is more important to emphasize his/her abilities than his/her disability. For example, the statement "John, who has a spinal cord injury, uses a wheelchair for mobility" is more appropriate than "Because he has a broken back, John is confined to a wheelchair." The use of the term person with a disability is preferable to the term disabled person to promote the person's self-esteem and recognition as a person first.

Some suggestions to improve your communications with persons with disabilities follow (Box 1–7). You should speak directly with the person rather than with his/her companion and should be prepared to shake hands. In some instances you may need to grasp the person's forearm or use your left hand rather than your right hand as you meet or greet him/her. The person who is visually impaired will appreciate knowing who is speaking with him/her, so you should identify yourself, similar to the way in which you identify yourself when using a telephone. It will be necessary to identify each individual in a group, and each individual should identify himself/herself as they speak. Remember it is not necessary to increase the volume of your voice when speaking with a person who is visually impaired. To improve your communications, position yourself in front of and at eye level when speaking; stoop or squat when talking with a person seated in a wheelchair or on a mat platform or a mat on the floor. A person who is hearing impaired will need to have tactile (touch, tap) or visual (hand wave, gesture) cueing from you before you initiate speaking with him/ her. If the person is able to lip read, you should stand so the person can see your lips clearly, speak slowly, and enunciate carefully. Again, increasing the volume of your voice is unnecessary in most communication situations. When you communicate with a person who has difficulty speaking, intensify your listening skills and provide feedback to the individual to indicate your understanding of the message. Avoid correcting the person, interrupting him/her, anticipating what he/she will or may say, or speaking for him/her. Be patient during the conversation and wait for confirmation of your feedback before continuing. The use of questions that require brief responses or that can be answered by a head nod or shake may assist this person. At times you may sense or realize a person with a disability will require assistance. If this occurs, you should ask the person whether he/she desires assistance, and if it is desired ask him/her for specific instructions or directions.

Occasionally even the experienced caregiver may feel awkward or embarrassed when communicating with a person with a disability, especially if an expression related to his/her disability is used during the conversation. Examples are "I am looking forward to seeing you again," "I'll see you later," "Did you hear about the big fire?" and "Let's go over the plan one step at time." In most instances the person with a disability will recognize these statements as expressions and components of the usual communication pattern, so there is no need to apologize or bring attention to the statement, but you may want to consider how you can limit the use of these expressions, and others, in the future. You should avoid the use of terms such as victim, stricken, and afflicted because they tend to indicate an unhealthy status.

Being aware of and applying these suggestions will enable you to communicate with a person with a disability appropriately, to maintain his/her self-esteem, and to recognize him/her as a person with abilities, rather than to stereotype him/her as being "disabled."

Communication between the caregiver and the patient is a critical aspect of patient care. The caregiver will be challenged to be aware of the importance of communication and to make every effort to communicate effectively. This can be accomplished through proper use of verbal, nonverbal, visual, and written communication.

BOX 1–7

Guidelines for Communicating With Persons With Disabilities

Speak and interact directly with the person with the disability.

Greet the person as you would greet persons without a disability; shake hands or forearm, and use your left hand as appropriate.

Identify yourself and other persons in a group to the person who is visually impaired.

Stoop or squat to communicate with a person in a wheelchair; position yourself in front and at eye level.

Avoid leaning or sitting on a person's wheelchair; use care when handling assistive aids.

Avoid statements, gestures, or actions that patronize; interact in the same manner you would interact with persons who do not have a disability.

Tactilely or visually cue the person who is hearing impaired so he/she is aware of your presence.

Be patient and listen carefully when interacting with a person who has difficulty speaking; use questions that require brief responses.

Place the person first in your words and thoughts; emphasize his/her abilities.

Determine whether the person desires assistance before assisting him/her; wait for instructions.

SAFETY CONSIDERATIONS

The caregiver bears primary responsibility for the safety of each patient, regardless of the treatment provided and, in some situations, who provides it. Patient transfers, changes in position, exercise activities, and the transport of equipment or patients all have the potential to cause injury; therefore, the caregiver must maintain a safe environment and equipment that functions properly. Family members must be instructed on how to assist the patient safely and should be informed of any specific precautions related to the patient's care. The patient also has to assume some responsibility to maintain his/her personal safety. Proper hygiene, skin care, changes in his/her position, proper handling techniques, bowel and bladder management procedures, and transfer patterns may have to be performed or directed by the patient. The patient frequently knows what is best for himself/herself, and the caregiver should listen and follow the patient's suggestions if they are reasonable and safe. The patient must be informed that he/she is responsible for his/her health and safety within the limitations of his/her condition.

Incidents leading to patient injuries can be linked to the use of improperly functioning or poorly maintained equipment, a physical setting with hazardous obstacles or congested space, an excessive number of patients in the treatment area in relation to the personnel available to treat them, and the limited availability of personnel (e.g., in the early morning or late afternoon or during lunch). The caregiver should be especially alert when treating a patient who is elderly, debilitated, or mentally disoriented; who is very young or has decreased mental capacity or a decreased physiologic status (e.g., severe burns, spinal cord injury, diabetes, or cardiopulmonary deficits); or who is emotionally disturbed. A patient with one or more of these conditions may experience difficulty tolerating the treatment or may be more easily injured than other patients. The prudent caregiver will consider all the information related to the patient and will modify or revise the patient's treatment to reduce the likelihood of injury. The caregiver should also be aware of his/her own safety and should follow established guidelines regarding body mechanics and personal health as described in Chapter 2. Some recommendations for promoting safety are listed in Box 1–8.

Accidents and subsequent injuries tend to occur when health care personnel or family members are careless, inadequately trained, inattentive, or excessively busy. Additional information and suggestions regarding patient safety are contained in the chapters on transfers (Chapter 6), ambulation (Chapter 8), and infection control (Chapter 10).

BOX 1–8

Safety Recommendations

1. Perform hand washing before and after treating each patient to reduce cross-contamination and transmission of disease. This is the best method to reduce cross-contamination.

2. Maintain sufficient space to maneuver equipment or perform a task. Store equipment that is not in use so it will not interfere with patient care. Avoid positioning a patient so that he/she is at risk of being struck by passing personnel or equipment.

3. Do not perform transfers or ambulation in an area where your view is obstructed, such as near a door or the corner of a hallway, or where space is inadequate or too congested for the activity.

4. Routinely evaluate equipment and be certain it functions properly; establish a maintenance program for each item.

5. Position equipment, furniture, and assistive aids so the items are stable, secure, and accessible when they are being used. Remove them when they are not in use so they do not interfere with patient and caregiver movements.

6. Keep the floor clear of electric cords, litter, loose rugs or floor mats, water, dirt, and other similar hazards.

7. Do not leave patients unattended, especially if they are compromised physiologically or mentally. Protect the patient with restraint straps, bed rails, or similar items when they are not closely attended, according to established state or federal restrictions and guidelines.

8. Obtain the equipment and supplies needed and prepare the treatment area before the patient arrives to avoid the need to leave the patient unattended.

9. Be certain the personnel who provide patient care are trained, qualified, and competent in their assigned duties.

10. Avoid storing potentially hazardous equipment or materials in a location where they are hidden from view or where there is a risk of a patient obtaining them. Do not store chemicals or heavy objects on a shelf above shoulder level. Clearly label the contents and weight of boxes or other containers.

SUMMARY

It is important to inform the patient of the planned treatment and about his/her responsibilities or participation in the activity. The explanation should contain the anticipated results or outcomes of the treatment and any potential adverse effects. The patient should have the opportunity to consent to or reject treatment based on the receipt of sufficient information to make an informed decision. The presence of the patient in the treatment area should not be assumed to be an expression of his/her consent for treatment. Communication between the caregiver and each patient can be improved if the caregiver reduces or avoids certain communication barriers and if he/she develops the skills associated with being an attentive listener.

The safety of the patient must be the first priority of all persons involved in all treatment activities performed. The responsibility for patient safety remains with the primary caregiver, even when the patient is treated by supportive personnel whom the caregiver supervises.

■ SELF-STUDY/DISCUSSION ACTIVITIES

1. Describe the criteria associated with short- and long-term goals.

2. Describe at least three reasons a patient's family members may need to be educated by a primary caregiver and provide the rationale for each reason.

3. Explain the types of communication you would use to instruct a patient to ambulate with crutches, perform a standing assisted transfer, instruct a family member to guard a patient who uses crutches, and perform active assistive exercise.

4. List at least four factors you should consider related to the general aspects of patient safety.

5. Explain why it is important and necessary to evaluate or assess each patient before initiating treatment or developing a treatment plan.

6. Describe how each evaluative procedure may assist you to make decisions or resolve clinical problems about the plan of care you develop with the patient.

7. Explain why it is important to develop a treatment plan *with* the patient rather than *for* the patient.

8. Describe why persons with the same diagnosis or disability or condition should be evaluated individually and have individual treatment programs developed.

9. Describe the steps or actions you could take to improve communication between you and your patient.

Body Mechanics

After studying this chapter, the reader will be able to:

1 Define the term *body mechanics.*

2 Describe proper body mechanics to be used for lifting, reaching, pushing, pulling, and carrying objects.

3 Instruct or teach another person to use proper body mechanics.

4 Explain specific precautions to be used when lifting, reaching, pushing, pulling, and carrying objects.

5 Provide basic information to educate another person to care for his/her back.

6 Use proper body mechanics for lifting, reaching, pushing, pulling, and carrying objects.

■ ■ ■ K E Y   T E R M S

Anterior: Situated at or directed toward the front of a body or object; the opposite of *posterior*.

Base of support (BOS): The area on which an object rests and that provides support for the object.

Center of gravity (COG): The point at which the mass of a body or object is centered.

Dysfunction: Disturbance, impairment, or abnormality of functioning of a body part.

Friction: The act of rubbing one object against another.

Gravity: The force that pulls toward the center of the earth and affects all objects.

Isometric: Maintaining or pertaining to the same length.

Lateral: Pertaining to a side; away from the midline of the body or a structure.

Lever arm: A component of a mechanical lever; it may be the force arm or the weight (resistance) arm; when the length of the force arm is increased or the length of the weight arm is decreased, a greater mechanical advantage is created for the lever system.

Lordosis: An increase in one of the forward convexities of the normal vertebral columns; a lumbar or cervical lordosis can occur.

Lumbar: Pertaining to the loin; lower region of the back superior to the pelvis.

Medial: Pertaining to or situated toward the midline of the body or a structure.

Pelvic tilt (inclination): Movement of the pelvis so that the anterior-superior iliac spines move anteriorly or posteriorly to produce an anterior or a posterior tilt or inclination of the pelvis.

Posterior: Situated at or directed toward the back of a body or object; the opposite of *anterior*.

Recumbent: Lying down.

Sagittal plane: Anteroposterior plane or body section that is parallel to the median plane of the body.

Torque: The expression of the effectiveness of a force in turning a lever system; it is the product of a force multiplied by the perpendicular distance from its line of action to the axis of motion ($T = F \times D$).

Vector: A quantity possessing magnitude and direction, such as a force or velocity.

Vertical gravity line (VGL): An imaginary vertical line that passes through the center of gravity of an object.

INTRODUCTION

Persons who are required to lift, reach, push, pull, and carry objects should be instructed to use proper body mechanics. Proper use of body mechanics will conserve energy, reduce stress and strain on body structures, reduce the possibility of personal injury, and produce movements that are safe.

Body mechanics can be described as the use of one's body to produce motion that is safe, energy conserving, and anatomically and physiologically efficient and that leads to the maintenance of a person's body balance and control. Thus, the person who teaches and uses proper body mechanics judiciously will better protect the patient and himself/herself from injury. Stress and strain to many anatomic structures and body systems are reduced so work activities and the patient can be managed with greater safety. In addition, energy expenditure can be reduced by developing proper habits that encourage comfort and ease or efficiency of movement (Box 2–1).

PRINCIPLES AND CONCEPTS OF PROPER BODY MECHANICS

Gravity and *friction* are forces that add resistance to many activities associated with the lifting, reaching, pushing, pulling, and carrying of an object (Table 2–1). Therefore, it is important to select and apply techniques that will, in some situations, reduce the adverse effects of gravity or friction or, in other situations, enhance the positive effects of these two forces to reduce expenditure of energy, avoid undue stress or strain to body systems, and maintain control of your body. You should review the concepts associated

---

BOX 2–1

Value of Proper Body Mechanics for the Caregiver

Conserve energy.

Reduce stress and strain to muscles, joints, ligaments, and soft tissue.

Promote effective, efficient, and safe movements.

Promote and maintain proper body control and balance.

Promote effective, efficient respiratory and cardiopulmonary function.

Table 2–1
PRINCIPLES OF BODY MECHANICS

1. Remain close to the object; stoop or squat to lift.
2. Use the largest and strongest muscles of your arms, legs, and trunk to lift, push, pull, or carry an object.
3. Widen your base of support (BOS) so your vertical gravity line falls within your BOS.
4. Use short lever arms for better control and efficiency when lifting or carrying.
5. Avoid twisting your body when you lift.
6. Maintain your center of gravity (COG) close to the object's COG; raise or lower your COG or the object's COG.
7. When possible, push, pull, roll, or slide an object rather than lift it.

with mechanics, as originally described by Sir Isaac Newton, especially the three laws of motion, which can be found in any basic physics or kinesiology textbook. Other forces involved with movement and body control are muscle forces and forms of external resistance.

Before lifting, reaching, pushing, pulling, or carrying an object, or a patient, position yourself close to the object or adjust the position of the object so it is close to you. This will allow you to use your upper extremities in a shortened position, or as short *lever arms.* Your muscles will function more effectively and with less strain to the structures of your trunk because a lower *torque* will be necessary in the muscles of the upper extremity when the object is held close to your body. When the upper extremity is positioned away from the body when attempting to lift, push, pull, reach, or carry an object, a larger torque is required by the muscles of the extremity to perform the task. This larger torque causes more energy to be expended and increases the strain to structures of your body.

When you are applying manual resistance, another way to use torque to your advantage—that is, to reduce the force you would generate by muscle contraction—is to require the patient to exercise as you apply resistance to a long lever arm. For example, during active manual resistive exercise or manual muscle testing, you will expend less energy if you provide resistance to a patient's distal forearm as he/she performs shoulder flexion with the elbow extended. The longer the lever arm the patient is required to use, the less force you will need to provide resistance. To illustrate this concept, apply resistance at various locations to another person's upper extremity as he/she sits and performs shoulder flexion with the elbow straight. Apply the resistance at the wrist, then at the elbow, and then at the proximal humerus, and sense the difference in the force you must develop to provide resistance as the other person performs shoulder flexion. This concept can be applied to other body segments.

In addition to being close to the object, it is important to position your *center of gravity (COG)* as close

to the object's COG as possible. The COG is where the mass of your body or an object is concentrated. Thus, it is the heaviest area to move or the most difficult to adjust to a new position. Your COG is located approximately at the level of the second sacral segment in the center of your pelvis. Maintenance of the two COGs in close proximity to each other will also help reduce the torque required to move or carry the object. Thus your muscles will require less energy to contract, experience less strain, and function more efficiently. You should recognize that it may be easier to adjust the object's COG than your own. Raising or lowering a patient's bed to adjust his/her COG in relation to your COG, before performing exercise with him/her, is one example of this concept.

It is important to increase your stability before lifting, reaching, pushing, pulling, or carrying an object. This can be accomplished by increasing your *base of support (BOS),* lowering your COG, maintaining your *vertical gravity line (VGL)* within your BOS, and positioning your feet according to the direction of movement you will use to perform the activity. When you place your feet farther apart in an *anterior-posterior* stance (i.e., one foot ahead of the other foot) or in a *medial-lateral* stance (i.e., with the feet farther apart in a sideward direction), you increase your BOS, because your BOS is dependent on the position of your feet. Either of these positions will help maintain your VGL within your BOS to further increase your stability.

The VGL is an imaginary line that bisects your body in the *sagittal plane* beginning at your head and continuing through your pelvis and specifically through your COG. It indicates the vertical positioning of your COG. The VGL must be within your BOS (i.e., between your feet) for balance and stability. Your VGL is affected by activities that alter your COG. For example, when you attempt to stand on one foot, you must initially shift your COG over that lower extremity and foot before you can lift the other foot. Failure to shift your body weight (COG) will result in a loss of balance, because your COG will not be located in your BOS. A patient's BOS can be improved by providing crutches, canes, or a walker to aid his/her ambulation.

Another example of a change in the position of your COG is when you reach for an object. When you reach with your arms, the relative position of your COG is changed, and you will have to adjust your BOS or use your muscles to maintain your balance and stability. One way to accomplish this is to widen your BOS by spreading your feet apart. Remember, the closer your feet are to each other, the less stable and the more unbalanced you will be. When you squat, stoop, or kneel, you lower your COG, which increases your stability. Objects with a high COG tend to be unstable. Tall, columnar types of equipment (e.g., ultraviolet or infrared lamps, intravenous poles) frequently have a weighted BOS to lower the object's COG.

PROCEDURE 2 – 1
Principles of Proper Body Mechanics for the Caregiver

1. Mentally and physically plan for the activity.
2. Position yourself close to the object to be moved to use short lever arms.
3. Maintain the vertical gravity line within the object's base of support to maintain stability and balance.
4. Position your center of gravity close to the object's center of gravity to improve control of the object.
5. Use the major muscles of the extremities and trunk to perform movements or activities.
6. Roll, push, pull, or slide an object rather than lifting it.

In addition, the item is apt to have an enlarged or wide base so the VGL of the object is located within its BOS.

In summary, position yourself close to an object or position the object close to you, increase your BOS, and approximate the COG of your body close to the object's COG before attempting to lift, pull, reach, or carry an object.

Prepare yourself mentally and physically and plan for the series of events or movements that will be required to perform the activity. For example, before moving an object, its approximate weight can be estimated by attempting to slide, tilt or tip, or partially lift it; by looking inside its container to determine its composition; or by reading the information about the contents and their weight, which is frequently printed on the container. A patient's weight can be determined simply by asking the patient. The size, configuration or shape, and position of the object should be evaluated and considered to determine whether the object can be moved or controlled safely and with relative ease.

You should determine the best method to move the object before you attempt to move it. For example, will it be easier and safer to roll or slide an object rather than lift it? The move itself should be planned so all obstacles are removed and a clear path from point A to point B is established. The distance of the move and the need for and availability of assistance should be determined and the final location or placement of the object decided. Gravity and momentum can be useful adjuncts and should be used whenever possible. It may be helpful to rock an object back and forth to generate some momentum, or an incline or ramp may be used to lower a heavy object from one

height to another. To conserve energy, you should roll, slide, push, or pull an object rather than lift it when any of those options are appropriate for the activity and the object (Procedure 2–1).

Persons who assist you and patients must be instructed about their responsibilities and tasks before the activity. They must be taught or trained what to do, how to do it, and when to do it. Requesting them to repeat your instructions will help confirm their level of understanding and their comprehension of their roles and expected performance. In addition, you should ask them if they have any questions about their role or the expected outcome. If you are the primary caregiver, you should establish yourself as the leader or coordinator of the activity. Your instructions and directions should be brief, concise, and action oriented (e.g., "lift now," "push down," "stand up"). You may find it helpful to lead into the action command by using phrases such as "ready"; "one, two, three"; "first, I want you to . . ."; or "on the count of three, lift."

It is important that you give your full attention to the activity, which includes anticipating the unusual or unexpected. When you are assisting a patient to transfer, be prepared to increase your assistance to a maximal effort at any time, even though the patient may have previously performed the transfer successfully with minimal assistance. You must guard and protect the patient until he/she is able to perform the activity safely and consistently.

Both your safety and that of the patient can be enhanced by prepositioning and securing the equipment required for the activity. An evaluation of the patient to determine his/her ability to assist with or need for assistance during a transfer will also improve

Precautions for the Caregiver when Lifting, Pushing, Pulling, Reaching, and Carrying Objects

Avoid simultaneous trunk bending (flexion) and twisting (rotation).

Stoop or squat to reach for and lift an object below waist level.

Stand on a stable foot stool or ladder to reach for an object above shoulder level.

Apply pushing and pulling forces parallel to the surface over which the object is being moved.

Carry objects close to your COG and close to the midline of the body.

Carry a one-hand item alternately with your upper extremities.

Avoid using long lever arms to push, pull, lift, reach, and carry.

Perform push, pull, lift, reach, and carry activities within your physical capacity and limits.

safety. The use of mechanical devices or equipment (e.g., a hoist, transfer or sliding board, wheeled stretcher, or cart) and following other previously described actions (e.g., raising or lowering the object, decreasing the distance of the move, or using gravity or momentum) can make the transfer safer and easier to perform. Assistance should be obtained before initiating any activity that you determine you cannot perform safely alone.

There are several precautions that you should be aware of before lifting, reaching, pushing, pulling, or carrying. You must avoid simultaneous trunk flexion (bending) and rotation (twisting) when you lift or reach for an object. Prolonged trunk flexion will lead to stress and strain to muscles, ligaments, and articulations of the posterior trunk and spine and perhaps the lower extremities. Therefore, when an object is below the level of your waist and must be lifted, you should stoop or squat rather than flex your trunk or raise the object so you can avoid trunk flexion. A footstool or ladder should be used to reach an object located above the level of your head. Be very cautious if you elect to use a chair or other similar object that is not designed for standing upon. If you do elect to use a chair, be certain to stand on the seat within the BOS of the legs of the chair. Finally, you must be fully aware of your personal abilities and the limits of your strength, stamina, and motor control as they relate to lifting,

reaching, pulling, pushing, and carrying. You must perform within the known limits of your physical abilities to avoid injury to yourself or the patient (Box 2–2).

Your primary goal is to perform the activity safely, efficiently, and with minimal stress or strain. The use of proper body mechanics, clear and concise instructions to the patient or to his/her caregivers (i.e., family, friends, or other medical personnel), and adherence to the precautions contained in this chapter will benefit you and the patient.

LIFTING MODELS

Five lifting models are described. There are many differing opinions about which model is most appropriate or best to use. Research studies have not shown or proven that one method is superior to, safer than, or more effective than another method; therefore, you may desire to practice each of the models and select one or more for your use. It has been hypothesized the lumbar lordosis models provide greater protection to the *lumbar* region of the spine, particularly during the lifting of a heavy object.

TRADITIONAL MODEL

The traditional model recommends that you lift an object below waist level by stooping or squatting, grasping the object, and lifting with a relatively straight lumbar and thoracic spine (Fig. 2–1). Incorporated in this posture is the concept of a posterior *pelvic tilt (inclination)*, which is produced in part by an *isometric* contraction of the abdominal musculature. The quadriceps and gluteus maximus muscles of the lower extremities and the biceps, pectoralis major, and deltoid muscles of the upper extremity are the primary muscles involved in lifting and controlling the object. The posterior pelvic tilt is performed to position the pelvis under the lumbar spine for improved stability. Contraction of the abdominal muscles also increases intra-abdominal pressure, which further stabilizes the lumbar spine by forming the thorax into a pneumatic cylinder (Procedure 2–2).

LUMBAR LORDOSIS MODELS

Patient education programs related to protective lifting and preventive back management techniques (i.e., "back schools") suggest three models that use a lumbar *lordosis* posture for lifting. The three lifting models are the deep squat, power lift, and straight leg

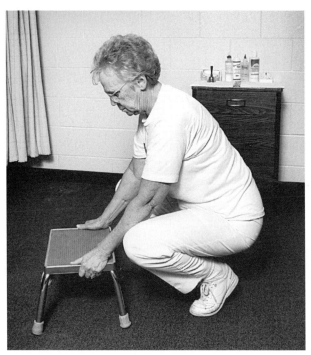

■ **FIGURE 2–1**
Traditional lifting model.

lift. The key element of each model is the maintenance of the lumbar spine in its usual position of slight lordosis.

1. **Deep Squat Lift** A full squat is performed to position the hips below the level of the knees. The lifter's feet straddle the object, and his/her upper extremities are positioned parallel to each other. The lifter's hands grasp the opposite sides, the handles, or under the bottom of the object. The lifter's trunk is maintained in a vertical position, and the lumbar spine remains in lordosis with an anterior pelvic tilt (Fig. 2–2).

2. **Power Lift** Only a half squat is performed so the hips remain above the level of the knees. The lifter's feet are positioned parallel to each other and remain behind the object, with the upper extremities positioned parallel to each other. The lifter grasps the opposite sides, the handles, or under the bottom of the object. The lifter's trunk is maintained in a more horizontal than vertical position, and the lumbar spine remains in lordosis with an anterior pelvic tilt (Fig. 2–3).

3. **Straight Leg Lift** The lifter's knees are only slightly flexed or may be fully extended. The lower extremities are either parallel to each other or straddle the object, and the upper extremities are either parallel to each other or grasp the opposite sides of the object. The trunk may be positioned either vertically or horizontally, and the lumbar spine remains in lordosis (Fig. 2–4).

The rationale used by proponents of lifting using lumbar lordosis is related to several anatomic and mechanical factors. It has been hypothesized that mechanical stresses are reduced to the posterior longitudinal, interspinous, and ligamentum flavum ligaments and to the posterior portion of the annulus fibrosus of the intervertebral disk when a person lifts while maintaining lumbar lordosis. In addition, the compression pressure to the nucleus pulposus of the disk may be directed more anteriorly. These factors may protect the posterior area of the disk and may reduce the tendency toward disk herniation or bulging in a posterior-lateral direction. Furthermore, it has been theorized that the lumbar lordosis position allows the vertebral facets to engage each other more fully, which tends to increase the stability of the lumbar spine. Finally, through proper positioning

---

PROCEDURE 2 – 2
Traditional Lift Model

1. Stoop or squat to lower your center of gravity closer to the object's center of gravity.
2. Perform a posterior pelvic tilt, with an isometric contraction of the abdominals, to position the pelvis, stabilize the lower spine, and increase intra-abdominal pressure.
3. Use the major muscles of the upper extremities to lift the object to waist level.
4. Rise to an upright position using the major extensors of the lower extremities; maintain the lumbar spine straight.
5. Hold the object close to the body at waist level.

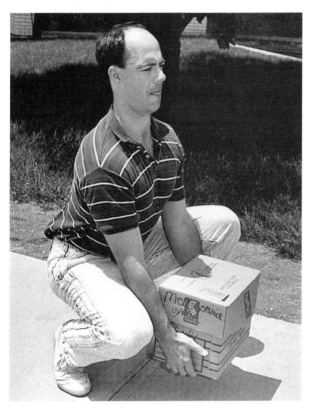

■ FIGURE 2–2
Deep squat lift.

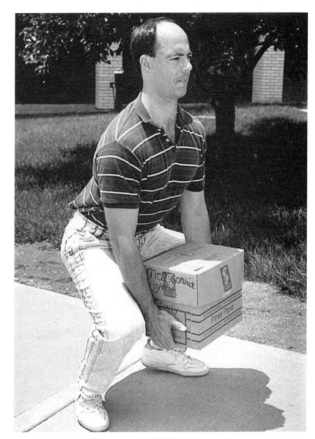

■ FIGURE 2–3
Power lift.

and the use of the squat, the lumbar paravertebral, abdominal, quadriceps, and gluteus maximus muscles are better able to function, leading to improved function of the lumbopelvic force couple. The same techniques can be used to return an object from waist level to the floor. These techniques may feel awkward or even uncomfortable to the person who has always used the traditional model; therefore, the lumbar lordosis models may require practice before they can be performed with comfort and ease (Box 2–3).

ONE-LEG STANCE LIFT ("GOLFER'S LIFT")

The one-leg stance lift can be used for light objects that can be lifted easily with one upper extremity. The lifter faces the object to be lifted, with the body weight shifted onto the forward lower extremity. To pick up the object, the weight-bearing lower extremity is partially flexed at the hip and knee, while the non–weight-bearing lower extremity is lifted into extension to counterbalance the forward movement of the trunk (Fig. 2–5). The lifter picks up the object in a manner similar to the way a golfer removes a golf ball from the cup and returns to an upright position.

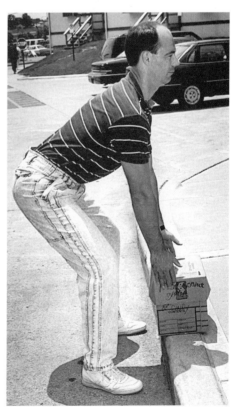

■ FIGURE 2–4
Straight leg lift.

Rationale for Lumbar Lordosis Lift Model

Lordosis reduces mechanical stress to the lumbar ligaments and IV disk.

Compression forces to the IV disk are directed anteriorly rather than posteriorly, which reduces the potential for a posterior-lateral rupture of the disk.

Lumbar spine stability is increased due to the approximation of the vertebral facets.

Function of the lumbopelvic force couple is maximized.

Anterior and posterior lower trunk muscles and hip and thigh extensor muscles are positioned to function more effectively.

PUSHING, PULLING, REACHING, AND CARRYING

Many of the same principles described for lifting also apply to pushing and pulling activities. You should use a crouched or semisquat position to push or pull (Fig. 2–6). This position lowers your COG nearer to the object's COG, which increases stability,

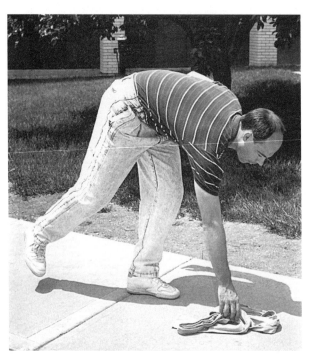

■ FIGURE 2–5
One-leg stance lift ("golfer's lift").

reduces energy expenditure, and improves control of the object. The force of the push or pull should be applied parallel to the surface over which the object is to be moved and in the line of movement desired. This reduces the effects of friction and moves the object in the proper direction. Consideration should be given to how to adjust to the effects of inertia and friction and the influence of *vector* forces. Inertia and friction are forces that impede the movement of an object. More force is required to initiate the movement of a stationary object than to continue its movement; therefore, you should prepare yourself to exert greater effort when beginning to push or pull an object than you will need to continue to push or pull it. You may find that rocking the object to generate some motion helps to overcome its inertia; similarly, tipping or partially lifting the object to reduce contact between the object and the surface on which it rests reduces the friction between the object and the underlying surface. You can turn or redirect the direction of movement of the object by the use of a force that alters the vectors of motion. This can be accomplished by pushing harder with one upper extremity than with the other, by pulling with one upper extremity and pushing with the other upper extremity, or by positioning your body at one corner of the object and pushing or pulling at an angle to the line of forward motion. Remember that in most situations, energy will be conserved if an object is moved by sliding, rolling, or turning it rather than by lifting or carrying it.

Reaching for an object that is above your shoulder or head will be less strenuous if the object is lowered or you raise your position by standing on a wide-based footstool or ladder (Fig. 2–7). These actions approximate the COG of the object and your COG, allow the use of shortened extremity lever arms, and decrease strain to back structures. An object at arm's length should be brought closer to one's body before lifting it to reduce the torque produced by long lever arms. For example, move a patient from the center of his/her bed or mat to one edge of the bed or mat before performing exercises, or help the *recumbent* patient to move up or down or to sit up. When carrying an object, hold it close to your body, using your arms as short lever arms, and maintain its COG near your COG. Localize the COG of bulky objects by folding or otherwise positioning extended portions of the object toward its center. If you carry an object in a backpack or chest pack, be certain both shoulder straps are used and the weight is distributed in the pack with the weight close to your COG. You should avoid carrying the pack over one shoulder because it will affect your COG and require you to alter your posture, leading to increased strain of several structures.

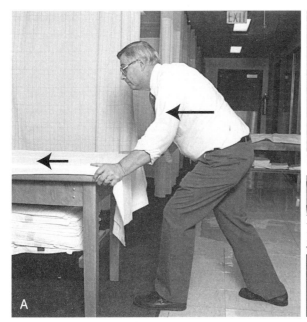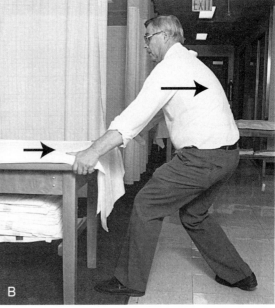

■ **FIGURE 2–6**
A, Pushing an object. *B,* Pulling an object.

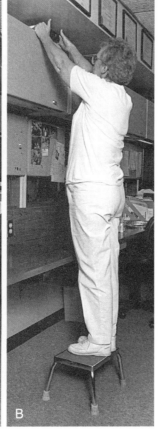

■ **FIGURE 2–7**
A and *B,* Reaching for an object above the shoulder.

POSTURE AND BODY CONTROL

Persons with a history of low back pain or *dysfunction* and those whose lifestyle or occupation predisposes them to trauma to structures of the back should be educated in ways to prevent back injuries.

BOX 2–4

Common Causes of Back Problems or Discomfort

Faulty posture

Faulty, improper use of body mechanics

Repetitive, sustained microtrauma to structures of the back and trunk

Poor flexibility of muscles and ligaments of the back and trunk

Decline in general physical fitness

Episodes of trauma that culminate in one specific or final event ("the final straw"):
Stress, strain, or tear of muscle or ligament occurs.
Disk may change shape and impinge on nerve roots.
Vertebral joints may become irritated.
Improper lift, push, pull, reach, or carry motion may cause trauma to back structures.

BOX 2–5

Principles for Proper Posture

1. Maintain the normal anterior (forward) and posterior (backward) curves of the spine for proper balance and alignment.

2. Stand and sit with your body erect so your shoulders and pelvis (hips) are level; avoid slouch or "round back" positions.

3. Stand with your body weight evenly placed on each leg; keep your knees flexed (bent) slightly, and allow your pelvis to roll forward to maintain lumbar lordosis.

4. Sit with your knees and hips flexed to 90 degrees with your feet flat on floor or stool. Your knees should be at the same level as your hips with the pelvis rolled forward. Avoid slouch or "round back" posture, especially during prolonged sitting.

5. Avoid standing or sitting in one position for a prolonged time period; occasionally alter the position. Move your head, neck, shoulders, back, hips, knees, and ankles periodically.

6. Stand with your ankles, knees, hips, and shoulders aligned; keep your head over your body, not in front of the shoulders.

7. When in lying position, lie on your back or side with your hips and knees partially flexed (bent). Use a pillow under or between the knees for support, and avoid lying prone (face down). Use a small or medium-size pillow to support your head but do not position it under the shoulders. Use a bed mattress that is firm and provides support to the natural curves of the spine.

An initial assessment or evaluation of the individual should be performed before the education process. Assess the individual's posture, his/her previous history related to the present condition, the mechanisms of his/her current injury, and his/her lifestyle and work activities, including the work environment (Box 2–4).

Most patients, regardless of their condition or cause of injury, will benefit from some basic education related to care of the structures of the back. This education is usually performed through a formal program frequently referred to as a "back school." However, some simple instructions and reminders can provide the patient or family member with information to protect the back structures. In this text, only the most basic information is presented.

Initially the patient should receive information about the basic anatomy of the body, especially the structures that affect his/her back. Instruction in the use of proper body mechanics and how to correct faulty standing, sitting, or recumbent postures should be presented. Suggestions on ways to identify and correct improper work, recreational, or daily life habits will be beneficial. All of the information about body mechanics presented in this chapter should be given to the patient. Instruction in ways to maintain the proper condition and function of muscles, ligaments, and joint structures through the use of relaxation, flexibility, and strengthening activities or aerobic exercise are important components of patient education. Methods that can be used to protect or relieve back stress, such as the placement of one foot on a footstool while standing or the use of a lumbar roll while sitting, should be provided (Box 2–5).

The person should be cautioned to balance his/her work, recreational, and rest activities to avoid chronic overuse syndromes or the development of specific dysfunction. It may be necessary to evaluate the person's work or home environment so specific suggestions related to those settings can be given. The person should be advised to reduce, eliminate, or occasionally change sustained or repetitive positions, postures, and activities that cause back stress,

BOX 2–6

Patient Guidelines to Reduce Stress-Producing Positions or Activities

Alter your posture or position frequently; avoid prolonged standing or sitting.

Place one foot on a footstool when standing for long periods of time (e.g., when ironing, washing dishes, and so on).

Avoid bending at the waist while working, washing your face, brushing your teeth, or performing activities that are below your waist (e.g., bathing children in a bathtub, removing clothes from the washer or dryer, and so on).

Stand on a cushioned mat and wear low-heeled shoes for activities that require prolonged standing.

Enter and leave an automobile with a sideward rather than a twisting motion of the trunk.

Adjust your car seat so your knees are at the same level as your hips. Use a footrest while seated at a typewriter or computer to keep your knees and hips level and bent at 90 degrees; your feet should be flat on the floor or footrest.

Chapter 3

Positioning and Draping

After studying this chapter, the reader will be able to:

1 Describe appropriate positioning of the trunk, head, and extremities with the patient supine, prone, side lying, or sitting.

2 Describe appropriate draping of the patient.

3 Discuss precautions related to positioning a patient who is supine, prone, side lying, or sitting.

4 Give reasons for using and applying proper patient positioning.

5 Present a rationale for the use and application of proper draping of a patient.

Abduction: Movement away from an axis or from the median plane of the body; movement of a body part away from the middle of the body.

Adduction: Movement toward an axis or toward the median plane of the body; movement of a body part toward the middle of the body.

Blanch: To become pale.

Comatose: Pertaining to or affected with coma; a state of unconsciousness.

Contracture: Shortening or tightening of the skin, muscle, fascia, or joint capsule that prevents normal movement or flexibility of the involved structure.

Extension: Movement that increases or straightens the angle between two adjoining body parts or bones.

Flexion: Movement that decreases the angle between two adjoining body parts or bones.

Hyperextension: Extension of a limb or part beyond the normal limit; overextension of a limb or part.

Ischemia: Deficiency of blood in a part due to functional constriction or actual obstruction of a blood vessel.

Ischial tuberosity: The protuberance of the ischium; the inferior, distal portion of the pelvis.

Necrosis: Morphologic changes indicative of cell death.

Occipital tuberosity: The protuberance of the occipital bone; the posterior skull.

Perineum: The pelvic floor and associated structures occupying the pelvic outlet.

Prone: Lying face downward on the vertical ("front") surface of the body; lying on the abdomen and chest.

Reverse "T" position: The position of the upper extremities when they are abducted to 90 degrees and externally rotated at the shoulders and with the elbows flexed to 90 degrees.

Rotation: The pivoting of a body part around its axis.

Shear: An applied force that tends to cause an opposite but parallel sliding motion of the planes of an object; stress is created to the object.

Spasticity: Continuous resistance to stretching by a muscle owing to abnormally increased tension.

Supine: Lying with the face upward or on the dorsal ("back") surface of the body; lying on the back.

"T" position: The position of the upper extremities when they are abducted to 90 degrees and internally rotated at the shoulders and with the elbows flexed to 90 degrees.

INTRODUCTION

Patient positioning must be considered before, during, and at the conclusion of treatment and when a patient is to be at rest for an extended period of time. Although patient comfort must be considered and constitutes one reason to carefully position a patient, the caregiver must be aware that the position of comfort may be the position that could lead to the development of a soft tissue *contracture;* therefore, frequent changes in the patient's position, approximately every 2 hours, may be necessary to prevent contractures or to relieve pressure to his/her skin and subcutaneous, circulatory, neural, lymphatic, or other structures. The greatest pressure occurs to the tissues that cover bony prominences. Table 3–1 provides an outline of the areas that receive the greatest pressure when the patient is in a specific position.

The caregiver should use caution when positioning a patient who has decreased sensation to pressure, is unable to alter his/her position independently and safely, has minimal soft tissue protection over bony prominences, and is unable to express or communicate his/her discomfort. The patient's trunk, head, and extremities should be supported and stabilized, and proper alignment of the axial and appendicular skeletal segments should be maintained to provide a position that will promote efficient function of the patient's body systems. The patient should be positioned to enable the caregiver to administer treatment effectively, efficiently, and safely; therefore, the caregiver should determine how the patient's position may affect his/her body mechanics and treatment program before initiation of treatment.

PRINCIPLES AND CONCEPTS

The patient should be draped, using clean linen, to expose only the areas or body parts to be treated, with the remainder of the patient's body covered to maintain his/her modesty and warmth. Precautions must be taken to avoid unnecessary exposure of sensitive areas of the patient's body. For example, draping of the anterior chest (breasts) of females and the *perineum* (genitalia) of both males and females must be performed carefully and may need to be adjusted periodically to ensure the drape is secure. The linen used to drape each patient should be clean and unused before being applied to the patient. Because the drape material may become soiled with perspiration, lubricants, or wound drainage, the patient's clothing should not be used as a drape. In many instances, undergarments as well as outer garments may need to be

Table 3–1
BONY PROMINENCES THAT OFTEN CAUSE PRESSURE INJURIES

Area	Supine Position	Prone Position	Side-Lying Position (lowermost extremity)	Side-Lying Position (uppermost extremity)	Sitting Position
Head and trunk	• Occipital tuberosity • Spine of scapula • Inferior angle of scapula • Vertebral spinous processes • Posterior iliac crest • Sacrum	• Forehead • Lateral ear • Tip of acromion process • Sternum • Anterior-superior iliac spine	• Lateral ear • Lateral ribs • Lateral acromion process	—	• Ischial tuberosity • Scapular and vertebral prominences (if leaning against back of chair)
Upper extremity	• Medial epicondyle of humerus	• Anterior head of humerus	• Lateral head of humerus • Medial or lateral epicondyle of humerus	• Medial epicondyle of humerus (if resting on a hard surface)	• Medial epicondyle of humerus (if resting on a hard surface)
Lower extremity	• Posterior calcaneus • Greater trochanter, head of fibula, and fibular malleolus with excessive hip external rotation	• Patella • Ridge of tibia • Dorsum of foot	• Greater trochanter of femur • Medial and lateral condyles of femur • Malleolus of fibula and tibia	• Medial condyle of femur • Malleolus of tibia	—

removed from the patient to prevent soiling and to add to the patient's comfort. Before removal of any garments, explain to the patient the need for their removal and receive the patient's permission. You may need to assure the patient that his/her modesty will be maintained throughout the treatment session or activity.

Remove or reduce folds or wrinkles in the linen beneath the patient to avoid increased skin pressure. Folded or wrinkled linen creates a greater thickness than the other areas of the linen and may cause localized pressure. Linen that is used to protect the patient's axilla, perineum, or gluteal cleft must be disposed of as soon as it is removed from the patient because it is likely to be soiled. This linen should never be reapplied to the patient or used for any other patient until it has been laundered.

Be certain to instruct or direct the patient how to position and initially drape himself/herself. A gown or other suitable item should be given to the patient if he/she is required to remove clothing and expose sensitive areas of the body. The treatment table or mat should be prepared with linen and pillows before positioning the patient. The caregiver's instructions and directions should inform the patient exactly what he/she is to do, how he/she is to lie on the table, and how he/she is to apply the gown and drape.

Pillows, rolled towels, or commercially available devices can be used to support or stabilize body segments, thus relieving strain to the patient's joints, liga-

ments, muscles, tendons, connective tissue, and nerves. A firm mattress usually enhances proper positioning, but the patient's condition and ability to alter his/her position should be considered when determining the type of surface on which he/she will sit or lie (Procedure 3–1).

POSITIONING

The recommendations provided for short-term positioning should be appropriate for most patients. However, there are differing opinions about the use (or nonuse) and placement of pillows, towel rolls, bolsters, and similar items. Specific patient needs and the treatment to be given will affect the position the caregiver selects, and the recommended positions should be modified based on criteria the caregiver determines to be appropriate for each patient. Specific patient conditions, such as the loss of or decreased sensory awareness, paralysis, decreased skin integrity, poor nutrition, impaired circulation, and a predisposition to contracture development, will require special attention to positioning. For a patient with any of these conditions, it will be necessary to inspect the patient's skin, especially over bony prominences, immediately after the treatment session. Areas that are red indicate areas of pressure, and pale, or *blanched*, areas may indicate severe, dangerous pressure. Complaints of numbness or tingling are indicators of excessive

PROCEDURE 3–1
Guidelines for Positioning and Draping

1. Introduce yourself to the patient; provide your name and status (i.e., physical therapist, physical therapist assistant, physical therapy student, aide, technician, occupational therapist, certified occupational therapist assistant) and confirm the patient's name and current, relevant information about him/her (i.e., diagnosis, complaints, previous treatment and response, physician).

2. Inform him/her of the planned treatment; apply the principles of informed consent, and obtain his/her consent for treatment.

3. Specifically describe how he/she is to be positioned; provide assistance if he/she requires it.
   a. If the person is wearing "street clothes," indicate the specific articles of clothing he/she is to remove or request permission to remove them if assistance is provided.
   b. Provide temporary clothing or linen to protect his/her modesty and provide warmth.
   c. Have sufficient linen, pillows, and equipment needed for the treatment available in the cubicle or treatment area.
   d. Provide safe and secure storage for his/her valuable items.

4. Specifically describe how you desire him/her to use linen items, gown, robe, or exercise clothing to cover (drape) himself/herself; provide privacy while he/she disrobes.

5. Instruct him/her to inform you when he/she is positioned and draped, or ask him/her if he/she is clothed or draped so you may enter the cubicle.

6. At the conclusion of the treatment:
   a. Instruct him/her to remove drape items and temporary clothing and to reapply his/her "street clothing"; provide assistance if he/she requires it.
   b. Provide linen so he/she can remove perspiration, massage lotion, electrotherapy gels, water, or other substances.
   c. Return valuables.
   d. Dispose of used linen in proper container.
   e. Prepare the cubicle or treatment area for future use or assign the task to a staff member.

Note: Depending on the gender of the caregiver and the patient and the area or areas of the patient that are to be exposed for treatment, it may be necessary for the caregiver to request another person to assist the patient in undressing, positioning, draping, and redressing himself/herself to protect his/her modesty.

pressure, as is localized edema or swelling. *Caution:* Pressure to a localized area of soft tissue, especially when there is an underlying bony prominence, produces local *ischemia*, which over time can lead to tissue *necrosis.* You must be particularly aware of these possible consequences when you treat a patient whose condition involves the contributing factors described previously in this paragraph.

Restraints or straps may be used to protect the patient from rolling or falling and to prevent injury. They are recommended for short-term use only and not to hinder or restrain the patient for several

Rationale for Proper Positioning

Prevent soft tissue and joint contractures.

Provide patient comfort.

Provide support and stability of patient's trunk and extremities.

Provide access and exposure to areas to be treated.

Promote efficient function of patient's organ systems.

Provide position changes to relieve excessive, prolonged pressure to soft tissue, bony prominences, and circulatory and neurologic structures.

hours. The patient who is *comatose*, experiences *spasticity*, has extensive paralysis, or is unable to mentally or physically maintain a safe position may require some form of temporary restraint or protective positioning. These protective measures are to be differentiated from the use of prolonged restraints, which may allow a patient to be unattended for several hours. Use of restraints in this manner for the elderly patient who is institutionalized is restricted by law.

The decision as to whether protective positioning is a necessary component of quality care rests with the caregiver who is responsible for the care of the patient at the time that care is being provided. When a patient in a hospital or nursing home is restrained at the conclusion of treatment, nursing personnel should be informed. Continued use of the restraint or release of the restraints then becomes the decision of nursing personnel, who should follow the policies and procedures of the facility or other entity that regulates the use of prolonged restraint, especially for the elderly (Box 3–1).

Supine Position   Place a small pillow or a cervical roll under the patient's head, but avoid excessive neck and upper back *flexion* or scapular *abduction* ("round shoulders") (Fig. 3–1). A small pillow, rolled towels, or small bolster can be placed in the popliteal spaces (i.e., behind the knees) to relieve lumbar lordosis and promote comfort. Some patients may prefer to use a small lumbar roll or pillow. *Caution:* The item behind the knees will encourage hip and knee flexion and may contribute to lower extremity contractures of the iliopsoas (hip flexor) and hamstring (knee flexor) muscles. This position should not be maintained for a prolonged period of time. A small, rolled towel or small bolster can be placed at the patient's posterior

ankles to relieve pressure to the calcaneus (heel), but knee *hyperextension* should be avoided.

In some situations, it may be acceptable to move the end of the mat or table pad over the edge of the mat or table and allow the patient's feet to project over the end of the mat or table. *Caution:* If the patient's feet project over the end of the mat or treatment table, they could be injured if they are struck by a large piece of equipment or other object. Therefore, do not position the patient so his/her feet project over the end of the mat or treatment table, especially if they are screened by a cubicle curtain or sheet and would extend into an area used by personnel to move equipment or walk. The patient's upper extremities may be elevated on pillows or positioned in whatever way the patient desires for comfort (e.g., by the patient's side, in a *reverse "T" position*, or folded on his/her chest). The patient's body and extremities should be totally supported on the mat or table; no part or portion of his/her body or extremities should project beyond its surface.

Remember: The areas of greatest pressure when the patient is *supine* are the *occipital tuberosity*, spine and inferior angle of the scapula, spinous processes of the vertebrae, posterior iliac crests, sacrum, and posterior calcaneus (see Table 3–1). Other possible pressure areas, depending on how the patient is positioned, are the medial epicondyle of the humerus, head of the fibula, and lateral malleolus if excessive external *rotation* of the hip occurs. A rolled towel or sandbag can be used to maintain the hip in a neutral position. The hip should be moved toward internal *rotation* and the towel or sandbags placed against the lateral aspect of the soft tissue of the thigh and lower leg.

Prone Position   Place a small pillow or towel roll under the patient's head or he/she may turn his/her head to the left or right (Fig. 3–2). Some patients may be more comfortable if they rest their forehead on a folded towel or special headrest. A pillow placed under the patient's lower abdomen will reduce his/her lumbar lordosis. (*Note:* For some patients, maintenance of his/her normal lumbar lordosis may be desired, and a pillow may be placed under his/her upper or middle chest or positioned lengthwise from his/her pelvis to the thorax to maintain the lordosis.) A rolled towel should be placed under each anterior shoulder to *adduct* the scapulae and reduce the stress to the interscapular muscles. The use of a pillow, towel roll, or small bolster under the patient's anterior ankles will relieve stress on his/her hamstring muscles and will allow the pelvis and lower back to relax. *Caution:* The pillow placed at the ankles causes knee flexion and may contribute to contracture of the hamstring (knee flexor) muscles. To avoid the development of a contracture, this position should not be maintained for a prolonged period of time. The patient's upper extremities may be positioned for his/her comfort (e.g.,

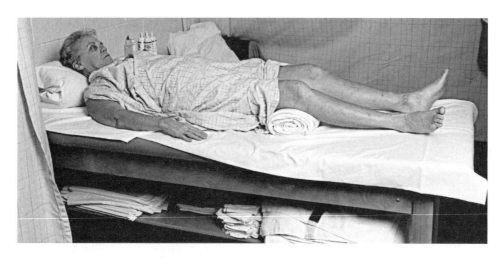

■ **FIGURE 3–1**
Supine position.

along his/her sides, in a *"T" position*, or with the hands under the head).

Remember: The areas of greatest pressure when the patient is *prone* are the anterior head of the humerus, sternum, anterior-superior iliac spine, patella, crest of the tibia, and dorsum of the foot (see Table 3–1).

Side-Lying Position   Initially, the patient should be positioned in the center of the bed, mat, or table with his/her head, trunk, and pelvis aligned (Fig. 3–3). Both of the patient's lower extremities should be flexed at the hip and knee. The uppermost lower extremity should be supported on one or two pillows and positioned slightly forward of the lowermost extremity. The lowermost lower extremity provides stability to the patient's pelvis and lower trunk. One or two pillows should be used to support the patient's head. A folded pillow placed at the patient's chest is used to support his/her uppermost upper extremity and prevent him/her from rolling onto his/her abdomen. It may be necessary to place a folded pillow along the patient's posterior trunk to prevent him/her from rolling onto his/her back.

If you determine that the patient will not be able to maintain a side-lying position independently and

safely, restraint straps should be applied. The lowermost upper extremity can be positioned to promote patient comfort and stability. If the lowermost greater trochanter requires protection, place a pillow distal to the trochanter under the patient's lowermost lower extremity and a second pillow under the trunk proximal to the trochanter. *Caution:* The patient whose condition predisposes him/her to the development of a pressure ulcer should be positioned to avoid direct pressure to the downmost trochanter. This can be accomplished by placing him/her in a slightly reclined position.

Remember: The areas of greatest pressure when the patient is in a side-lying position are the lateral aspect of the patient's lowermost ear, lowermost acromion process, lowermost greater trochanter, medial condyle of the uppermost femur, lateral condyle of the lowermost femur, malleolus of the uppermost tibia, malleolus of the lowermost fibula, and medial condyles of the femurs and the malleolus of the lowermost tibia if the uppermost lower extremity is positioned directly over the opposite lower extremity.

Sitting Position   The patient should be seated in a chair with adequate support and stability for his/her

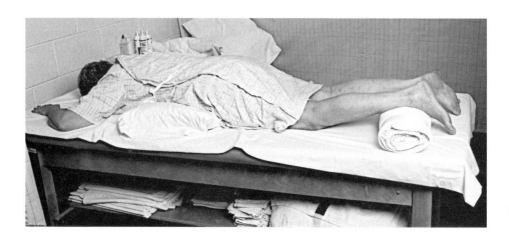

■ **FIGURE 3–2**
Prone position.

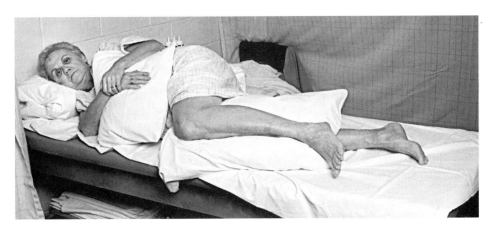

■ **FIGURE 3–3**
Side-lying position.

trunk, which can be provided by pillows, belts, or straps or the back of the chair or by leaning forward onto a treatment table. The patient's lower extremities should be supported by placing his/her feet on a footstool, on the footrests of a wheelchair, or on the floor. The distal and posterior thigh tissue and deeper structures should be free of excessive pressure from the edge of the chair or wheelchair seat. When the patient receives treatment with the trunk leaning forward against the treatment table, one or more pillows can be used to support the anterior trunk. Use one or more pillows behind the patient when he/she sits with the trunk leaning back against the chair. The patient's upper extremities can be supported on pillows, on the chair armrests, on the treatment table, or on a lap board or by placing them on a pillow in the patient's lap. To improve access to the patient's back, he/she can sit in an armless chair with the chair back directed to the left or right.

Remember: The areas of greatest pressure when the patient is sitting are the *ischial tuberosities* and the posterior thigh. Other possible areas of pressure are the sacrum and the spinous processes of the vertebrae if the patient leans against the chair back, and the medial epicondyle of the humerus if the elbow rests on a hard surface such as a lap board.

In general, a patient should not be positioned for an extended period of time (more than 30 minutes) in any position that causes or produces the following:

1. Excessive rotation or bending of the spine
2. Bilateral or unilateral scapular abduction or a forward head position
3. Compression of the thorax or chest
4. Plantar flexion of the ankles and feet
5. Hip or knee flexion
6. Adduction and internal rotation of the glenohumeral joint
7. Elbow, wrist, or finger flexion
8. Hip adduction or internal/external rotation

These positions promote excessive stress or strain to various structures and may promote the development of a soft tissue contracture or patient discomfort (Box 3–2). You must observe the areas of pressure in those patients who are susceptible to skin irritation or breakdown (e.g., the elderly, those who lack sensation, and those who are paralyzed). A reddened or blanched area that does not return to a normal appearance within an hour after the treatment session must be monitored. The use of the position that

---

BOX 3–2

Common Soft Tissue Contracture Sites Related to Prolonged Positioning

Supine
    Hip and knee flexors
    Ankle plantar flexors
    Shoulder extensors, adductors, and internal rotators
    Hip external rotators
Prone
    Ankle plantar flexors
    Shoulder extensors, adductors, and internal/external rotators
    Neck rotators, left or right
Side lying
    Hip and knee flexors
    Hip adductors and internal rotators
    Shoulder adductors and internal rotators
Sitting
    Hip and knee flexors
    Hip adductors and internal rotators
    Shoulder adductors, extensors, and internal rotators

Note: Forearm, elbow, wrist, and finger contractures can develop depending on the position used.

Precautions for Patient Positioning

Avoid the presence of clothing or linen folds beneath patient.

Observe skin color before, during, and after treatment.

Protect bony prominences from excessive and prolonged pressure.

Avoid positioning the patient's extremities beyond the support surface.

Avoid excessive, prolonged pressure to soft tissue and circulatory and neurologic structures.

Use additional caution when positioning patients who are mentally incompetent or confused, comatose, very young or elderly, paralyzed, or lacking normal circulation or sensation.

caused the problem should be avoided in the future. Various positioning aids (e.g., elbow and heel protectors, footboards, seat cushions, lap boards, slings, splints, cones, or bolsters) can be helpful to reduce soft tissue stress, support or stabilize a joint or segment, relieve pressure, or immobilize a segment. However, these items must be applied carefully and removed or adjusted periodically to avoid secondary problems. Straps on protective devices or splints may occlude peripheral circulation if applied too tightly; an unpadded lap board may cause excessive pressure to the medial humeral epicondyle; and bolsters, cushions, or cones may create a source for the development of perspiration, which, if it is not dissipated, may lead to skin maceration. Therefore, cautious and judicious use of these aids is recommended (Box 3–3).

Remember to be particularly careful when positioning the patient who is elderly, mentally confused, mentally incompetent, very young, comatose, paralyzed, agitated, or known to have an impaired cardiopulmonary system. These persons may not tolerate remaining in one position for more than a few minutes. Their circulation or respiration may become impaired, and their skin may develop a lesion more readily as a result of pressure or *shear* forces created by the position. They may have more difficulty complying with instructions to maintain a given position, they may lack the ability to sense the need to change their position, or they may be unable to alter their position without assistance. These patients should be monitored frequently to avoid the adverse complications associated with positioning.

PREVENTIVE POSITIONING

It is recommended that a patient's position be altered frequently to avoid excessive or prolonged pressure, reduce the development of contractures, avoid postural malalignment, and prevent other adverse effects. In addition, there are specific positions that should be avoided for certain patients because their diagnosis or condition predisposes them to complications related to short-term or prolonged positioning. The functional ability or capacity of the patient may be compromised because of problems caused by improper positioning techniques, which may affect the patient's independence or quality of life. Some conditions in which selected positions should be avoided are discussed in the sections that follow.

Thigh Amputation For the patient with an above-the-knee or partial thigh amputation, prolonged hip flexion should be avoided. The residual limb (RL) or "stump" should not be elevated on a pillow while the patient is supine for more than a few minutes of each hour. The amount and length of time the patient is permitted to sit should be limited to no more than 30 minutes of each hour. Each of these positions promotes the development of a contracture of the patient's hip flexor muscles. If those muscles become contracted, the patient is apt to experience difficulty using a prosthesis for ambulation. In addition, it may not be possible to fit the patient with a prosthesis if contractures occur.

Hip abduction of the RL should be avoided to prevent a contracture of the hip abductor muscles. If this contracture develops, the patient will experience difficulty ambulating with a prosthesis. The patient should be encouraged to maintain his/her pelvis in a level position and to maintain his/her trunk in proper alignment while recumbent to avoid developing back discomfort and an abnormal posture. When the patient stands or is recumbent, he/she should maintain the RL in *extension*. Periodic prone lying is recommended.

Lower Leg Amputation For the patient with a below-the-knee or partial leg amputation, prolonged hip and knee flexion should be avoided. The RL or "stump" should not be elevated on a pillow while the patient is supine for more than a few minutes of each hour. If the RL is elevated, the knee should be maintained in extension. The amount and length of time the patient is permitted to sit should be limited to no more than 30 minutes of each hour. Each of these positions promotes the development of a contracture of the patient's hip flexor and knee flexor muscles. If those muscles become contracted, the patient will experience difficulty using a prosthesis for ambulation. In addition, it may not be possible to fit the patient with a prosthesis if contractures occur. When the patient sits, stands, or is recumbent, he/she should maintain his/her knee in extension. Periodic prone lying is recommended.

Hemiplegia When the patient's upper extremity is involved, prolonged shoulder adduction and internal rotation; elbow flexion; forearm supination or pronation; wrist, finger, or thumb flexion; and finger and thumb adduction should be avoided. These positions are the ones most likely to lead to soft tissue contractures owing to muscle spasticity, reduced function of the opposing muscles, and lack of active or passive motion. The use of a sling to support the involved extremity places the shoulder in adduction and internal rotation, the elbow in flexion, and the forearm in pronation, and the wrist and fingers may be flexed. This also is a position of comfort for many patients, but if contractures of the muscles of the upper extremity develop, the potential for functional use of the extremity will be reduced; therefore, the upper extremity should be positioned in varying amounts of shoulder abduction and external rotation, elbow extension, slight wrist extension, thumb abduction and extension, and finger extension and slight abduction.

When a patient's lower extremity is involved, prolonged hip and knee flexion, hip external rotation, and ankle plantar flexion and inversion should be avoided. These positions are those most likely to lead to soft tissue contractures due to muscle spasticity, reduced function of the opposing muscle, and lack of active or passive motion. The potential for function of the lower extremity will be reduced if contractures develop; therefore, the lower extremity should be positioned in varying amounts of hip and knee extension, hip abduction and internal rotation, and ankle dorsiflexion and eversion.

However, static positioning of the extremities may not be the most effective treatment technique depending on the patient's neurologic condition and response to positioning. The extremities should be exercised several times per day and should not remain in a single position for a prolonged period of time.

The normal alignment of the patient's head and trunk should be maintained when he/she is sitting or lying. Frequent adjustments of his/her posture or position may be necessary to ensure proper alignment.

Rheumatoid Arthritis Rheumatoid arthritis is a systemic disease and one of the major systems involved by the disease is the musculoskeletal system, especially the joints. Prolonged immobilization of the affected extremity joints should be avoided, particularly if the joint is maintained in flexion. Gentle, careful,

and frequent active or passive movement of the involved joints should be performed several times per day unless the joints are in a state of acute inflammation. The uninvolved joints should be exercised actively.

Contractures may develop even when various therapeutic measures are used. Carefully applied exercise can benefit most patients, but each patient should be given a treatment plan specifically designed for him/her. The patient will need to assume a great deal of the responsibility to maintain his/her body at its maximal level of function once he/she has been instructed by the appropriate caregiver or practitioner.

Split Thickness Burns and Grafted Burn Areas
Healing or regenerating skin is apt to develop scar tissue, and contractures are likely to occur. It is important to avoid prolonged positioning of the joints that have been affected by the burn or graft used to repair the wound. It is particularly important to avoid positions of comfort. A position of comfort for the patient with a burn is the position that does not produce stress or tension to the wound or graft. Prolonged flexion or adduction of most peripheral joints should be avoided when the burn is located on the flexor or adductor surface of a joint. The patient should be encouraged to perform gentle, careful, and frequent active movement of the involved joints and should exercise his/her uninvolved joints actively. When the patient is unable to perform active exercise, passive exercise should be performed.

Usually the patient should not be permitted to assume the position that provides the greatest comfort for an extended period of time because contractures are more apt to develop when the position of comfort is maintained. Once a contracture has developed, time, exercise, and perseverance by the patient and health care providers will be necessary to return the joint to a normal position and functional use. The patient is likely to experience a great deal of pain and discomfort during the process used to restore normal joint motion. Everyone involved with the care and management of the patient, including the patient, must understand that prevention of a contracture is far more desirable and less costly than the treatment required to overcome one.

These examples of patient conditions illustrate the need for proper positioning techniques for selected patients. Many other patient problems require thoughtfulness and planning to prevent the development of contractures or maintain function. The general rule to remember is that prolonged immobilization and failure to change positions frequently are precursors to the development of contractures and decreased function.

DRAPING

The primary reasons to appropriately drape or clothe a patient are to expose or free the area to be treated while the patient's modesty is protected and a comfortable body temperature is maintained. The caregiver must be aware that each patient has his/her own concept of modesty. Some patients may be embarrassed or consider their body excessively exposed when only the upper or lower extremity is uncovered. Others may seem to have a disregard for their modesty and may expose themselves, to the embarrassment of other patients or the caregiver. Each patient should be informed of the type of clothing he/she should wear for the treatment session, or the facility may provide suitable clothing. Before treatment, the caregiver should inform the patient that clothing may need to be removed and why such removal is necessary. The patient should be told that his/her body will be protected by linen or substitute garments, except for the areas to be treated. In some instances the caregiver will need to inform the patient that his/her clothing may become soiled even though clean linen is used as protection.

The area to be treated must be exposed and have freedom of motion so treatment can be performed effectively and observation and palpation of the area can occur. However, if the patient senses or experiences exposure of a sensitive area of his/her body (e.g., the perineum, gluteal region, or anterior chest area in female patients), it is doubtful the treatment session will be effective.

Another person may have to assist the patient to apply proper clothing or drape material in preparation for treatment (Box 3–4). If it is necessary to undress the patient, you should request his/her permission to do so. To avoid or reduce the transference of disease or infection from one patient to another, only clean and previously unused linen and garments should be used for each patient. Soiled linen and garments must be properly disposed of at the conclusion

of each treatment session. If an undergarment is removed, it is imperative that the patient's modesty be preserved throughout the treatment session.

Remember that some patients may be reluctant to remove their clothing, even though you have indicated that their modesty will be preserved. You can help to reduce their apprehension by providing sufficient and appropriate drape materials, by instructing the patient how to apply or use the items, by being certain the treatment cubicle is shielded by a closed curtain or door, by asking the patient's permission to enter the cubicle and whether he/she is draped, and, if necessary, by having a caregiver of the same gender as the patient assist the patient to undress and dress. Access to the treatment area should be permitted only for those persons required to provide treatment. Whenever the caregiver leaves the treatment cubicle, the patient should be dressed or draped so his/her body is not unduly exposed in case another person enters or looks into the cubicle.

With the patient supine, the upper extremities can be exposed for treatment (Fig. 3–4). Either the caregiver or patient should remove any restrictive clothing, splints, or other devices to expose the areas to be treated. It may be necessary to provide a gown for him/her and to be certain that any clothing that was not removed does not restrict movement or access to the extremity. A towel, gown, or sheet can be used

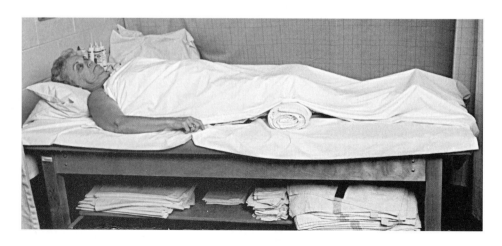

■ **FIGURE 3–4**
Draping of a supine patient for treatment of the upper extremity.

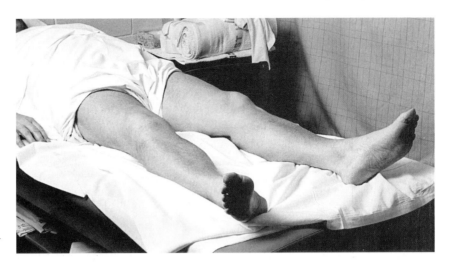

■ **FIGURE 3–5**
Draping of a supine patient for treatment of the lower extremities.

to drape the patient's anterior chest and lower extremities. The drape should not restrict joint motion or access to the area to be treated. In some instances it may be necessary to apply the drape into the axilla to shield the anterior and lateral chest.

With the patient supine, the lower extremities can also be exposed for treatment (Fig. 3–5). Either the caregiver or the patient should remove any restrictive clothing, splints, or other devices to expose the areas to be treated. Any clothing that is not removed should not restrict motion or limit access to the area to be treated. A towel or sheet can be used to drape the patient's perineum (groin); this must be applied high in the groin and under the thigh to shield the perineum fully. Be certain the drape remains secure throughout the treatment and that it does not restrict joint motion of the hip or knee. The patient's upper body and opposite lower extremity should be covered for warmth and to preserve his/her modesty.

Draping material is frequently used to absorb perspiration, water, and various lubricants or to prevent these fluids from contacting the patient's clothing. It is also used to protect the patient's modesty and maintain body warmth. Therefore, this material must not be used on another patient and must be disposed of at the termination of treatment. The patient should be instructed or assisted to dress at the end of the treatment. The caregiver should evaluate the patient's response to treatment before releasing him/her. Specific draping techniques necessary for massage are beyond the scope of this text and are not presented; however, they are available in other textbooks.

SUMMARY

Proper techniques to position and drape a patient are important because they protect the patient from injury, provide stabilization to an area, provide access while exposing only the specific area to be treated, maintain the person's body temperature, and protect him/her from unnecessary exposure of body areas, especially the breasts and perineum.

Prolonged use of any one position should be avoided to reduce the development of a soft tissue contracture. Pillows, towel rolls, or similar devices can be used to promote comfort and stability, but these should be used with caution to avoid contractures. The caregiver should be aware of the body areas that will be affected most by pressure, depending on the position selected, so they can be protected or the pressure relieved periodically.

■ SELF-STUDY/DISCUSSION ACTIVITIES

1. List at least three possible adverse effects of improper or prolonged positioning on the musculoskeletal, neuromuscular, and cardiopulmonary systems.

2. Describe why proper patient positioning and draping are important for the practitioner.

3. Explain why or how the patient positions presented in the text provide comfort for the patient.

4. Outline the precautions you would use if it were necessary for you to position a patient who has decreased sensation, who is elderly, who is mentally confused, who is unable to independently change position, who has impaired respiration, or who has impaired peripheral circulation.

5. Explain how you would position and drape a patient for treatment to his/her right upper and lower extremities while he/she is supine and for treatment to his/her left upper and lower extremities while he/she is side lying.

Chapter 4

Vital Signs and Body Composition Assessments

OBJECTIVES

After studying this chapter, the reader will be able to:

1 Provide the rationale for the need to measure, monitor, and record a patient's vital signs.

2 Locate and palpate a patient's arterial pulse at various sites.

3 Describe and define blood pressure.

4 Accurately measure and record a patient's blood pressure, pulse and heart rates, respiration rate, and body temperature.

5 Describe the expected normal and abnormal changes in blood pressure, heart rate, and respiration rate resulting from exercise and other factors.

6 Explain to a patient or family member the significance of measuring and monitoring vital signs.

7 Accurately measure an individual's body composition using skinfold, girth, and volumetric measurements.

■■■ KEY TERMS

Anoxia: Absence of oxygen in the tissues.

Apical pulse: The pulse that is found by placing a stethoscope on the chest wall over the apex of the heart; may also be found by palpation.

Apnea: The absence of breathing.

Auscultation: Listening for sounds produced within the body using the unaided ear or the stethoscope.

Bradycardia: A slow heart beat (i.e., pulse rate less than 60 beats per minute); may be a normal finding in a well-conditioned person or an abnormal finding.

Cardiac output: The amount of blood that is pumped from the heart during each contraction.

Diaphoresis: Profuse perspiration.

Diastole: The period of time when the least amount of pressure is exerted on the walls or the arteries during the heart beat; usually indicates the resting phase of the heart.

Dyspnea: Labored or difficult breathing.

Expiration: The passive phase of respiration when the person breathes out; also referred to as *exhalation*.

Fever: Body temperature that is above the normal level; also referred to as *pyrexia*.

Hypertension: Abnormally high blood pressure.

Hypotension: Abnormally low blood pressure.

Inguinal: Pertaining to the groin.

Inspiration: The active phase of respiration when the person breathes in; also referred to as *inhalation*.

Intubation: The insertion of a tube, as into the larynx to maintain an open airway.

Korotkoff's sounds: Sounds heard during auscultatory determination of blood pressure; thought to be produced by vibratory motion of the arterial wall as the artery suddenly distends when compressed by a pneumatic blood pressure cuff. The origin of the sound may be within the blood passing through the vessel or within the wall itself.

Occlude: To fit close together; to close tight; to obstruct or close off.

Orthopnea: A condition in which breathing is easier when the person is seated or standing.

Pulse: A palpable wave of blood produced in the walls of the arteries with each heart beat or contraction.

Rale: An abnormal discontinuous nonmusical sound heard on auscultation of the chest, primarily during inhalation; also called a *crackle*.

Rectal: Pertaining to the rectum, or the distal portion of the large intestine.

Respiration: The act of breathing.

SOB: Shortness of breath.

Sphygmomanometer: An instrument used to measure blood pressure; it may use a mercury column or an enclosed air pressure spring system.

Stethoscope: An instrument used to convey sounds produced in the body of a person to the ears of the examiner; it is composed of a diaphragm, tubing, and ear pieces.

Stridor: A shrill, harsh sound, especially the respiratory sound heard during inspiration in laryngeal obstruction.

Syncope: A temporary suspension of consciousness due to cerebral anemia; fainting.

Systole: The period of time when the greatest amount of pressure is exerted on the walls of the arteries during heart beat; usually indicates the contractile phase of the heart beat.

Tachycardia: An abnormally fast heart beat (i.e., pulse rate greater than 100 beats per minute).

Vital signs: Measurement of a person's body temperature, heart and respiration rates, and blood pressure; also referred to as *cardinal signs*.

INTRODUCTION

The patient's *vital signs*—blood pressure (BP), heart rate, respiration rate, and body temperature—are important because they are indicators of his/her general health or physiologic status. Normal values or ranges have been established for vital signs, and significant deviations from these norms may indicate an abnormal condition. It is important for the caregiver to know the normal values and determine the normal and abnormal changes that may occur as a result of illness, trauma, exercise, or physical conditioning.

For most patients, a baseline measurement of his/her vital signs at rest should be established so changes in the values due to exercise or other activity factors can be determined. It is particularly important to establish baseline values for the following types of patients:

Elderly patients (i.e., older than 65 years)

Very young patients (younger than 2 years)

Debilitated patients

Patients who have performed limited aerobic activities for several weeks or months

Patients with a previous or current history of cardiovascular problems

Patients with traumatic injuries, a disease that adversely affects the cardiopulmonary system (e.g., spinal cord injury, cerebrovascular accident, hypertension, peripheral vascular disease, or chronic obstructive pulmonary disease), or who have had surgery

If abnormal values are found when the person is at rest, the cause of these abnormal values should be determined before the initiation of any activity that could affect his/her vital signs. Frequently, the patient with abnormal resting values will be less able to tolerate physical activity or stress-producing events.

Measurements of the patient's vital signs can be used to establish goals of treatment, assist with the development of a treatment plan, and assess a patient's response to treatment (i.e., determining the effectiveness of treatment).

General factors that usually cause a change in a person's vital signs (i.e., increasing or decreasing them) are the level or amount of physical activity, environmental temperature, person's age, emotional status of the person, and physiologic status of the person (i.e., the existence of illness, disease, or trauma).

Some possible adverse and potentially dangerous responses to activity are mental confusion; fatigue; exhaustion; lethargy; slow reactions of movement or response to commands; decreased response to verbal and tactile stimuli; complaints of nausea, *syncope*, or vertigo; *diaphoresis;* a change in appearance (e.g., pallor, erythema); pupil constriction or dilation; and loss of consciousness. Many of these responses may be due to *anoxia*. The caregiver should monitor the patient during and after treatment for any indication of these undesirable signs and symptoms. Prompt and appropriate care may have to be provided to reduce or relieve them, and modifications in the treatment program may be necessary to avoid them.

BODY TEMPERATURE

Body temperature is an indication of the intensity or degree of heat within the body. It represents a balance between the heat that is produced in the body and the heat that is lost. In humans, body temperature remains relatively constant regardless of the environmental temperature. However, there are some exceptions, such as when someone is exposed to extremes of heat or cold or when other factors such as humidity and physical exertion are involved.

Depending on the source, an accepted normal range for human oral core or body temperature is 96.8°F to 99.5°F (36°C to 37.5°C). The average temperature of 98.6°F (37°C) is the most generally accepted single value. The normal range for human rectal temperature is 97.8°F to 100.5°F (36.6°C to 38.1°C). Slight variations from these norms may occur

---

BOX 4–1

Factors Affecting Body Temperature

1. *Time of day.* Body temperature is usually lower in the early morning and higher in the afternoon.
2. *Age.* Body temperature tends to decrease slightly with age and is increased slightly in the very young.
3. *Environmental temperature.* Body temperature tends to increase slightly in a hot environment and decrease slightly in a cold environment.
4. *Infection.* Body temperature increases when a major infectious process occurs.
5. *Physical activity.* Body temperature usually increases slightly with physical activity but reaches a plateau as the person becomes better conditioned.
6. *Emotional status.* Body temperature increases slightly during stressful or emotional periods (e.g., crying or anger).
7. *Site of measurement.* Body temperature values are slightly higher if measured rectally and slightly lower if measured in the axilla when compared with oral values.
8. *Menstrual cycle.* Body temperature is slightly higher at the time of ovulation, and a pregnant female's body temperature tends to be slightly higher than usual.
9. *Oral cavity temperature.* Body temperature measurement may be inaccurate if measured orally within 15 to 30 minutes of ingestion of warm or cold substances or smoking. The body core temperature probably is not affected by these factors, but a false reading is obtained as a result of the temporary changes in the temperature of the oral cavity.

---

in patients, and therefore it is important to establish a norm for each patient by repeatedly measuring his/her temperature. A person whose normal core temperature is 98.6°F is considered to have a *fever*, or to be pyrexic, with a temperature above 100°F (38°C) and to be hyperpyrexic with a temperature above 106°F (41.1°C). Factors that affect body temperature are listed in Box 4–1.

ASSESSMENT OF BODY TEMPERATURE

Sites used to assess a person's body temperature are the oral cavity, rectum, axilla, ear canal, and, occa-

P R O C E D U R E 4 – 1
Measuring Body Temperature Orally With a Glass Thermometer

1. Wash your hands and obtain a thermometer, recording form, pen, alcohol, and a wipe to clean the thermometer.

2. Position the patient and explain the procedure. Observe the patient and evaluate signs or symptoms related to body temperature: skin color, temperature (hot, warm, cool), and condition (moist, dry). Clean the thermometer bulb with an alcohol wipe or wipe it dry if it has been stored in alcohol or a similar solution.

3. Check the level of the mercury in the thermometer to be certain it is below 96°F or 35°C. If it is higher than those values, hold the end of the thermometer opposite to the bulb and shake the thermometer with several quick wrist movements.

4. Instruct the patient to open his/her mouth, position the thermometer bulb under the person's tongue, and instruct the patient to hold the thermometer in place with the lips, not with the teeth, and to breathe through the nose.

5. Leave the thermometer in place for approximately 3 to 5 minutes, although some sources indicate that 7 to 8 minutes may be necessary to obtain an accurate value.

6. Remove the thermometer using your thumb and index finger and lightly clean the thermometer by wiping from the top to the bulb end. Do not hold the bulb end of the thermometer when you clean it or when you attempt to read the scale.

7. Read the thermometer by holding it horizontally at eye level so that the mercury column is clearly visible. Each long line on the scale is one degree and each small line is two tenths of a degree. A special line usually marks 98.6°F or 37°C.

8. Clean and place the thermometer in its container and wash your hands.

9. Record the results, using even increments to report tenths (e.g., 97.6°F, 98.6°F, or 99.2°F).

---

sionally, *inguinal* fold. The most common and a convenient location to measure a person's temperature is the oral cavity, but the most accurate measurement of body temperature is obtained from the *rectal* cavity. Rectal or ear canal measurement can be used in infants or young (i.e., preschool) children who are unable to maintain the thermometer under the tongue or to safely hold it between the lips. It also can be used in unconscious patients or patients who are unable to maintain the thermometer in the mouth (e.g., a patient who is *intubated*). The axillary or inguinal folds are the least desirable sites because the measurement will not be accurate due to air currents, which tend to reduce the measurement. Therefore, measurement at these sites should be used only when measurement at either of the other two sites is neither possible nor safe. If the temperature is measured by the rectal or axillary method, it should be so noted on the patient's record.

Equipment available to measure body temperature includes the clinical glass thermometer or the oral electronic thermometer with a probe, both of which are reusable; the chemical thermometer, which is disposed of after one use; or the ear canal electronic thermometer.

A thermometer is available that measures body temperature on the basis of heat generated by the ear canal and its surrounding tissue. It is especially useful for infants, toddlers, and older persons for whom it is difficult to use an oral thermometer. Most ear thermometers require a 9-volt battery as the power source, and disposable lens filters are used to protect the ear canal and lens cone. The lens filter should be cleaned thoroughly or discarded after each use to prevent cross-contamination or a false reading of the unit. The temperature value is obtained from a liquid crystal display (LCD) in a window on one side of the thermometer. The unit has two settings—rectal and oral. The rectal setting is used for infants and toddlers, and the oral setting is used for other persons. These setting selections allow the unit to measure and report a temperature that is consistent with the sites for which a glass thermometer is used. Regardless of the setting selected, the lens cone is placed in the person's ear canal. It is suggested that a normal or baseline temperature be established for an individual before the need to measure his/her temperature during an illness, especially when the person is an infant or a toddler. Two or three serial measurements should be taken for infants younger than 3 months and for toddlers younger than 3 years when the presence or absence of a fever is a critical finding or when the operator is unfamiliar with the unit. When the individual has been lying on his/her ear for a period of time, that ear should not be used for measurement until it has been exposed to the air for 2 to 3 minutes so the ear canal temperature can become stable. If the temperature of the ear canal is not permitted to acclimate, a falsely high reading may occur. A temperature differential may exist between the person's left and right ear, so the same ear should be used for all measurements during each period the thermometer is used. When you document the results of the measurement, you should indicate in which ear the thermometer cone was placed.

Steps to measure body temperature orally using a glass thermometer are listed in Procedure 4–1. Use of an oral electronic thermometer is described in Procedure 4–2, and the use of the ear canal electronic thermometer is described in Procedure 4–3.

Nursing personnel usually measure temperature, but other health care personnel should be prepared to perform this task. In addition, treatment decisions may need to be made based on the patient's body temperature or response to exercise. Exercise should not be initiated in a person whose body temperature is elevated before treatment. The cause of this abnormal temperature should be determined before exercise is initiated. The person whose body temperature is lower than normal before treatment should be monitored to be certain he/she tolerates the treatment and determine whether his/her temperature changes during or at the conclusion of the activity. The person with a normal body temperature before treatment can be monitored during or at the conclusion of the treatment to determine whether normal responses occur; if an excessive temperature value is measured or any signs/symptoms of excessive temperature are observed, the patient should have adequate periods of rest to allow his/her body temperature to stabilize at the normal value. The patient whose body temperature becomes lower than normal during treatment may also be demonstrating an abnormal response to the treatment. In any of these abnormal situations, caution should be used if the treatment is continued. It may be necessary to have the patient examined by an appropriate medical practitioner.

PULSE

The *pulse* is an indirect measure of the contraction of the left ventricle of the heart and indicates the rate at which the heart is beating. It consists of the movement of blood in an artery, which can be palpated at various sites of the body or measured through *auscultation* over the apex of the heart with the use of a *stethoscope*. The rate or frequency of ventricular contractions of the heart is reported in beats per minute (bpm).

Depending on the source that is used, the accepted normal range for the resting pulse is 60 to 100 bpm in the adult, 100 to 130 bpm in the newborn, and 80 to 120 bpm in the child 1 to 7 years old. The normal resting pulse can be established for each patient by repeatedly measuring his/her pulse at the same site and under the same conditions. Wide variations in pulse rate are apt to be found among patients and may or may not be indicative of abnormalities. However, unusual or abnormal findings in a specific patient should be carefully evaluated to determine their potential cause and the potential effect the treatment may have on the patient.

Factors that affect the pulse are listed in Box 4–2.

ASSESSMENT OF PULSE

Sites used to measure pulse are the temporal, carotid, brachial, radial, femoral, popliteal, dorsal pedal, and posterior tibial arteries (Fig. 4–2) and the apex of the heart, with the use of a stethoscope. The most common sites used are the radial and carotid arteries because of their ease of access. The temporal or carotid sites can be used when access to the radial site is restricted. The carotid site is usually preferred by persons when measuring their own pulse (Fig. 4–3A). The *apical pulse* site is used when the peripheral sites are

PROCEDURE 4–2
Measuring Body Temperature Orally With an Electronic Thermometer

1. Wash your hands and obtain an electronic thermometer, probe cover, recording form, and pen.

2. Position the patient and explain the procedure. Observe the patient and evaluate signs and symptoms related to body temperature: skin color, temperature (hot, warm, cool), and condition (moist, dry).

3. Turn the unit on and apply the disposable probe cover to the probe (Fig. 4–1A).

4. Instruct the patient to open his/her mouth, position the probe under the patient's tongue, and instruct the patient to hold the probe in place with the lips, not with the teeth, and to breathe through the nose (Fig. 4–1B).

5. Leave the probe in place until the digital readout or alarm indicates that a normal temperature level has been reached; note the value.

6. Remove the probe from the patient's mouth, discard the probe cover, turn the unit off, and wash your hands.

7. Record the results, using even increments to report tenths of a degree.

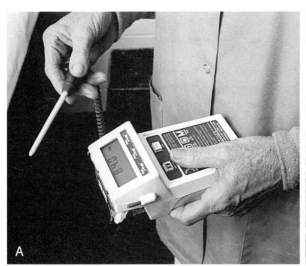
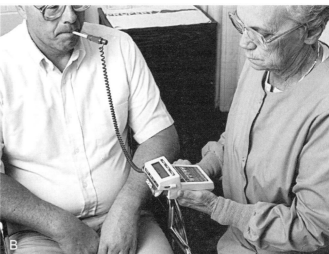

■ **FIGURE 4–1**
A and B, Use of an electronic thermometer for oral body temperature.

PROCEDURE 4 – 3
Measuring Body Temperature
With an Ear Thermometer

1. Wash your hands and obtain the ear thermometer, lens filter, recording form, and pen.

2. Position the patient to expose one ear; an infant or a toddler may be held on your lap so his/her head can be stabilized; other persons may lie or sit.

3. Apply a clean lens filter and select either the oral or rectal setting; select rectal for an infant or toddler and oral for an older child or adult. Regardless of the setting you select, the thermometer lens will be placed in the person's ear canal.

4. Gently but firmly pull and hold the ear to straighten the ear canal. Pull straight back on an infant's ear, and pull up and back on a person's ear who is older than 1 year.

5. Insert the thermometer lens cone, with a clean filter applied, into the ear opening. It may be necessary to gently rock the lens cone back and forth to insert it far enough to seal the ear canal from the external air.

6. Maintain the lens cone in the ear canal and depress and hold the activation button for 1 second. The temperature reading will appear in the LCD window; mentally record the value.

7. Remove the lens cone from the person's ear, and discard or thoroughly wash the lens filter if it is to be used again. *Note:* In the home, it may be appropriate to wash and reuse a lens filter, but in other environments the used lens filter should be discarded. Wash your hands.

8. Record the results using the value from the LCD reading; indicate whether the rectal or oral setting was used, and indicate the ear that was used.

---

inaccessible or the pulse is difficult to palpate at those sites. The inguinal, popliteal, tibial, and pedal arterial sites are used to evaluate the pulse in the lower extremity. These measurements are important when treating patients with peripheral vascular disease or a disorder affecting peripheral blood flow.

The pulse is often subjectively described according to its rate, rhythm, and volume. Examples of descriptive terms include the following:

1. "Strong and regular" indicates even beats with a good force to each beat.
2. "Weak and regular" indicates even beats with a poor force to each beat.
3. "Irregular" indicates that both strong and weak beats occur during the period of measurement.
4. "Thready" indicates a weak force to each beat and irregular beats.

5. *"Tachycardia"* indicates a rapid heart rate (greater than 100 bpm).
6. *"Bradycardia"* indicates a slow heart rate (less than 60 bpm).

A timepiece that will allow the evaluator to easily count the pulse for 1 minute or part of a minute (e.g., 10, 15, 20, or 30 seconds) is necessary to accurately measure the pulse rate. A stopwatch, clock, or wristwatch with a sweep second hand or a second digital readout are the most convenient and readily available timepieces. Materials to record the measured value and a stethoscope (if the apical pulse is to be measured) are other items that may be needed to measure the patient's pulse rate.

Steps to measure pulse are listed in Procedure 4–4.

In most persons, the apical and radial pulse rates

Text continued on page 53

BOX 4–2

Factors Affecting Pulse

1. *Age.* Persons older than 65 may exhibit a decreased pulse rate, while young persons (adolescents and younger) usually exhibit an increased rate.
2. *Gender.* Male pulse rates are usually slightly lower than female rates.
3. *Environmental temperature.* The pulse rate tends to increase with high temperature and decrease with low temperature.
4. *Infection.* The pulse rate tends to increase when a major infectious process occurs.
5. *Physical activity.* Normally the pulse rate should rise rapidly in response to vigorous physical activity, plateau or stabilize as the intensity or severity of the exercise plateaus, and then decline as the intensity of the exercise declines. The postexercise pulse rate should revert to the person's resting pulse rate within 3 to 5 minutes after cessation of exercise. A person with a conditioned cardiopulmonary system will probably exhibit less change in his/her pulse rate, and the rate should return to its normal resting level in a shorter time period than that required by an unconditioned or debilitated person.
6. *Emotional status.* The pulse rate increases during episodes of high stress, anxiety, or emotion (e.g., anger or fear) and may decrease when the person is asleep or in a state of extreme calm.
7. *Medications.* Various medications may cause the pulse rate to increase or decrease, depending on their effect on the cardiovascular system.
8. *Cardiopulmonary disease.* The condition of the heart and the peripheral vascular system and their ability to function normally both affect the pulse rate. For example, a patient with hypertension may exhibit a slower (lower) pulse rate, while a patient with hypotension may exhibit a faster (higher) pulse rate to compensate for the higher or lower blood pressure.

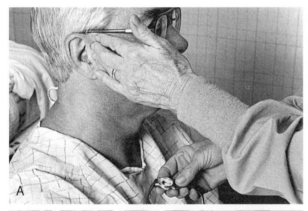
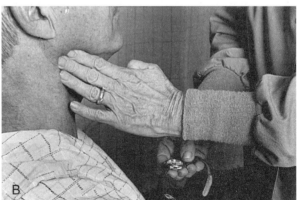
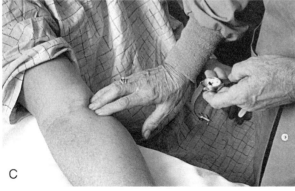

■ **FIGURE 4–2**
Pulse measurement sites. *A,* Temporal. *B,* Carotid. *C,* Brachial.

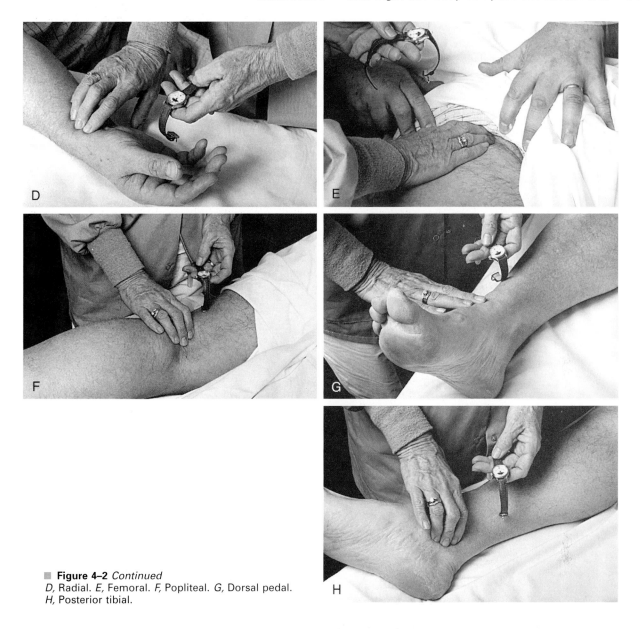

■ **Figure 4–2** *Continued*
D, Radial. *E,* Femoral. *F,* Popliteal. *G,* Dorsal pedal. *H,* Posterior tibial.

■ **FIGURE 4–3**
Person measuring his own pulse at the carotid *(A)* and radial *(B)* sites.

PROCEDURE 4 – 4
Measuring the Pulse

1. Wash your hands, obtain a timepiece that measures seconds, and explain the procedure to the patient. Observe the patient for signs or symptoms of stress, anxiety, or cardiovascular distress. The patient may be recumbent, sitting, or standing.

2. Select an arterial site and firmly but gently place two or three fingertips over the artery. Avoid using your thumb, as you may perceive your own pulse rather than that of the patient and the thumb's pad is less sensitive than that of the other fingers. Avoid excessive pressure, because it may *occlude* the artery. An exception to light pressure is when you attempt to palpate the popliteal artery. Very firm, deep pressure may be required to locate the artery and palpate its pulse. When determining a patient's resting heart rate for the first time, allow him/her to rest supine or seated for approximately 5 minutes immediately prior to the measurement. Measure the pulse rate for a full minute to reduce the potential for error and improve the accuracy of the measurement.

3. Mentally count each beat that you palpate. If you measure the rate for 10 seconds and multiply that value by 6, the margin of error is ±6 bpm; if you measure the rate for 15 seconds and multiply that value by 4, the margin of error is ±4 bpm; if you measure the rate for 30 seconds and multiply that value by 2, the margin of error is ±2 bpm.

4. Record the results in beats per minute, indicate any variations in rhythm or volume, and identify the location you used to palpate and measure the pulse (e.g., 68 bpm, regular, R brachial pulse; 86 bpm, irregular (every fourth beat absent in 1 minute), L radial pulse, patient sitting).

5. Measurement of the apical pulse usually requires a stethoscope, but manual palpation is possible. Wash your hands and explain the procedure to the patient. The patient must be positioned so that the left anterior chest is accessible.

    a. *Manual palpation.* Place two or three fingertips on the patient's skin on the left lateral side of the base of the sternum at approximately the 4th–5th or 5th–6th rib interspace; then count and record the pulse rate as previously described.

    b. *Auscultation.* Clean the stethoscope's diaphragm and ear pieces with an alcohol wipe. Position the ear pieces in your ears with the ear pieces directed forward. This position will be the most comfortable, and the ear pieces will be in line with the auditory canal. Warm the diaphragm with your hand or by rubbing it with a cloth. Then place the diaphragm on the patient's skin in a location similar to the one described previously. In an adolescent or adult female patient, it may be necessary to position the diaphragm slightly medially or laterally and inferior to the left breast. Count and record the pulse rate as described previously. Remove the ear pieces from your ears and clean them and the diaphragm with an alcohol wipe. (*Note:* If the stethoscope is a personal one, only the diaphragm needs to be cleaned before and after use with a patient. If the stethoscope is loaned to other persons or belongs to the department, the ear pieces should be cleaned using an alcohol wipe before and after use. This action will decrease the possibility of contamination of the ear pieces and diaphragm and help prevent the spread of disease or infection from one person to another.)

will be equal. However, in patients with cardiac disease or peripheral arterial disease, these two values may differ. Therefore, the radial and apical pulse rates should be evaluated simultaneously during the initial evaluation of the patient. Two persons should monitor the two pulses simultaneously (i.e., one monitors the radial pulse for 1 minute, while the other monitors the apical pulse for 1 minute), and the results are compared. Any difference in the two values is referred to as the "pulse deficit." Further evaluation of the patient is necessary to determine the cause of the difference between the two pulse rates. Both the left and the right radial pulses should be compared with the apical pulse. If there is a difference between the apical and radial pulse rates, then only the apical pulse should be used to evaluate the patient. Such differences should be documented in the patient's medical record.

The expected normal responses of the pulse rate to exercise have been described (refer to item 5, Box 4–2). A patient with resting tachycardia or bradycardia should be carefully evaluated by an appropriate practitioner (i.e., physician, nurse, or cardiovascular exercise specialist) to determine his/her limitations or tolerance to exercise or treatment before treatment is initiated.

During the monitoring of the patient's pulse, the evaluator should be aware of abnormal pulse responses to exercise or other treatment activities. It may be necessary to modify or terminate treatment when these abnormalities are severe or persistent. Additional caution or a consultation with other medical personnel may be necessary before proceeding with treatment to protect the patient from harm or undue stress.

Abnormal responses of the pulse rate during or after exercise or physical activity are listed in Box 4–3.

BLOOD PRESSURE

Systemic arterial BP is a physiologic variable that reflects the effects of *cardiac output*, peripheral vascular resistance, and other hemodynamic factors. BP is measured with a *sphygmomanometer* (i.e., a BP cuff) and is an indirect measurement of the pressure inside an artery caused by blood flow through the artery. Specifically, it is the force exerted by the blood against any unit area of the vessel wall. BP is composed of the systolic and diastolic pressures. The systolic pressure is the BP at the time of contraction of the left ventricle (*systole*), and the diastolic pressure is the BP at the time of the rest period of the heart (*diastole*).

The various phases of a person's BP can be identified by listening for *Korotkoff's sounds* with a stethoscope. These sounds have been described as occurring in phases, as shown in Table 4–1. A great amount of

---

BOX 4–3

Abnormal Responses Exhibited by the Pulse

1. The pulse rate slowly increases during active exercise.
2. The pulse rate does not increase during active exercise.
3. The pulse rate continues to increase or decreases as the intensity of exercise or activity plateaus.
4. The pulse rate slowly declines as the intensity of the exercise or activity declines and terminates.
5. The pulse rate does not decline as the intensity of the exercise or activity declines.
6. The pulse rate declines during the exercise before the intensity of the exercise or activity declines.
7. The increased pulse rate or the amount of the increase exceeds the level expected to occur during the exercise period.
8. The rhythm of the pulse becomes irregular during or after the exercise or activity (e.g., dysrhythmia, arrhythmia, or ectopic beats occur).

---

practice and a quiet environment are necessary for the evaluator to differentiate these five phases. Phases I and V are the two most important phases to identify in most patients. However, in patients with a known or suspected cardiovascular condition, it may be important to identify most or all of the phases.

Table 4–1
KOROTKOFF'S SOUNDS

Phase	Description
I	The first faint, clear tapping sounds are detected and gradually increase in their intensity. These sounds are the initial indication of systolic pressure in an adult, according to the American Heart Association.
II	The sounds heard have a murmur or swishing quality to them.
III	The sounds become crisp and louder than previously heard.
IV	There is a distinct and abrupt muffling of the sounds until a soft, blowing quality is heard. This phase is the initial indication of the diastolic pressure and is the best indicator of diastolic pressure in adults, according to the American Heart Association.
V	The sounds essentially disappear totally; the phase is also referred to as the "second diastolic pressure phase."

PROCEDURE 4 – 5
Measuring Blood Pressure by Auscultation

1. Wash your hands and obtain a stethoscope and a sphygmomanometer (Fig. 4–4A). Explain the procedure and rationale for measurement to the patient. Observe the patient for signs or symptoms of stress or recent exercise. If the patient has exercised, ambulated, or experienced emotional stress, he/she should rest for 15 to 30 minutes before his/her blood pressure is measured. Position the patient sitting with his/her forearm supported on a firm object approximately at the level of his/her heart, with the thighs parallel to each other and the feet flat on floor. Position yourself so that you are comfortable and can view the manometer gauge easily. If the patient is sitting or recumbent, you should sit and face him/her. If the patient is standing, you should elevate his/her arm and support it between your arm and lateral chest while you face the patient.

2. Expose the antecubital space of either the left or right arm; do not roll the shirt or blouse sleeve too tightly, as it may partially occlude the artery. Palpate the brachial pulse so you will know where to place the diaphragm of the stethoscope.

3. Apply the deflated cuff to the arm with the center of the bladder over the medial aspect of the arm so it will occlude the artery when it is inflated. The cuff should be applied approximately 2½ cm above the antecubital space (about 1½ fingerbreadths) with the manometer attached to the cuff or placed so that the needle and scale can be observed easily without being held in your hand (Fig. 4–4B).

4. After cleaning the earpieces and diaphragm with an alcohol wipe, apply the stethoscope to your ears with the earpieces directed forward. Place the diaphragm on the skin where the brachial artery was palpated, but avoid contact with the patient's clothing or with the cuff. Apply firm but light pressure on the diaphragm to maintain contact with the skin (Fig. 4–4C).

5. To initially determine the amount of pressure needed in the cuff to occlude the brachial artery, palpate the radial pulse and inflate the cuff by closing the valve on the inflation bulb and squeezing the bulb until the radial pulse is no longer palpable. This value can be used as a baseline for the cuff pressure inflation level (Fig. 4–4D). Note this value and deflate the cuff. After waiting 30 to 60 seconds, reinflate the cuff to 15 to 20 mm Hg above the pressure that previously occluded the artery to ensure that the artery is fully occluded. (*Note:* Once the patient's systolic pressure has been determined several times and a normal systolic value has been established, the cuff can be inflated to approximately 15 to 20 mm Hg above that value each time the blood pressure is measured.)

6. To deflate the cuff, release the valve on the inflation bulb so the needle drops at the rate of 2 to 3 mm Hg per second. Listen for normal Korotkoff's sounds and mentally note the needle position (reading) when the initial sound is heard through the stethoscope. This is the systolic pressure value.

PROCEDURE 4–5, *continued*

7. Continue to deflate the cuff, listening for the absence of the sound of a pulse or beat, and mentally note the needle position. This is the diastolic pressure value.

8. Allow the cuff to deflate completely, remove it from the patient, and remove the stethoscope from your ears.

9. Record the values, including the patient position and extremity used (e.g., 130/70 RUE, sitting; 140/80 LUE, sitting [RUE, right upper extremity; LUE, left upper extremity]).

10. Clean the stethoscope earpieces and diaphragm with an alcohol wipe.

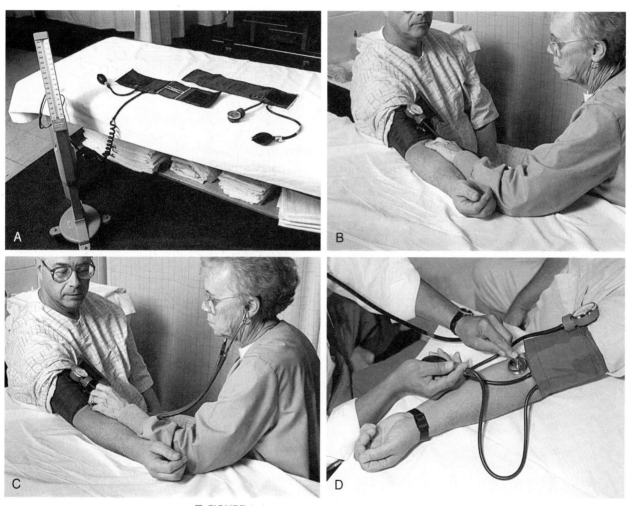

■ **FIGURE 4–4**
Measurement of blood pressure by auscultation.

Depending on the source, accepted normal BP ranges in adults are systolic, 90 to 135 or 140 millimeters of mercury (mm Hg); and diastolic, 60 to 80 mm Hg. A systolic/diastolic value of 120/80 mm Hg is frequently used as the normal value.

Persons whose resting systolic pressure consistently measures more than 135 to 140 mm Hg or whose resting diastolic pressure consistently measures more than 90 mm Hg are frequently considered to be hypertensive. Factors that are associated with or contribute to *hypertension* are obesity; physical inactivity; excessive use of nicotine, alcohol, or salt; arteriosclerosis; diabetes mellitus; oral contraceptives (in women); advanced age (i.e., middle age or older); kidney

---

BOX 4–4

Factors Affecting Blood Pressure

1. *Age.* Younger patients (adolescents and younger) exhibit lower systolic and diastolic values. Elderly patients (65 and older) may exhibit slightly higher systolic and slightly lower diastolic pressure.

2. *Physical activity.* Systolic pressure should gradually increase with exercise, plateau as the exercise intensity plateaus, and then gradually decline as the exercise intensity declines. It should return to its normal resting value within 5 to 7 minutes after termination of the exercise. The diastolic pressure should remain essentially unchanged throughout the exercise period, although an increase of approximately 10 to 15 mm Hg is usually not considered abnormal. However, an increase of more than 10 to 15 mm Hg as a result of exercise is considered abnormal.

3. *Emotional status.* Blood pressure will increase during episodes of high stress, anxiety, or emotion (e.g., anger or fear).

4. *Medications.* Various medications may cause blood pressure to increase or decrease, depending on their effect on the cardiovascular system. Medications are frequently used to control hypertension and may result in a temporary state of hypotension in some patients.

5. *Size and condition of arteries.* Arteries that have a reduced lumen will produce an increased blood pressure value, and arteries that have decreased elasticity will produce an increased systolic value and a decreased diastolic value. These two factors tend to account for the changes that occur in the blood pressure values of the elderly.

6. *Arm position.* The standard arm position to measure blood pressure is as follows: the forearm is maintained at the level of the fourth intercostal space at the sternum, with the elbow extended when the person is seated or standing. No adjustment in arm position is required when the person is supine, because when it is supported on the bed, it is at the proper level. Blood pressure will increase 10 to 20 mm Hg as the arm is lowered from the level previously described and will decrease 10 to 20 mm Hg as the arm is raised above that level.

7. *Muscle contraction.* The patient should not maintain arm position by contraction of his/her upper extremity musculature, as this causes an increase in the blood pressure because of the increased resistance to blood flow caused by the muscle contraction.

8. *Blood volume.* Blood pressure decreases when there is a loss of blood and increases with an increase in blood volume (i.e., after transfusion of whole blood or plasma).

9. *Cardiac output.* Systolic blood pressure increases with increased cardiac output and decreases with decreased cardiac output.

10. *Site of measurement.* Blood pressure values are often higher in the left upper extremity than in the right upper extremity. If the thigh is used as the measurement site, the systolic pressure is usually higher than that found in the arm, partly because of the need to use a wider bladder in the cuff, but the diastolic pressure will be essentially the same as that found in the arm.

disease; race (i.e., greater incidence in blacks); and diet. In most persons, there are no signs or symptoms associated with hypertension, and unless the person has his/her BP measured periodically, the condition often goes unrecognized and undiagnosed. Persons with hypertension are more susceptible to coronary artery disease, cerebrovascular accident, peripheral vascular disease, and congestive heart failure. Therefore, it is important for all persons to have their BP evaluated several times a year.

Hypotension is defined as a systolic pressure that is consistently below 100 mm Hg. This condition is usually nonthreatening, but some hypotensive patients may experience dizziness or syncope when abruptly standing from a lying, sitting, or squatting position.

Factors that affect BP are listed in Box 4–4.

ASSESSMENT OF BLOOD PRESSURE

The most common site used to measure BP is the brachial artery. Occasionally, the femoral artery is used, particularly in patients with known or suspected lower extremity peripheral vascular diseases.

A stethoscope and sphygmomanometer, chairs, an object to support the patient's upper extremity, alcohol wipes, and recording materials are necessary to measure and record the patient's BP. The cuff must be the proper size to obtain an accurate measurement. If the bladder in the cuff is too narrow in relation to the circumference of the patient's arm, the reading will be erroneously high; if the bladder is too wide, the reading will be erroneously low. The width of the bladder should be 40% of the circumference of the midpoint of the limb. For an average size adult, the bladder should be 5 to 6 inches (13 centimeters [cm]) wide; for an infant, it should be 1 to 1½ inches (3 cm) wide; and for a large adult, it should be 6 to 8 inches (17 cm) wide. If the thigh is used for measurement, the bladder should be 8 to 9 inches (20 cm) wide. The length of the bladder is also important and should be approximately twice the width of the bladder, or 80% of the arm circumference.

Decisions regarding the size of the bladder should be based on the circumference of the patient's extremity, not on the patient's age or other personal factors. Steps to measure BP are shown in Procedures 4–5 (auscultation) and 4–6 (palpation).

If it is necessary to repeat the measurements, the cuff should be completely deflated and the patient allowed to sit quietly for 1 to 2 minutes before the measurements are retaken. This will allow any blood that may be trapped in the veins to be released and will allow the circulatory system to return to normal. The caregiver/practitioner should be alert to the potential sources of or reasons for errors in measurement of blood pressure so they can be avoided or eliminated.

You will need to develop your hearing, vision, and manual dexterity so you can accurately hear phases I and V of Korotkoff's sounds, read the value accurately, and properly operate the valve on the cuff-inflation bulb (i.e., close it, open it, and control the rate of deflation) with your thumb and index finger.

You should develop the habit of reporting the values without "rounding" them to the nearest higher or lower value. For example, if you read the systolic pressure as 137 mm Hg, report it as 137 mm Hg; do not report it as 135 mm Hg.

Do not bias the findings by expecting a certain value rather than listening for it. Some patients will tell you what their usual values are before you actually take a measurement; you may have read the values determined previously by another evaluator; or you may recall the values you measured during a previous treatment session. This information may bias you into predicting or expecting similar values rather than recording the values as you hear and measure them. When you eliminate, reduce, or avoid these potential sources of errors in the measurement of a patient's BP, you will increase the accuracy and precision of your measurement.

Reminders

1. The patient may sit, stand, or lie for this procedure, but his/her upper extremity must be supported with the forearm and arm at the approximate level of his/her heart to reduce inaccurate measurements (Fig. 4–5). If the extremity is positioned in a dependent (hanging) position, the hydrostatic

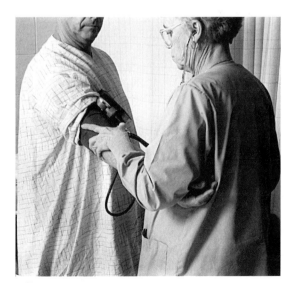

■ **FIGURE 4–5**
Blood pressure being taken for a standing patient.

PROCEDURE 4 – 6
Measuring Blood Pressure by Palpation

1. Perform steps 1 through 3 outlined in Procedure 4–5.
2. Palpate the brachial artery pulse in the antecubital space with two or three fingers and maintain your fingers over the pulse.
3. Inflate the cuff as described previously.
4. Deflate the cuff as described previously and observe the manometer. Mentally note the needle position when the first pulse in the artery is palpated. This is the systolic pressure value.
5. Continue to deflate the cuff while observing the manometer. Mentally note the needle position when the last distinct pulse is palpated. This is the diastolic pressure.
6. Completely deflate the cuff and remove it from the patient.
7. Record the values as described previously; indicate that the palpation method was used.

---

pressure of the blood will be increased, which will erroneously increase the value of the patient's BP. Do not allow the patient to position the upper extremity by contracting the muscles of chest, shoulder, and arm. Isometric muscle contractions will partially occlude secondary blood vessels and the patient's true BP may be distorted. In a normal subject, no significant difference in his/her blood pressure should be found, regardless of position, providing the upper extremity is properly positioned as described previously.

2. Stimuli that may influence the BP should be controlled, eliminated, avoided, or accounted for (see Box 4–4).

3. The measurement should be performed in a quiet, warm, comfortable environment, and the cuff size must be appropriate for the size (circumference) of the patient's arm. A cuff that is proportionately too small will produce a value higher than it should be, and a cuff that is proportionately too large will produce a value lower than it should be.

4. Unless you desire to evaluate the patient's BP in response to exercise, the patient should avoid vigorous physical activity for approximately 30 minutes before measurement, and postural position changes should be avoided in the 5 minutes before measurement.

5. You may need to practice measuring BP to improve your accuracy and efficiency.

The expected normal responses of BP during exercise have been described (refer to item 5, Box 4–4). A patient with a resting elevated BP (hypertension) or a resting depressed BP (hypotension) should be carefully evaluated by an appropriate practitioner to determine his/her limitations or anticipated tolerance to exercise or treatment before treatment is initiated.

During monitoring of the patient's BP, the evaluator should be aware of abnormal BP responses to exercise or other treatment activities. It may be necessary to modify or terminate the patient's treatment if these abnormalities are serious or persistent. Additional caution or a consultation with medical personnel may be necessary before proceeding with treatment to ensure patient safety.

Abnormal responses of BP during or after exercise or physical activity are listed in Box 4–5.

RESPIRATION (PULMONARY VENTILATION)

The physical components of *respiration* produce an inflow (*inspiration/inhalation*) and outflow (*expiration/exhalation*) of air between the environment and the lungs. Air moves into and is expelled from the lungs by muscle contraction and relaxation. One respiration consists of one inhalation and one exhalation.

Depending on the source used, the accepted normal range for respiration is 12 to 18 respirations per minute for adults and 30 to 50 respirations per minute for infants. Resting values above 20 or below 10 respi-

BOX 4–5

Abnormal Responses Exhibited by Blood Pressure

1. Systolic pressure slowly increases during active exercise.
2. Systolic pressure does not increase during active exercise.
3. Systolic pressure continues to increase or decreases as the intensity of the exercise or activity plateaus.
4. Systolic pressure slowly declines as the intensity of the exercise or activity declines and terminates.
5. Systolic pressure does not decline as the intensity of the exercise or activity declines.
6. Systolic pressure declines significantly below its resting level at the termination of exercise or activity.
7. Systolic pressure declines during exercise before the intensity of the exercise declines.
8. The systolic pressure rate or the amount of systolic pressure increase is excessive during the exercise or activity period.
9. Diastolic pressure increases more than 10 to 15 mm Hg during the exercise or activity period.

BOX 4–6

Factors Affecting Respiration

1. *Age.* Both very young (infant to age 5) and elderly (65 and older) patients tend to have higher respiration rates.
2. *Physical activity.* The rate and depth of respiration increase during exercise.
3. *Emotional status.* The rate and depth of respiration increase during episodes of high stress, anxiety, or emotion (e.g., anger or fear).
4. *Air quality.* Impurities in the atmosphere may cause the respiration rate to increase or decrease, depending on their effects on various components of the pulmonary system.
5. *Altitude.* High altitudes cause the respiration rate to increase until a person is acclimated.
6. *Disease.* Disease that affects various components of the pulmonary system usually increases the respiratory rate and may also affect the depth of respiration.

rations per minute are considered abnormal for adults.

Factors that affect respiration are listed in Box 4–6.

ASSESSMENT OF RESPIRATION

Measurement of the rate, rhythm, depth, and character of respiration is performed by observation or tactilely. "Rate" refers to the number of breaths per minute, "rhythm" refers to the regularity of the pattern, "depth" refers to the amount of air exchanged with each respiration, and "character" refers to deviations from normal, resting, quiet respiration. The evaluator observes or tactilely measures the rate of movement of the patient's thorax, abdomen, or both. Patients who are extremely ill and in respiratory distress may have to have their respiration measured by stethoscope. The amount of effort required and the sounds produced during resting respirations should be evaluated as part of the assessment.

Normal respiration requires minimal effort for inspiration and essentially no effort for expiration. Persons who have difficulty breathing while at rest experience *dyspnea*, or labored breathing. No sound should be heard during normal, resting respiration. Abnormal sounds include wheezing, *rales*, and *stridor*. Patients may also demonstrate *orthopnea*, or difficulty breathing while recumbent. This condition is relieved when the patient sits or stands. *Apnea*, or absence of breathing, and shortness of breath *(SOB)* also may be experienced by patients and may require the use of a ventilator if they persist.

A watch or clock that measures both seconds and minutes, or a stopwatch, and materials to record the results will be necessary to evaluate a patient's respiration rate.

Steps to measure respiration rate are shown in Procedure 4–7.

The expected normal responses of the respiration rate when a person exercises have been described (refer to item 2, Box 4–6). A patient who exhibits problems or difficulty with breathing while at rest should be carefully evaluated by a qualified practitioner to determine his/her limitations or tolerance to exercise or treatment before treatment is initiated.

During monitoring of the patient's respiration rate, the practitioner should be aware of abnormal respiration responses to exercise or other treatment activities. It may be necessary to modify or terminate treatment if these abnormalities impair function or are persistent. Additional caution or a consultation with other medical personnel may be necessary before proceeding with treatment. Frequent monitoring of the patient's respiration rate may be necessary during

PROCEDURE 4 – 7
Measuring Respiration Rate

1. Wash your hands and obtain a timepiece that measures seconds. Observe the patient for signs or symptoms of abnormal respiration (e.g., gasping, panting, open-mouth breathing, use of accessory neck muscles). The patient may be sitting, lying, or standing, as long as his/her abdomen or thorax can be observed. To avoid voluntary control of respiration by the patient, do not explain the procedure to the patient.

2. Simulate measurement of the radial pulse with the patient's forearm resting on his/her abdomen. Observe or tactilely measure the outward and inward movement of the patient's thorax or abdomen (Fig. 4–6).

3. Count either the inspirations or the expirations for 1 minute. (One inspiration and one expiration equals one respiration cycle.) The rate is reported in respirations per minute. Once the rate, rhythm, depth, and character of the person's respirations have been determined to be within normal parameters, the measurement period can be reduced to 30 seconds, but the number of inspirations or expirations must be multiplied by 2 to determine the rate for a full minute.

4. Reposition the patient's clothing or bed linen if it was removed or adjusted to expose the patient's abdomen or thorax.

5. Note and record the rate, depth, rhythm, and character of the person's respirations. Record the rate as respirations per minute and describe the depth, rhythm, and character of the pattern if they vary from normal.

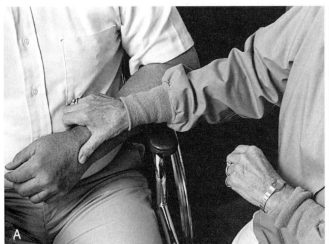 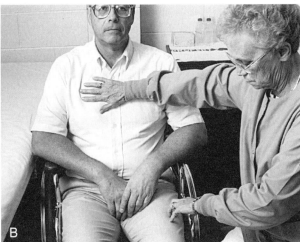

■ FIGURE 4–6
Measuring a patient's respiration rate.

Abnormal Responses Exhibited by Respiration Rate

1. The respiration rate slowly increases during exercise or activity.
2. The respiration rate does not increase during exercise or activity.
3. The respiration rate increases as the intensity of the exercise or activity plateaus.
4. The respiration rate slowly declines as the intensity of the exercise or activity declines and terminates.
5. The respiration rate does not decline as the intensity of the exercise or activity declines.
6. The respiration rate declines during exercise or activity before the intensity of the exercise declines.
7. The increase in the rate or the amount of increase in the patient's respiration rate is excessive during the exercise period.
8. The rhythm of the respiration pattern becomes irregular during or after exercise or activity.

his/her initial treatment sessions to ensure he/she is functioning within safe limits.

Abnormal responses to watch for while measuring respirations are listed in Box 4–7.

BODY COMPOSITION ASSESSMENTS

Assessment of a person's body composition is valuable to determine his/her percentage of body fat in relation to the other components of his/her body mass (i.e., bone, muscle). Athletes and individuals who are involved with weight control or weight loss programs, who have a metabolic disorder, or who have a condition that affects their cardiopulmonary systems may benefit from body composition assessment. Common methods or procedures for assessing body fat include hydrostatic weighing, skinfold measurements, bioelectric impedance, and girth measurements. A variation of girth measurements can be used to track changes in the circumference of an extremity when edema is present. In addition to girth measurements, volumetrics can be used to assess a change in the volume of a distal segment.

Hydrostatic weighing is considered to be the most reliable and accurate procedure by which to assess a person's percentage of body fat. This method requires the total immersion of the individual, including his/her head, into a tank of water or pool. When the person is lowered into a tank of water or pool, water is displaced. The person who has a low percentage of body fat (compared with his/her total body weight) will weigh more in water than a person with a high percentage of body fat because his/her body has greater density; thus, according to Archimedes' principle, the person with less body fat will displace more water.

Furthermore, a person will weigh much less in water than out of water, and the loss of weight in the water will be equal to a portion of his/her body volume. Therefore, to determine his/her body volume, subtract his/her body weight in water from his/her body weight out of water. Before the person's percentage of body fat can be calculated, his/her body density must be determined. When the body density has been calculated, the percentage of body fat, total mass of body fat, and lean body mass can be calculated (refer to Box 4–8 for equation formulas for these calculations).

There are several disadvantages of this method, including the need for sophisticated, expensive equipment, sufficient space for the equipment, adequate water supply, the difference in body density that exists among individuals, the need to estimate the residual lung volume for each person, the apprehension or intolerance of some persons to being totally immersed in water, and the fact that several trials may be necessary to obtain an accurate measurement.

Skinfold measurements can be used to indicate relative fatness among individuals and to predict a person's percentage of body fat. These measurements correlate well with the results obtained through hy-

Equation Formulas

1. Body volume = weight out of water − weight in water (*Note*: Correction values for water temperature and residual lung volume can be used to calculate the final body volume for greater accuracy.)
2. Body density = body mass ÷ body volume
3. Percentage body fat = 495 ÷ (body density − 450) (Siri's equation)
4. Fat mass = body mass × (percentage fat ÷ 100)
5. Lean body mass = body mass − fat mass

From McCardle WD, Katch FI, Katch VL. *Essentials of Exercise Physiology*. 4th edition. Philadelphia, PA: Lea & Febiger, 1994:459, 461.

drostatic weighing when they are performed by a trained, experienced evaluator. Measurements are made at several standardized body sites with calipers designed to measure skinfolds and calibrated in millimeters (Box 4–9). As few as three or as many as seven sites can be measured: chest, midaxillary, triceps, subscapular, abdomen, suprailiac, and thigh (Figs. 4–7 to 4–12). The biceps and calf are other sites, which are used less frequently. Training and practice with the use of the calipers, proper selection of each site, and careful separation of the skin and subcutaneous fat from the underlying muscle are necessary to ensure accurate and reliable measurements. Two or three measurements are made at each site, and an average

BOX 4–9

Sites for Skinfold Measurements

All sites are measured with the person standing with a relaxed but erect posture, and all measurements are made on the right side of the body.

Triceps. At the midpoint between the acromion and olecranon processes along the midline of the arm; a vertical fold is used.

Subscapular. One to 2 centimeters (approximately ½ to 1 inch) below the inferior angle at a 45-degree angle from the medial border; a diagonal fold is used.

Midaxillary. Along the midaxillary line at the level of the xiphoid process; a vertical fold is used.

Chest. For men, at the lateral aspect of the pectoralis major one half the distance between the anterior axillary line and the nipple; a diagonal fold is used. For women, at the lateral aspect of the pectoralis major one third the distance between the anterior axillary line and the nipple; a diagonal fold is used.

Abdomen. One inch to the right of the umbilicus; a vertical fold is used.

Suprailiac. Just above the iliac crest along the midaxillary line; a diagonal fold is used.

Thigh. At the midpoint between the upper edge of the patella and the inguinal crease along the middle of the thigh; a vertical fold is used.

Biceps. At the midpoint of the muscle belly along the midline of the arm; a vertical fold is used.

Note: Some slight variations exist for some of these sites depending on the reference source used.

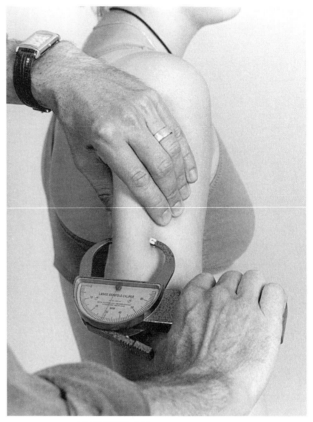

■ **FIGURE 4–7**
Skin fold measurement: triceps.

of the measurements is calculated for each site. The calipers will produce a constant pressure against the skin, which over time will compress the subcutaneous tissue (fat); therefore, the evaluator must read the caliper values within the first 3 seconds they are applied to the skin to enhance the accuracy and reliability of the measurements. All measurements are made on the right extremities and the right side of the body with

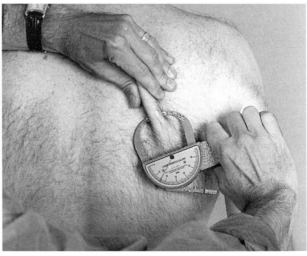

■ **FIGURE 4–8**
Skin fold measurement: subscapular.

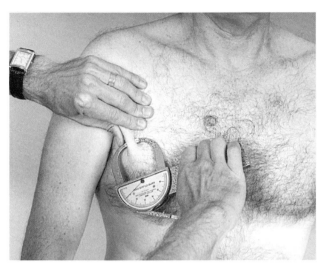

■ **FIGURE 4–9**
Skin fold measurement: pectoral (chest).

the person standing. When the values obtained from the sites selected are added together, an indication of a person's relative fatness, compared with other individuals, is available. When regression equations are used, the values can be converted into a predicted percentage of the person's body fat. Most of the equations are population specific, but some have been adjusted to provide comparisons with a generalized popula-

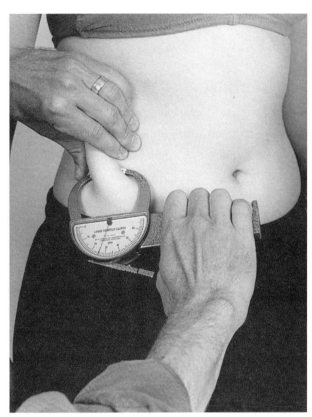

■ **FIGURE 4–11**
Skin fold measurement: suprailiac.

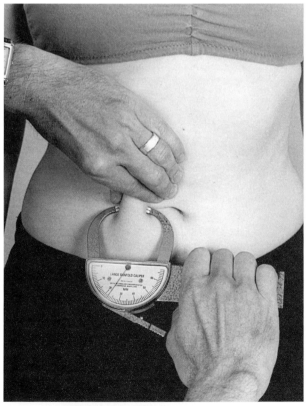

■ **FIGURE 4–10**
Skin fold measurement: abdomen.

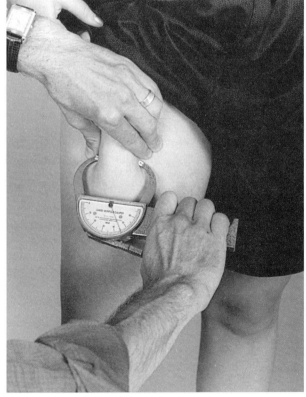

■ **FIGURE 4–12**
Skin fold measurement: thigh.

PROCEDURE 4–8
Skinfold Measurement

1. Expose the site on the right side of the body as the person stands with an erect but relaxed posture; explain the procedure and obtain consent.

2. Specifically locate the site; use your thumb and forefinger to gently but firmly pinch and lift the skin and subcutaneous tissue away from the underlying muscle; form a vertical or diagonal fold depending on the site.

3. Apply the calipers approximately 1 centimeter from your thumb and forefinger as you maintain your pinch-grasp; apply the caliper perpendicular to the skin fold approximately halfway between the crest and base of the fold.

4. Read the value on the caliper display or scale within the initial 2 to 3 seconds during which the caliper is applied; do not delay obtaining the measurement to avoid sustained compression of the tissue.

5. Make two or three measurements at each site; remeasure the site if your measurements vary more than 2 millimeters, or add them together and calculate an average value.

6. When duplicate measurements are made, it is recommended that you rotate through the sites to allow the skin and subcutaneous tissue at each site to return to its normal texture and thickness.

7. Use a regression equation to convert the measured values to percentage of body fat; compare the person's results with the values listed in a table of body fat estimates for males or females.

8. Record the results and document your activity.

---

tion. Separate tables are available for men and women to estimate percentage of body fat based on the sum of selected skinfolds or the result of an equation. Two of these tables (which are named for the investigators who developed them) are the Jackson-Pollock and the Durnin-Womersly (Procedure 4–8).

Girth measurements can be used to predict a person's percentage of body fat when measurements are performed at specific locations. All measurements are made on the right extremities, with the person standing, and the use of a plastic or metal anthropometric measuring tape is recommended. These types of tapes will not deteriorate, are easy to clean, and their calibration marks will be able to be read easily. The measurement sites are outlined in Box 4–10.

The anthropometric measuring tape is wrapped horizontally around the body part or area using sufficient pressure to maintain contact with the skin without causing an excessive indentation in the skin. Two measurements to the nearest ¼ inch should be made at each site, and the average of the two is used as the reporting value. Equations are available to use to convert the measurements into predictions of a person's percentage of body fat. However, these

BOX 4–10
Girth Measurement Sites for Body Fat

Right upper extremity
  Arm—Midway between the shoulder and elbow; extremity in anatomic position and relaxed at side.
  Forearm—Proximal third of the forearm at which the greatest girth appears; extremity positioned as described previously.

Abdomen—One inch above the umbilicus.

Buttocks—At the level of the greatest protrusion; the heels are in contact.

Right lower extremity
  Thigh—Upper thigh just below the gluteal fold.
  Calf—Proximal third of the calf at which the greatest girth appears.

Note: All measurements are made with the person standing erect and relaxed (Figs. 4–13 to 4–17).

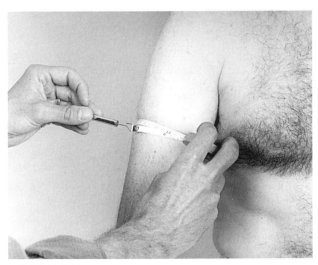

■ **FIGURE 4–13**
Anthropometric measurement: biceps (arm) girth; note the use of a spring tension measurement tape.

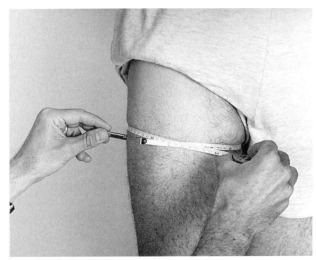

■ **FIGURE 4–16**
Anthropometric measurement: upper thigh girth.

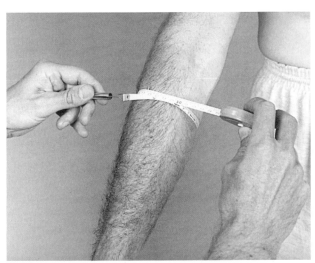

■ **FIGURE 4–14**
Anthropometric measurement: upper forearm girth.

equations are population specific, and the person must be matched to a particular population. (See Figs. 4–13 to 4–17.)

Girth measurement of an extremity to serially measure its circumference is a technique used to evaluate the presence of edema. A plastic or metal anthropometric measuring tape is recommended for these measurements for the reasons cited previously.

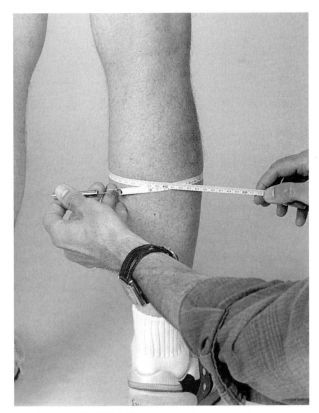

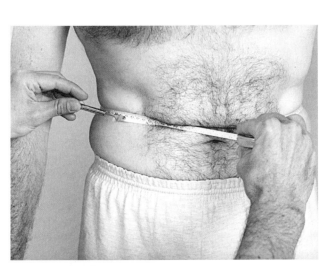

■ **FIGURE 4–15**
Anthropometric measurement: abdominal girth.

■ **FIGURE 4–17**
Anthropometric measurement: calf girth.

PROCEDURE 4 – 9
Girth Measurements

1. Expose the extremity; position the patient so his/her extremity is relaxed, supported, and elevated from the underlying surface, and explain the procedure.

2. Use a plastic or metal anthropometric measuring tape with well-defined easily visible calibrations; it will be helpful if the tape can be locked at any length so it will not retract but can be lengthened.

3. Palpate and mark the bony landmark to be used as the base for the series of measurement sites on the extremity; position the free end of the tape on the mark and extend it along the extremity.

4. Use a skin-marking pencil to mark the sites at which the circumferential measurements are to be made; the sites should be equidistant from each other.

5. To measure the circumference of the extremity, apply the tape around the extremity so it contacts the skin firmly and lies flat, but without causing an excessive indentation in the soft tissue; use consistent pressure as you apply the tape at each mark, and apply the tape so each measurement is parallel to the one above and below.

6. Observe the measurement value at which the free end of the tape meets the portion of the tape that was wrapped around the extremity; use the same procedure for each measurement.

7. Record the results for each site (mark); document your activity, and identify significant findings.

Note: Girth measurements are difficult to perform on irregularly shaped areas such as the hand/wrist and foot/ankle; volumetric measurements are suggested for those areas.

A bony landmark is used to establish a consistent site from which the locations of a series of measurements can be established along the extremity. The free end of the tape is held on the landmark, and the tape is extended along the extremity. A skin-marking pencil is used to mark the levels or locations for the circumferential measurements so they are the same distance from each other (i.e., as measured in centimeters or inches) and parallel to the mark above and below. Accuracy and reliability of the measurements are enhanced when the same person performs the measurements, the patient is in the same position, measurements are made at the same time of day, and the same tape measure is used. The caregiver should apply the tape horizontally around the extremity with the same tension applied at each measuring session. Serial measurements, performed over a period of time, will provide some objective evidence of the changes in the circumference of the extremity, which indirectly indicates the effect of edema on the girth (Procedure 4–9).

Bioelectric impedance analysis is another technique that can be used to assess body composition. Electricity will flow more readily through body tissues that have a normal level of fluid and low levels of fat. The electrolyte content in those tissues is greater than that in fat tissue and reduces the resistance to current flow. To measure the impedance (or resistance) to the flow of a painless electrical current, electrodes are positioned on a person's hands and feet, and the amount of impedance is measured. Through the use of mathematical equations, the impedance value is converted to body density; then, the body density can be converted to percentage of body fat with use of the Siri equation. Two major factors that affect the accuracy and reliability of bioelectric impedance measurements are air temperature and the person's level of hydration.

PROCEDURE 4-10
Volumetric Measurements

1. Expose the area to be assessed, seat the patient to assess the foot/ankle, have him/her sit or stand to assess the hand/wrist, inform him/her about the procedure, and obtain the two water and one calibrated containers.

2. Fill the main container to overflowing with warm water, and use the overflow container to collect the water. When water no longer drips from the spout, empty the overflow container and dry it. Replace it beneath the spout, and be certain both containers are on a firm, level surface.

3. Instruct the patient to slowly and carefully immerse his/her foot/ankle or hand/wrist, with the hand open and fingers relaxed, into the water until his/her foot rests on or his/her fingers touch the bottom of the container. Instruct him/her to leave the part immersed, without movement, until water no longer drips from the spout.

4. Remove the overflow container before he/she lifts his/her foot or hand from the water so any water that would drip from the part does not drip into the container. Dry his/her foot or hand.

5. Carefully pour the water from the overflow container into the calibrated container. Place the container on a firm, level surface, and position yourself to read the scale at eye level.

6. Record the results, document your activities, and identify significant findings.

Skin temperature affects resistance to the current, and hydration affects the electrolyte concentration. A decrease in body water decreases the resistance (or impedance) to the current, so a false lower percentage of fat value is found; an increase in water retention produces the opposite result. A warm environment provides a lower predicted percentage of body fat; a cool environment produces the opposite result. Therefore, the air temperature and person's level of hydration must be standardized each time bioelectric impedance measurements are made.

Volumetric displacement, with the use of a volumeter, is a method to measure changes in the distal aspect of an extremity due to edema, swelling, or muscle atrophy. The technique is more accurate and easier to use than girth measurements due to the irregular shape of the hand and foot, but it requires some equipment. A container, with a spout, that is large enough to immerse a foot and ankle or a hand and wrist; a collection container; and a measurement container with a calibrated scale are necessary. The large container with the spout is filled with warm water so it overflows. The container is not ready for use until the water ceases to drip from the spout. The collection container is positioned so it will catch the water that overflows when the person immerses his/her hand or foot into the water-filled container. The person should be instructed to immerse his/her hand or foot slowly and carefully into the water and to remain motionless as the displaced water flows through the spout; the two containers should rest on a firm, level surface. The collected water is poured into the calibrated container, which is usually in the form of a column. This container should be placed on a firm, level surface and at a height that allows the caregiver to read the scale at eye level. When a series of measurements are made of the same extremity, conditions such as the water temperature, time of day, equipment, patient position, and evaluator should be replicated at each session to enhance accuracy and reliability of the findings. Differences of several millimeters of water displacement may occur between a person's left and right hand and between his/her dominant and nondominant hand. Despite these differences, it may be helpful to measure the displacement of water caused by the unaffected hand or foot to establish a baseline or comparison value for the affected hand or foot. Repetitive measurements can be reviewed and compared to determine the change in volume of the segment being measured (Figs. 4–18 and 4–19 and Procedure 4–10).

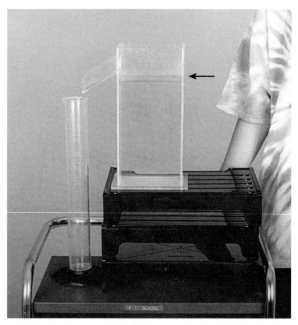

■ **FIGURE 4–18**
Equipment for volume displacement measurement of the hand and wrist. Note: Water level indicated by arrow.

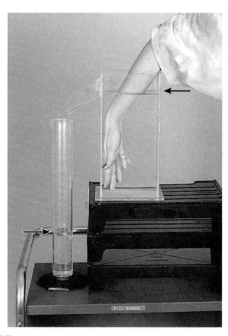

■ **FIGURE 4–19**
Immersion of the hand and wrist for volume displacement measurement. Note: Water levels indicated by arrow.

SUMMARY

It is important to monitor a patient's vital signs (i.e., body temperature, pulse, BP, and respiration rate), because they are indicators of the patient's general health or physiologic status. The caregiver should be able to differentiate between normal and abnormal findings and should have some knowledge of the possible causes of abnormal findings.

It may be necessary to measure the vital signs before, during, and after exercise or physical activity. The use of proper techniques during the measurement of vital signs will produce the most accurate findings. Adverse responses or reactions to exercise or activity should be reported to the patient's physician or to nursing personnel and documented by the caregiver. It may be necessary to adjust or modify the exercise or activity at future sessions to reduce or eliminate undesirable reactions. If it is apparent that the patient is in acute distress or his/her condition is life threatening, then emergency procedures should be implemented immediately. Contact skilled personnel using the 911 emergency exchange or emergency number within the facility before you initiate emergency care.

■ SELF-STUDY/DISCUSSION ACTIVITIES

1. List the normal values for adult heart rate, blood pressure, and respiration rate.
2. Explain the reactions a normal adult should exhibit to aerobic exercise or activity in terms of heart rate, blood pressure, and respiration rate.
3. Discuss the factors that may affect a person's heart rate, blood pressure, and respiration rate; indicate why it is important for the caregiver to be knowledgeable about these factors.
4. Describe three factors or procedures that can adversely affect the accuracy of blood pressure values.
5. List six specific sites at which a patient's heart rate (pulse) can be accurately palpated and measured.
6. Perform skinfold measurements of an individual's triceps, subscapular, and suprailiac sites and calculate his/her percentage of body fat.
7. Perform girth measurements of an individual's right upper and lower extremities.

Chapter 5

Basic Exercise–Passive and Active

After studying this chapter, the reader will be able to:

1 Differentiate among passive exercise, active assistive exercise, active exercise, and active resistive exercise.

2 Provide rationale for the use or objectives of each form of exercise.

3 Discuss the principles of preparation for these forms of exercise.

4 Discuss the principles of application of these forms of exercise.

5 Demonstrate the application of passive, active assistive, and active resistive exercise.

■■■ K E Y   T E R M S

Active assistive exercise: Exercise performed by a person with manual or mechanical assistance; can be static or dynamic.

Active exercise: Exercise performed by a person without any mechanical assistance from another person.

Active resistive exercise: Exercise performed by a person against manual or mechanical resistance.

Atrophy: A decrease or reduction in the size of normally developed cells, tissues, organs, or body parts.

Capsular pattern: A characteristic pattern for a given joint that limits joint motion and indicates that a problem exists within that joint.

Concentric contraction: An overall shortening of a muscle as it develops tension and contracts; positive work is performed, or movement is accelerated.

Contraction: A drawing together or a shortening or shrinking (for example, a muscle contracts).

Dorsal: Directed toward or situated on the back surface.

Eccentric contraction: An overall lengthening of a muscle as it develops tension and contracts to control motion performed by an outside force; negative work is performed, or movement is decelerated.

End feel: The quality of the movement a person senses when pressure is applied passively to a joint at the end of its available range of motion.

Extrinsic: Being, coming, or acting from the outside; not inherent.

Hypertrophy: An increase in the cross-sectional size of a fiber or cell.

Isokinetic exercise: A form of active resistive exercise; the speed of movement of the limb is controlled throughout the arc or range of motion, and the resistance offered is in direct proportion to the force offered by the patient throughout the range of motion of the exercise.

Isometric contraction: A muscle contraction that develops tension but does not perform any mechanical work; there is no appreciable joint motion, and the overall length of the muscle remains constant.

Isotonic contraction: A muscle contraction whereby tension is developed and movement of a joint or body part occurs; an eccentric or concentric contraction may be used, and the muscle may lengthen or shorten.

Joint play: The laxity or elasticity of a joint capsule that allows movement of the joint surfaces within the capsule.

Length-tension curve: The curve that accounts for the active and passive elements of muscle tension and dictates that optimal tension is developed at one point known as *rest length,* the point in its range where peak torque is developed.

Passive exercise: Exercise performed on a person by manual or mechanical means; no voluntary muscle contraction occurs.

Phlebitis: Inflammation of a vein.

Pronation: The position of the forearm that places the hand palm downward; medial rotation of the forearm. The motion occurs in the forearm.

Proprioceptive neuromuscular facilitation (PNF): A treatment technique that uses various stimuli to affect the muscle or joint proprioceptors to facilitate or alter movement responses.

Range of motion (ROM): The normal extent of movement in a joint; the amount of motion allowed between two bony levers.

Resistance: A force external to the body that creates additional work for a muscle when it contracts.

Soft tissues: Tissues that lack bony or skeletal components; these include muscle, ligament, joint capsule, tendon, skin, and fascia.

Stretching: Any therapeutic technique or procedure designed to lengthen or elongate shortened soft tissue structures and to increase the range of motion.

Supination: The position of the forearm that places the hand palm upward; lateral rotation of the forearm. The motion occurs in the forearm.

Thrombophlebitis: Inflammation of a vein associated with the formation of a thrombus.

Thrombus: An aggregation of blood factors, primarily platelets and fibrin, with entrapment of cellular elements that frequently leads to a clot and obstruction of a blood vessel.

Valsalva phenomenon or maneuver: Increased intrathoracic pressure caused by forcible exhalation against a closed glottis.

Volar: Pertaining to the palm; indicating the flexor surface of the forearm, wrist, or hand.

INTRODUCTION

Exercise is an important therapeutic modality that is used to improve the functional capacity of many patients. Some general goals of exercise are to enhance the metabolic and physiologic function or capacity of muscle, maintain or improve joint motion and range, and enhance efficiency of the cardiopulmonary system and independent function of the body. Exercise can affect strength, endurance, joint flexibility, coordination, and one's general sense of well-being.

There are two basic types of exercise: active and passive. Each type has several subdivisions or categories. In general terms, *active exercise* requires the patient to assist with or independently perform the exercise with the use of active, voluntary *contraction* of muscle. In contrast, *passive exercise* is used for the patient who is unable or not permitted to contract his/her muscles or to avoid undesired muscle contraction, pain, or adverse effects to the cardiopulmonary, musculoskeletal, or neuromuscular systems that may be associated with muscle contractions. When exercise is performed, the caregiver should consider the effect of gravity, the amount and type of stability and support necessary for the patient during the exercise, the purpose of the exercise, the ability of the patient to perform or participate in the activity, and the safety measures or protection required to avoid injury or an increase in the patient's symptoms or condition.

Support should be provided to relieve stress to a joint or body area, control the weight of an extremity or a body part, or compensate for the loss of muscle strength. The caregiver may need to use one or both hands to provide support to the segment or area. Support is used to promote motion or movement while stabilization is used to avoid, limit, or prohibit movement. Stabilization is appropriate to protect the site of a recent, healing fracture; extensive soft tissue trauma or damage; or recently injured, healing musculotendinous structure and where movement of an uninvolved joint or body part is to be avoided. The caregiver will need to use both hands to stabilize the area by grasping above and below the site of the problem or securing one structure (e.g., scapula) while moving or mobilizing another structure. In some instances, an external splint or bandage can be used as the stabilizing force providing it does not restrict or prevent movement that is desired. The hand positions used by the caregiver may need to be revised as the exercise is performed to maintain proper control, support, or stability. Reference to the photographs in this chapter will assist in identifying where to apply your hands to provide support and stabilization. Future decisions about hand placements should be based on the caregiver's knowledge, skill, experience, and competence.

The caregiver must integrate his/her knowledge of the musculoskeletal, neuromuscular, and cardiopulmonary systems to properly determine and apply an exercise program. In addition, concepts and principles such as torque, force, force couples, levers, axis of motion, joint structures and components, muscle contractility and elasticity, stresses to skeletal and soft tissue, joint biomechanics, ligamentous and muscular attachments, sensation, neural innervation patterns, and muscle tone should be considered and applied by the caregiver. An explanation of these terms, concepts, and principles is beyond the scope of this textbook, and the reader is referred to the Bibliography for appropriate resources. The desired outcome of exercise must be determined and measured throughout the treatment program. Patient progression toward pre-established objectives or goals is the key determinant of the effectiveness of the treatment program and its procedures, techniques, or activities. This progression should be measured frequently and recorded in the patient's medical record.

TYPES OF EXERCISE FOR RANGE OF MOTION

Passive exercise is the movement of a joint or body segment by a force external to the body, within an unrestricted and normal range of motion and without an active, voluntary muscle contraction by the patient. The external force may be applied manually by the patient or by another person, mechanically by using weights or pulleys or continuous passive motion (CPM) unit, or by gravity. Passive exercise or passive range of motion (PROM) differs from passive stretching. When PROM is used, no increase in joint range should be expected; the goal or objective is to maintain the unrestricted joint range. When passive stretching is used, the goal or objective is to increase the restricted joint range to the full joint range. Only PROM techniques will be described in this text.

Active exercise is the movement of a joint or body segment produced by active, voluntary muscle contraction by the patient within the unrestricted, normal range of motion. No increase in joint range should be expected, but strength and endurance can be increased.

Active assistive exercise is a form of active exercise whereby an external force is used to assist the patient to perform the exercise. The assistance may be applied manually, mechanically, or by gravity. The patient must still perform active, voluntary muscle contractions to the extent that he/she is able. This technique may be used when muscular weakness, fatigue, or pain limit the patient's performance and when active, voluntary muscle contractions are desired.

These forms of exercise are used to preserve or maintain the normal *range of motion (ROM)* of a joint or segment, to maintain or improve strength and endurance, and to prepare the patient for future activities.

INDICATIONS FOR PASSIVE EXERCISE

In general, passive exercise is used when a patient is unable to perform any form of active exercise. When there is paralysis, when the patient is comatose, when pain occurs if an active muscle contraction is attempted but not when PROM is performed, when recovery from a surgical procedure prohibits active muscle contraction, or to avoid exercise of an unhealed fracture whose healing would be disrupted with active muscle contraction are some specific examples of indications for passive exercise. PROM is also used to counteract the negative aspects of immobilization, to evaluate joint range and flexibility, to provide sensory stimulation and awareness, and to reduce stress on the cardiopulmonary system.

Passive exercise is usually contraindicated when the passive movement increases the patient's symptoms or intensifies the condition and when he/she is capable of and would benefit from some type of active exercise.

Several benefits can result from passive exercise: it can assist in preserving and maintaining existing ROM; it can minimize the development of muscle shortening or the development of capsular, ligamentous, or tendinous adhesions resulting from immobilization; and it can assist in maintaining the mechanical elasticity of muscle. Passive exercise also assists in maintaining local circulation and maintaining or developing a patient's awareness of joint motion by enhancing his/her kinesthesia, proprioception, mental imaging, and sensory awareness.

Passive exercise is beneficial to evaluate joint ROM, stability, flexibility, and muscle tone. Cartilage nutrition and movement of the synovial fluid in the joint capsule are enhanced by passive exercise. The movement the patient is expected to perform with active exercise can be demonstrated passively to assist him/her in learning the desired movement. Finally, passive exercise may reduce or inhibit pain when proper support is given to a specific joint or body segment.

Passive exercise also has some limitations of which the caregiver should be aware. It cannot prevent muscle *atrophy;* maintain or increase muscle tone, strength, or contractile endurance; or reduce adipose tissue. Although passive exercise can assist in maintaining local circulation, it is not as effective as active exercise. The caregiver will usually find that it is difficult to apply passive exercise when the patient's muscles are fully innervated and the patient is conscious, or when pain occurs with motion.

At times passive exercise may appear to the caregiver to be of little value, and it may become a boring task. The best results can be expected when passive exercise is performed by a conscientious individual who integrates what he/she palpates, senses, and observes during treatment. The progression to active assistive exercise, observation of changes in the joint range, and being alert to other patient responses to the exercise program are the responsibilities of the primary caregiver, particularly if the exercise activities are assigned to supportive persons (e.g., family members, aides, assistants).

INDICATIONS FOR ACTIVE EXERCISE

In general, active exercise is used when a patient is able to voluntarily contract, control, and coordinate muscular movements with or without assistance; when there are no contraindications to its use; and when its established benefits are desirable to fulfill the goals of the patient's treatment.

Active exercise may be contraindicated in patients with cardiopulmonary dysfunction, an unhealed and unprotected fracture site, an unhealed and unprotected recent surgical site, or severe soft tissue trauma. Caution in the use of active exercise is recommended when soft tissue or joint pain or joint swelling occur. If active exercise increases the patient's symptoms or his/her condition intensifies when improper or substitutive movement patterns are used, active exercise may be contraindicated.

Benefits associated with active exercise include maintaining the physiologic elasticity, strength, and contractile endurance of muscle and increasing the local circulation. Active exercise also provides increased sensory awareness of joint motion, which is associated with proprioception, kinesthesia, and coordination. The cardiopulmonary functions of cardiac output, capillary efficiency, stroke volume, oxygen uptake, gas exchange in the lungs, and overall cardiac efficiency can be maintained or improved when multiple muscles perform simultaneously and the patient is in a deconditioned physiologic state. Active exercise such as repetitive ankle dorsiflexion–plantar flexion ("ankle pumping") can be used to assist in preventing the development of a *thrombus, thrombophlebitis,* or *phlebitis* in the peripheral veins of the lower legs. The stimulus of stress, produced by muscle contraction, will assist the tendon–bone interface to maintain its structural integrity. Finally, active exercise can improve muscle strength in a patient whose strength is measured at a grade of "fair" (50% or less of normal) on a manual muscle test. Muscles that are initially stronger than "fair" need to contract against external resistance, in addition to the weight of the segment, to increase the strength of the muscle.

Active exercise will not develop strength in muscles whose initial strength was measured at a grade of "good" (75% or more) on a manual muscle test. Furthermore, cardiopulmonary efficiency in the normally conditioned or well-conditioned individual will not be increased unless vigorous aerobic exercise is performed.

Active exercise is usually more beneficial for a patient than passive exercise, but the caregiver must determine which type of exercise should be used. A treatment program may begin with passive exercise, progress to active assistive exercise and then to active free exercise, and eventually lead to active resistive exercise depending on the goals of treatment and the patient's physical abilities. This progression requires the skill and knowledge of the caregiver to determine when the exercise progression can or should occur. The patient should be encouraged to perform within his/her ability but at his/her maximal effort levels whenever possible. Patients should be taught to breathe normally when performing active exercise to avoid the potential adverse effects of the *Valsalva phenomenon or maneuver.* This phenomenon can occur when the patient holds his/her breath and air is trapped in the thorax, which increases intrathoracic pressure. This increased pressure can affect the circulatory system by decreasing the return of venous blood to the right side of the heart, which decreases cardiac output and increases peripheral blood pressure. These events could result in the rupture of a cerebral vessel, which could lead to death or a cerebrovascular accident. This phenomenon is most likely to occur when the patient is performing heavy resistive exercise but could occur at any time he/she performs active exercise.

Passive ROM and active ROM can be performed in the traditional anatomic planes or in diagonal planes of motion using the techniques of *proprioceptive neuromuscular facilitation (PNF)*. ROM may also be performed in specific arcs or planes of motion of any joint to better affect a given muscle or portion of the joint range. The caregiver will need to decide which motions to perform and whether to perform them through the full range or through a portion of the range. His/her decision should be based on evaluation and observation of the patient's responses to the exercise, as well as the patient's condition.

PREPARATION FOR APPLICATION OF PASSIVE AND ACTIVE RANGE OF MOTION

Initially you should evaluate the patient and obtain information from the medical record or other reliable sources to assist you in determining the goals of treatment and the type of exercise to be used. Intro-

duce yourself, and explain the rationale, or purpose, and the expected outcome of treatment. Obtain the consent of the patient to perform treatment before you begin. You should be prepared to respond to questions regarding the treatment before you initiate the exercise program.

Position the patient to have access to his/her extremities, align and support his/her trunk and extremities, enhance your body mechanics, and provide patient comfort to the extent that it is compatible with the treatment. Restrictive clothing, orthoses, and linen should be removed or loosened. Be certain there is sufficient space to perform the treatment, and drape the patient to protect his/her modesty, maintain warmth, and expose the area or segment to be treated. Remember to use proper body mechanics when performing the exercises; this can be done by adjusting the height of the bed or the position of the patient or by positioning yourself close to the person. Obtain assistance to move or position the patient if it is necessary (Procedure 5–1 and Box 5–1).

APPLICATION OF PASSIVE EXERCISE

Passive exercise can be used to maintain the mechanical length of muscles, tendons, and other *soft tissues;* to assist in maintaining local circulation; to evaluate ROM; to maintain joint flexibility; to provide sensory stimulation; and to assist in preventing the development of soft tissue contractures. Remember: Passive exercise differs from *stretching*, and the following information refers only to passive exercise (Box 5–2).

Passive exercise can be a beneficial treatment approach (1) when a patient is unable to actively move a body segment; (2) to avoid pain, undesired movements or patterns of motion, development of undesired muscle tone, and stress to a localized site of poor integrity; and (3) to reduce cardiopulmonary stress. The patient does not assist with the movements; instead, an external manual, mechanical, or gravitational force is used to provide motion of the segment. Examples of mechanical forces are free weights, a pulley system, and a CPM unit. A gravitational force, or the effect of gravity on a joint or muscle, can be used in conjunction with specific positioning of the segment to permit gravity to affect the structure. None of these forces is described or depicted in this text, but sources of such information can be found in the Bibliography.

Manual PROM can be performed by the patient (self-performed ROM), family member, or trained professional. Gentle, firm support and stabilization,

---

PROCEDURE 5-1
Procedures for Basic Exercise Activities

1. Evaluate the patient to determine his/her exercise needs and establish appropriate outcome goals; inform the patient of the purpose(s) of the exercise program.

2. Develop a treatment plan designed to meet the patient's needs and outcome goals (i.e., frequency, duration, sequence); obtain consent from the patient.

3. Select the treatment activities, techniques, and procedures that will be most apt to fulfill the predetermined needs and outcome goals effectively and within an acceptable period of time.

4. Be prepared to protect structures that are unstable or vulnerable to injury when the exercise program is performed (e.g., hypermobile joints, healing fracture and surgical sites, muscle and ligamentous strains or sprains).

5. Instruct the patient in his/her performance responsibilities and to maintain a breathing pattern during active exercise so the Valsalva maneuver will be avoided.

6. Exercise movements should be performed smoothly and slowly throughout the unrestricted range of motion; resistive exercises should be performed within the patient's physical limits.

7. Proper precautions should be used during the exercise program; equipment must be secure and free from damage, and the patient and caregiver should use proper body mechanics.

8. The caregiver should monitor the effects of the exercise with all patients, especially those with known cardiac dysfunction.

9. The exercise plan, activities, techniques, or procedures should be revised or modified depending on the patient's response and his/her progress toward the outcome goals; the program should be discontinued if adverse effects occur and persist for 24 hours or longer.

---

through proper hand placement and control, should be provided to avoid stress to the structures or segment being moved. Practice will assist the caregiver in determining the best hand placements (areas of grasp) to use to provide smooth, controlled, and complete motion with minimal adjustments. All planes of motion of the joint should be exercised, which may require moving the joint through a variety or combination of motions. Although it is possible to exercise or "range" several joints simultaneously, you should first evaluate the range of each joint individually. This will assist you in determining whether there is a limitation in the range of one or more of the joints. If all joint ranges of the segment or extremity are similar, time can be saved by "ranging" multiple joints simultaneously. However, one must be cautious to avoid under- or over-ranging one or more of the joints of the extremity.

PROM should be performed through the entire unrestricted, normal range of the joint and soft tissue. The caregiver must be aware of normal joint range parameters and must perceive or sense the resistance, or lack of it, from the soft tissue or joint capsule and other joint structures as the exercise is being performed. This is the concept of *end feel*, or the "feel" of the resistance of the tissue at the end or completion of the range. To determine the feel, an excess pressure known as "overpressure" is applied at the end of the range. End feels are described as "soft" when soft tissues are compressed or stretched (e.g., in elbow or knee flexion); "firm" when joint capsules or ligaments are stretched (e.g., in hip rotation); "hard" when a bony block or resistance is reached (e.g., in elbow extension); or "empty" when no end feel is elicited because the patient does not permit full motion to occur, usually because of acute pain. An abnormal end feel

Principles of Exercise Activities

1. The patient should not be challenged to exceed his/her maximal physical capabilities.
2. Instruct the patient to maintain a breathing pattern that allows him/her to avoid the Valsalva maneuver.
3. Avoid applying excessive stress to the patient's skin, soft tissues, joints, and bones when manual or mechanical resistance is used.
4. Protect structures that are unstable or vulnerable to injury, such as hypermobile joints, healing fracture sites, healing surgical sites, and muscle or ligamentous strains/sprains.
5. Monitor the effect of exercise closely for the patient who has a known history of cardiac dysfunction.
6. Evaluate the equipment used to be certain it is secure and stable and functions properly.
7. Use proper body mechanics as you participate in the exercise program.

may result from muscle guarding, muscle spasm, muscle spasticity, or an intra-articular block such as a torn meniscus or articular cartilage or a loose body in the joint. The caregiver should evaluate the ROM in relation to these normal and abnormal end feels or *capsular patterns* and adjust the treatment as necessary.

Muscles that cross more than one joint (i.e., multijoint muscles) must be identified and given special consideration when PROM is performed. Some examples of multijoint muscles are the biceps and triceps, *extrinsic* finger flexors and extensors, the quadriceps, the hamstrings, and the gastrocnemius. It is important to differentiate between the available or normal joint range and the muscle range when multijoint muscles are involved. To allow full joint motion to occur, multijoint muscles must be relaxed and must not be lengthened simultaneously over the joints they cross. Joint motion is important, because it assists in maintaining proper capsular and ligamentous flexibility. Motion over the full muscle range is performed to assist in maintaining the length or flexibility of the muscles and tendons that cross a given joint. Multijoint muscles must be lengthened simultaneously over each joint they cross to maintain their functional length. This concept is particularly important when applying PROM to the extrinsic flexors and extensors of the fingers. For example, to maintain the length of the extrinsic finger extensors, wrist flexion should be combined with finger flexion. Conversely, to maintain

the length of the extrinsic finger flexors, wrist extension should be combined with finger extension. There is at least one patient condition for which full lengthening of the extrinsic finger flexors usually is contraindicated: The patient with a spinal cord injury that has spared the C6 nerve root may benefit from tightness or limited range of the extrinsic finger flexors. Limited range of the finger flexors, when combined with active wrist extension, can provide the person with a passive grasp. As the wrist is extended, the finger flexors, already limited in length, are elongated or "stretched" over the *volar* area of the wrist, which further shortens them. When this occurs, a gross, passive grasp develops, known as a "tenodesis" grasp or movement. Relaxation of the wrist extensors allows the hand to lower and releases the passive tension on the finger flexors. This is the opening phase of the grasp-and-release action.

Other persons with a spinal cord injury may benefit if their erector spinae muscles are not elongated by passive exercise because their trunk stability when they sit may be improved by the limited length or range of those muscles. Stability of a hypermobile joint may be enhanced if the muscles that cross or support the joint are not elongated, but a contracture of the joint should be avoided.

Although most of the photographs in this text show the patient to be supine or prone when PROM is performed, other positions can also be used depending on the patient's condition. Many PROM activities can be performed with the patient sitting in a wheelchair (or other type of chair), side lying, or standing. Mechanical devices such as pulleys or CPM units can be used as replacements or adjuncts to manual PROM techniques.

Research studies have not specifically determined the frequency or number of repetitions necessary for PROM to be effective. Many factors affect joint or

Benefits of Passive Exercise

1. Preserve and maintain range of motion.
2. Minimize contracture formation.
3. Minimize adhesion formation.
4. Maintain mechanical elasticity of muscle.
5. Promote and maintain local circulation.
6. Promote awareness of joint motion (i.e., sensory awareness).
7. Evaluate joint integrity and motion.
8. Enhance cartilage nutrition.
9. Inhibit or reduce pain.

muscle range, and there is no assurance that PROM will, in and of itself, maintain the free, unrestricted range of a given joint or muscles. The use of protective equipment, positioning regimens, general medical and nursing care, and the type of illness or trauma all affect the results of PROM activities. The skill, knowledge, and judgment of the caregiver are required to reach decisions regarding the actual protocol that is applicable for each patient. Therefore, the caregiver must evaluate the patient's response to treatment frequently and consistently.

The caregiver must also understand and recognize which muscles or soft tissues are affected by the application of PROM. In general, a passive movement should be performed in the direction *opposite* to the movement the muscle would produce if it were to contract actively. For example, passive elbow extension is performed to lengthen the biceps, passive knee flexion is performed to lengthen the quadriceps, and passive ankle dorsiflexion is performed to lengthen the gastrocnemius-soleus muscle complex. This concept can be applied to movement of other muscles, soft tissues, and joints. A muscle or soft tissue that is limited in its ability to relax or lengthen will produce a contracture in the *same* direction as the movement the muscle would produce if it were to contract actively.

TRADITIONAL PROM MOVEMENTS

Before initiating PROM, you should determine the purpose or goal of each exercise and explain this goal to the patient. It is helpful to establish a sequence for the exercise program so you will be more likely to perform each motion and less likely to omit a motion. For example, perform all shoulder movements; then move to the elbow and to the forearm, wrist, and fingers. For the lower extremity, perform all hip, then all knee, and then all ankle and foot movements. In some situations, it may be desirable or beneficial to perform two or more movements simultaneously; in other situations, it may be undesirable to combine movements. These situations will be explained as they arise in the progression of the exercise program.

You must be alert during the application of PROM so you can perceive and determine the patient's response to the exercises. These exercises are passive for the patient, but the caregiver must be physically and mentally involved. Position yourself in such a way that you are able to observe the patient's face as you perform each exercise; you should also be positioned so you can exercise the extremity nearest to you. By avoiding reaching across one extremity or the patient's trunk to exercise the more distant extremity, you will use better body mechanics, thereby reducing strain to your body and decreasing the expenditure of energy.

All motions should be performed slowly, and there should be a brief pause or hold at the point of greatest joint range or elongation of a muscle. You should sense or perceive when the terminal, unrestricted joint range or muscle elongation has occurred and stop the exercise at that point. Remember: Passive exercise is different from stretching, and no increase in joint range or muscle length should be anticipated with PROM.

Proper support and stabilization of segments and joints must be incorporated into the exercise. The patient must develop trust and confidence that the caregiver will not cause further injury or pain during the performance of the exercises. This trust and confidence can be established through the manner in which the caregiver physically handles the patient and by explaining the intent or purpose of each exercise. After several exercise sessions have been completed, it should not be necessary to explain the intent or purpose of each exercise unless new exercises are initiated (Procedure 5–2).

Cardinal or Anatomic Planes of Motion

The cardinal planes of motion are associated with and described according to the anatomic position. A person who is standing upright is considered to be in the anatomic position with the upper extremities relaxed along the sides of the trunk, shoulders externally rotated, forearms supinated, and fingers extended and adducted; lower extremities parallel and in neutral rotation, heels approximately 4 inches apart, and toes directed forward; and the face directed forward with the head in neutral flexion-extension, rotation, and lateral bending.

The three cardinal planes are the sagittal, frontal or coronal, and transverse. The sagittal plane is a vertical plane that divides the body into left and right components; flexion and extension occur in this plane. The frontal plane is a vertical plane that divides the body into front (anterior) and back (posterior) components; abduction and adduction occur in this plane, with the exception of the thumb. The transverse plane is a horizontal plane that divides the body into upper and lower components; rotation occurs in this plane.

Upper Extremity Movements

Traditional Anatomic Planes The primary patient position is supine on a firm surface; he/she should be draped and close to the near edge of the treatment table. Other positions can be used depending on the patient's condition and the caregiver's preference.

PROCEDURE 5 – 2
Application of Passive Exercise (PROM)

1. Position the patient for support, stability, and access to the area or segment to be exercised; drape as necessary.
2. Explain the purpose and goals of exercise; obtain consent for treatment.
3. Position the patient to promote use of proper body mechanics by the patient and caregiver.
4. Grasp the part to be treated to provide support, stability, and control during exercises. Refer to the photographs and instructions in this chapter for specific information.
5. Perform exercises through the complete, unrestricted range of motion.
6. Perform the predetermined number of repetitions and frequency of exercises based on patient needs and goals.
7. Perform the exercises smoothly and slowly; pause at the start and end positions of the exercise.
8. At the conclusion of treatment, position the patient for proper alignment, support, and safety; drape or replace clothing for modesty and body temperature control.
9. Evaluate the patient's response to treatment; document important findings.

Articulation: Scapulothoracic.

Movement: Scapular elevation and depression (Fig. 5–1).

Hand placement and motion: Cup the inferior angle with one hand while resting the other hand on the superior border of the scapula; move the scapula upward and downward.

Articulation: Scapulothoracic.

Movement: Scapular protraction (abduction) and retraction (adduction) (Fig. 5–2).

Hand placement and motion: Rest one hand over the medial (vertebral) border while resting the other hand over the acromion process of the scapula; move the scapula toward and away from the spinous processes.

Articulation: Scapulothoracic.

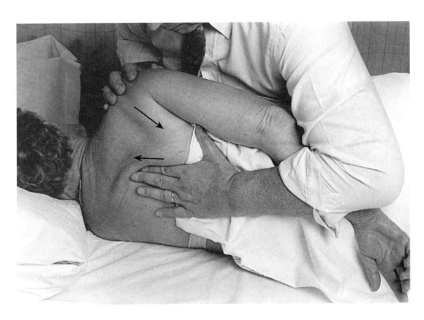

■ **FIGURE 5–1**
Scapular elevation and depression.

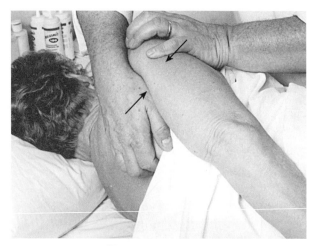

■ **FIGURE 5–2**
Scapular protraction.

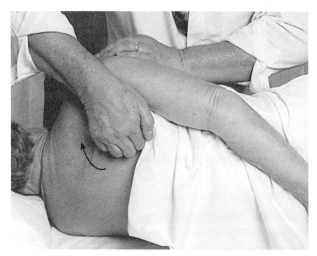

■ **FIGURE 5–3**
Scapular vertebral border lift.

Movement: Scapular vertebral border lift ("winging") (Fig. 5–3).

Hand placement and motion: Slide the fingertips of one hand under the medial (vertebral) border of the scapula; gently lift the scapula from the ribs. It will be easier to grasp the vertebral border if the patient's upper extremity is relaxed behind the trunk with him/her in a side-lying position.

Articulation: Glenohumeral.

Movement: Shoulder flexion and extension (Fig. 5–4).

Hand placement and motion: For the right upper extremity, grasp the right wrist and hand with your left hand and grasp the right elbow with your right hand; lift the extremity through the available range and return. Extension of the arm beyond the midline of the body produces hyperextension. This can be accomplished with the patient supine with the shoulder at the edge of the support surface or with the patient in a side-lying or prone position.

Articulation: Glenohumeral.

Movement: Shoulder abduction and adduction (Fig. 5–5).

Hand placement and motion: Grasp the wrist and elbow; move the extremity away from the trunk and return. The elbow may be extended or flexed, but avoid shoulder flexion and maintain the arm horizontal to the floor. It may be necessary to externally rotate the humerus to reduce impingement of the humeral head on the acromion process. In some instances it may be helpful to prevent excessive elevation of the scapula by

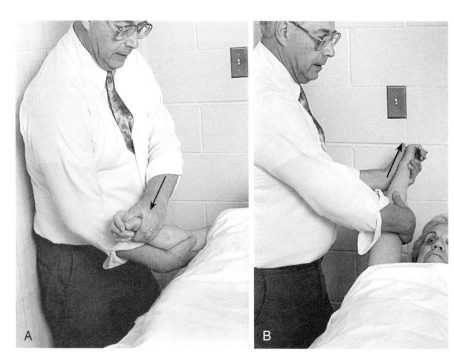

■ **FIGURE 5–4**
A, Hand position for shoulder extension. *B,* Shoulder flexion.

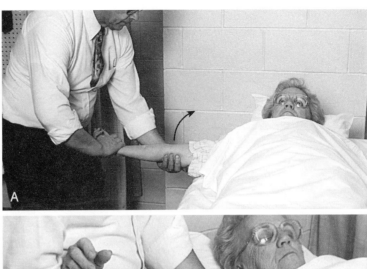

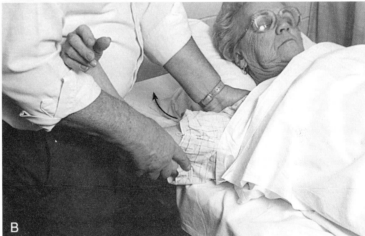

■ **FIGURE 5–5**
A, Shoulder abduction, elbow extended. *B,* Shoulder abduction, elbow flexed.

placing one hand over its superior border. When the exercise is performed with the elbow extended, you will have to adjust your position by moving toward the patient's head.

Articulation: Glenohumeral.

Movement: Shoulder horizontal adduction and abduction (Fig. 5–6).

Hand placement and motion: Grasp the wrist and elbow; begin with the patient's shoulder abducted to 90 degrees and parallel to the floor. Lift the arm up and across the upper chest and return. To attain full abduction, the patient's shoulder must be at the edge of the supporting surface to allow the humerus to clear the edge of the table. The elbow may be flexed or extended.

Articulation: Glenohumeral.

Movement: Shoulder internal (medial) rotation (Fig. 5–7).

Hand placement and motion: Abduct the shoulder to 90 degrees, and flex the elbow to 90 degrees. Position yourself opposite the patient's elbow and facing him/her. Grasp the patient's wrist with one hand and support the hand; rest the other hand on the acromion process or use it to support the distal humerus. Move the forearm forward toward the floor, causing the humerus to rotate.

Stop the motion when the acromion process tips forward, indicating that the head of the humerus has been blocked by the acromion.

Articulation: Glenohumeral.

Movement: Shoulder external (lateral) rotation (Fig. 5–8).

Hand placement and motion: Use the same hand placement described for internal rotation. Move the forearm backward toward the floor, causing the humerus to rotate. Stop the motion when the forearm is horizontal to the floor. (*Note:* Shoulder internal/external rotation can be performed with the elbow extended and the extremity positioned along the patient's side. Grasp the humerus just above the epicondyles, and grasp the forearm at wrist; turn or roll the entire extremity inward and outward. As an alternative method, start with the humerus next to the trunk and the elbow flexed to 90 degrees. Grasp the distal forearm, support the patient's hand, and move the forearm toward and away from the chest without abducting/adducting the shoulder. When this technique is used, internal rotation will be incomplete, because the forearm will strike the chest before complete range is attained.)

Articulation: Humeral-ulnar.

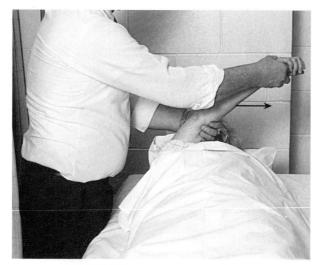

■ **FIGURE 5–6**
Shoulder horizontal adduction.

Movement: Elbow flexion and extension (Fig. 5–9).

Hand placement and motion: For the right upper extremity, grasp the patient's distal forearm and support the hand with your left hand; use your right hand to support and stabilize the distal humerus. Flex and extend the elbow with the forearm neutral, *pronated*, and *supinated*, but avoid any shoulder motion.

Articulation: Radial-ulnar.

Movement: Forearm supination and pronation (Fig. 5–10).

Hand placement and motion: For the right forearm, grasp the distal forearm and support the patient's hand with either your left or right hand; use your other hand to support and stabilize the humerus. Supinate and pronate the forearm. This exercise can be performed with the elbow flexed or extended, but the motion must occur in the forearm. Avoid shoulder rotation, and reduce stress to the wrist by grasping the distal forearm. This motion can be combined with elbow flexion and extension.

Articulation: Carpal-radial-ulnar.

Movement: Wrist flexion and extension (Fig. 5–11).

Hand placement and motion: Grasp the patient's hand over its palmar and *dorsal* surfaces with one hand, and use the other hand to support and stabilize the forearm. Move the palm toward the forearm, and then move the dorsum toward the forearm. Allow the patient's fingers to relax, and do not stress the carpals. This motion can be performed with the elbow flexed or extended. After the range of the extrinsic finger flexors and extensors has been evaluated, you may desire to combine wrist and finger flexion and wrist and finger extension. Review the information on mul-

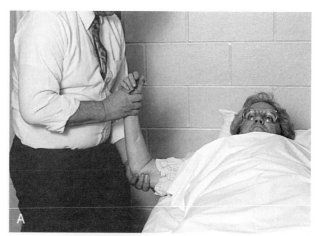

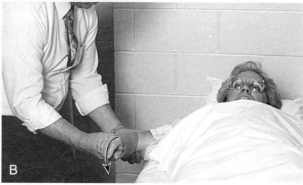

■ **FIGURE 5–7**
A, Hand positions for shoulder rotation. *B,* Internal (medial) shoulder rotation.

tijoint muscles before combining wrist and finger motions.

Articulation: Carpal-radial-ulnar.

Movement: Wrist radial and ulnar deviation (Fig. 5–12).

Hand placement and motion: Grasp the patient's hand as described for wrist flexion and extension, and maintain the hand in neutral flexion-

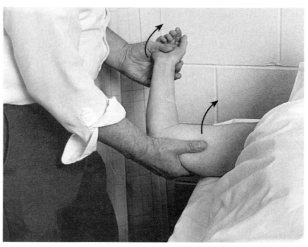

■ **FIGURE 5–8**
External (lateral) shoulder rotation.

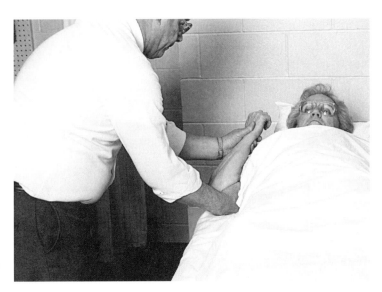

■ **FIGURE 5–9**
Elbow flexion.

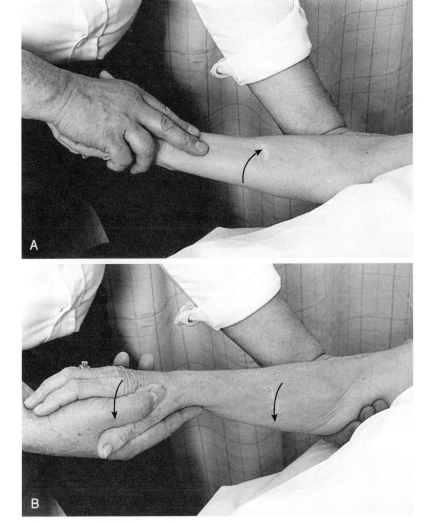

■ **FIGURE 5–10**
A, Elbow extension with forearm supination.
B, Forearm pronation.

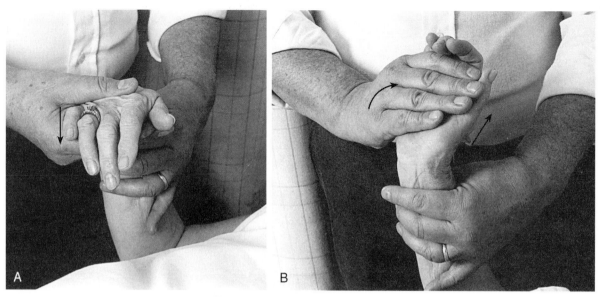

■ **FIGURE 5–11**
A, Wrist flexion. *B,* Wrist extension.

extension. Move the hand in a radial and ulnar direction, but avoid wrist flexion and extension.

Articulation: Metacarpal head *joint play.*

Movement: Elevation and depression of individual metacarpal heads (Fig. 5–13).

Hand placement and motion: Grasp the dorsal and palmar surfaces of the metacarpal of a finger just proximal to its head with the thumb and index finger of one hand, and use your other hand to stabilize the adjacent metacarpal with a similar grasp. Using the first hand, move the head of one metacarpal upward and downward, but do not allow the adjacent metacarpal to move. Progress to the next metacarpal until all four distal metacar-

pals have been moved. This technique should not be applied to the thumb.

Articulation: Metacarpophalangeal (MCP).

Movement: Flexion and extension (Fig. 5–14).

Hand placement and motion: Grasp the dorsal and palmar surfaces of a metacarpal just proximal to the metacarpal head with the thumb and index finger of one hand, and use the thumb and finger of your other hand to grasp the dorsal and palmar surfaces of a proximal phalanx. Stabilize the metacarpal while you move the phalanx upward and downward. Perform the motion for each articulation on each hand, and use the same techniques for the thumb.

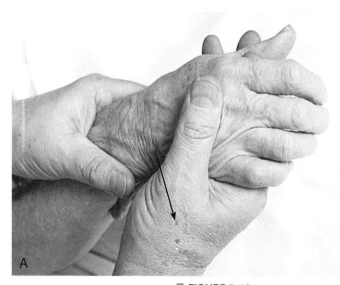

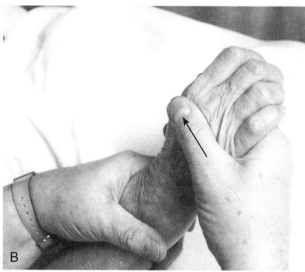

■ **FIGURE 5–12**
A, Ulnar deviation of the wrist. *B,* Radial deviation of the wrist.

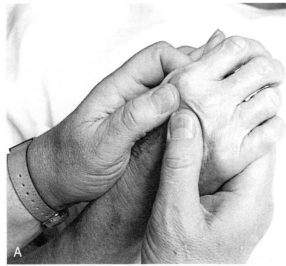

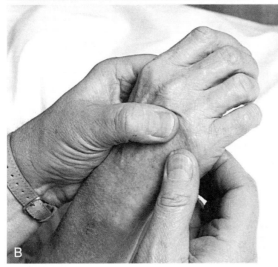

■ **FIGURE 5–13**
Elevation *(A)* and depression *(B)* of individual metacarpal heads.

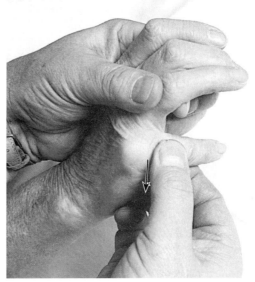

■ **FIGURE 5–14**
Flexion of the metacarpophalangeal (MCP) joint.

tain the wrist in a neutral position. This motion can be performed with the elbow flexed or extended.

Articulation: Metacarpophalangeal.

Movement: Abduction (Fig. 5–17).

Hand placement and motion: Use one hand to grasp and stabilize the DIP joints of the first, second, and third fingers, and use your other hand to grasp the fourth finger. Keeping the MCP and interphalangeal (IP) joints extended, gently move the fourth finger away from the third finger. Then stabilize the first and second fingers, and move the third finger away from the second finger. Next, stabilize the second, third, and fourth

Articulation: Distal and proximal interphalangeal (DIP and PIP, respectively).

Movement: Flexion and extension (Fig. 5–15).

Hand placement and motion: Use the grasp described for MCP flexion and extension. Stabilize the more proximal phalanx and move the more distal phalanx upward and downward. Perform the motion for each articulation on each hand, and use the same technique for the thumb.

Articulation: Metacarpophalangeal and interphalangeal (combined motions).

Movement: Finger flexion and extension (Fig. 5–16).

Hand placement and motion: Place one hand over the patient's extended fingers, and use your other hand to support and stabilize the forearm. Fold the fingers into a fist gently, and return them to an extended position; use the same technique for the thumb by flexing the thumb into the palm and returning it to an extended position. Main-

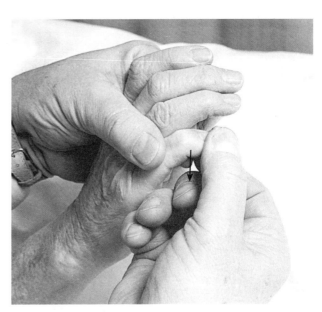

■ **FIGURE 5–15**
Flexion of the distal interphalangeal (DIP) joint.

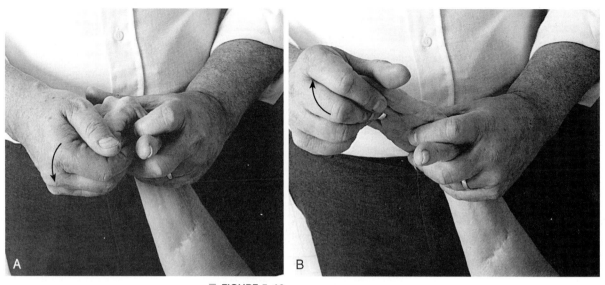

■ FIGURE 5–16
A, Finger flexion. *B,* Finger extension.

fingers, and move the first finger away from the second finger. The second finger can be moved to the left and to the right independently and without stabilizing any of the other fingers. (*Note:* These motions are performed independently of the thumb and are used to maintain the web spaces between the four fingers.)

Articulation: Thumb metacarpal-carpal and meta-carpophalangeal.

Movement: Thumb opposition (Fig. 5–18).

Hand placement and motion: Grasp the patient's thumb with the thumb and fingers of one hand, and use your other hand to grasp the fifth metacarpal and finger. Roll the thumb toward the fifth finger, maintaining the MCP and IP joints in ex-

tension. Return the thumb to a position of full extension to maintain its web space.

Articulation: Metacarpal-carpal of the thumb.

Movement: Thumb abduction and adduction (Fig. 5–19).

Hand placement and motion: Grasp the patient's thumb with the fingers and thumb of one hand, and use the other hand to stabilize the second metacarpal. Lift the thumb away from the palm so it is perpendicular to the palm, but maintain the MCP and IP joints in extension. Return the thumb to the palm parallel to the second metacarpal.

Articulation: Metacarpal-carpal of the thumb.

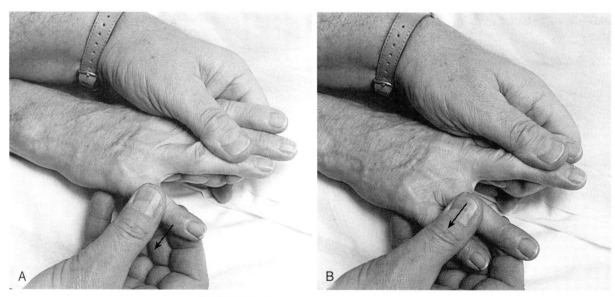

■ FIGURE 5–17
Abduction of the metacarpophalangeal joints.

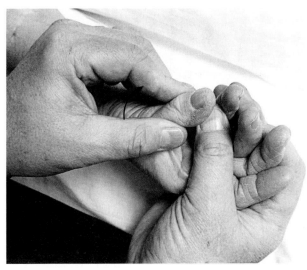

■ **FIGURE 5–18**
Thumb opposition.

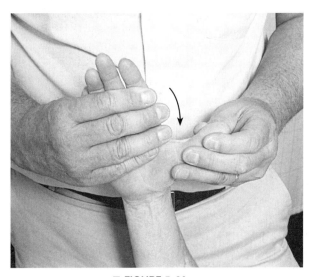

■ **FIGURE 5–20**
Thumb extension.

Movement: Thumb extension and flexion (Fig. 5–20).

Hand placement and motion: Grasp the patient's thumb with the fingers and thumb of one hand, and use the other hand to stabilize the second metacarpal. Move the thumb away from the index finger and horizontal to the palm; widen the web space to its maximum. Return the thumb so it rests next to the side of the second metacarpal.

Articulation: Thumb metacarpophalangeal and interphalangeal.

Movement: Thumb flexion and extension (Fig. 5–21).

Hand placement and motion: Grasp the patient's metacarpal with the thumb and fingers of one hand. Use the thumb and index finger of the

other hand to flex the distal joints of the thumb. Return the distal joints to extension.

Elongation of Multijoint Muscles   Review the information presented earlier in this chapter on the concepts related to joint range and the range of multijoint muscles. All motions should be performed individually initially so the multijoint muscle is elongated over only one joint. This will assist in determining the muscle's free unrestricted range and will prevent excessive elongation of the muscle or excessive stress to the joint and its capsule.

Biceps brachii: Start with the patient supine and the shoulder at the edge of the support surface, with the elbow extended and the forearm pronated. Lower the arm below the level of the support surface (i.e., hyperextend the shoulder) until you sense maximal tension in the muscle or the pa-

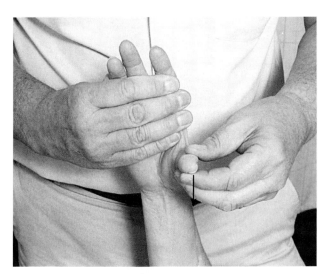

■ **FIGURE 5–19**
Thumb abduction.

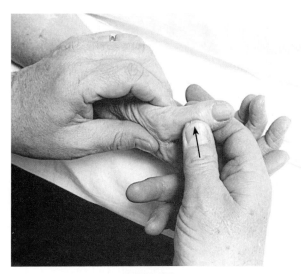

■ **FIGURE 5–21**
Thumb flexion.

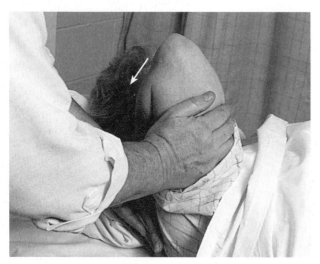

■ FIGURE 5–22
Elongation of the triceps brachii.

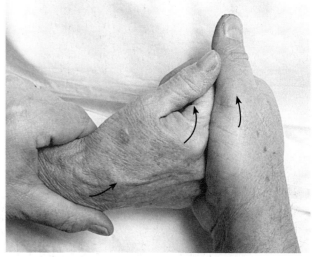

■ FIGURE 5–23
Elongation of the extensor digitorum.

tient complains of discomfort along the anterior (upper) aspect of the extremity.

Triceps brachii (long head): Start with the patient supine, side lying, or sitting. Grasp the wrist with one hand, and use the other hand to support the distal humerus. Flex the elbow maximally and simultaneously flex the shoulder. The patient will have to be side lying, sitting, or standing for maximal elongation to occur. Terminate the motion when you sense maximal tension in the muscle or when the patient complains of discomfort along the posterior aspect of the arm (Fig. 5–22).

Extensor digitorum: Place one hand over the dorsum of all the fingers of the patient's hand, and use your other hand to support and stabilize the forearm. Gently and sequentially flex the DIP, PIP, and MCP joints, and then carefully flex the wrist. Terminate the motion when you sense maximal tension in the muscle or when the patient complains of discomfort along the dorsal surface of the wrist, hand, or fingers. This motion can be performed with the elbow flexed or extended (Fig. 5–23).

Flexor digitorum superficialis and profundus: Place one hand over the palmar surface of all of the fingers of the patient's hand, and use your other hand to support and stabilize the forearm. Gently and sequentially extend the DIP, PIP, and MCP joints, and then carefully extend the wrist. Terminate the motion when you sense maximal tension in the muscles or when the patient complains of discomfort along the palmar surface of the wrist, hand, or fingers. Avoid hyperextension of the MCP joints. This motion can be performed with the elbow flexed or extended (Fig. 5–24).

Lower Extremity Movements

Traditional Anatomic Planes The primary patient position is supine on a firm surface; he/she should be draped and close to the near edge of the treatment table. Other positions can be used depending on the patient's condition and the caregiver's preference.

Articulation: Acetabular-femoral and tibial-femoral.

Movement: Hip and knee flexion and extension (Fig. 5–25).

Hand placement and motion: Use one hand to cradle the patient's heel, and place your other hand in the popliteal space. Lift the lower extremity, allowing the hip and knee to flex. Slide your hand

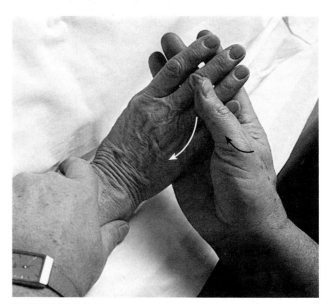

■ FIGURE 5–24
Elongation of the flexor digitorum superficialis and profundus.

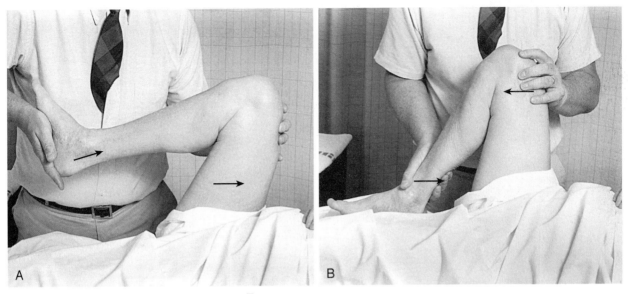

■ **FIGURE 5–25**
Hip *(A)* and knee *(B)* flexion.

from under the knee to the lateral thigh to prevent hip abduction as the hip and knee flex. Approximate the thigh to the chest and the leg to the posterior thigh; return to the starting position. The patient will need to have his/her hip at the edge of the support surface to perform hip hyperextension by lowering the extremity toward the floor. Terminate the movement when the pelvis rotates anteriorly or when lumbar lordosis is increased. (*Note:* Hip hyperextension can be performed more easily when the patient is in a side-lying or prone position.)

Articulation: Acetabular-femoral.

Movement: Hip flexion and extension with the knee extended (straight leg raising) (Fig. 5–26).

Hand placement and motion: Use one hand to support the patient's distal leg, and use your other hand to initially provide support in the popliteal space. Shift your hand from the popliteal space to the anterior knee as the hip is flexed to maintain knee extension and to lift the entire lower extremity to flex the hip. Terminate the motion when you sense maximal tension in the hamstring muscles or when the patient complains of discomfort along the posterior thigh or knee. Do not attempt to increase the range of the hamstrings by forceably flexing the hip with the knee extended. It may be necessary to stabilize the knee of the opposite lower extremity as you perform this motion. Some caregivers prefer to place the ankle of the exercised extremity on one shoulder and to lift the lower extremity by moving the body forward.

Articulation: Acetabular-femoral.

Movement: Hip abduction and adduction (Fig. 5–27).

Hand placement and motion: Use one hand to support the patient's distal leg, and use your other hand to provide support in the popliteal space and to maintain the knee extended. Move the extremity away from the opposite lower extremity, keeping it parallel to the floor and in neutral internal-external rotation. Return it to a position of adduction. To attain complete adduction of the exercised extremity, the opposite lower extremity must be adducted. Some individuals adduct the extremity by lifting it above the opposite extremity so that more adduction is attained.

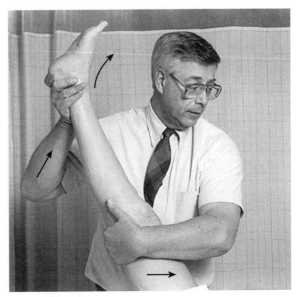

■ **FIGURE 5–26**
Hip and knee extension (straight leg raise).

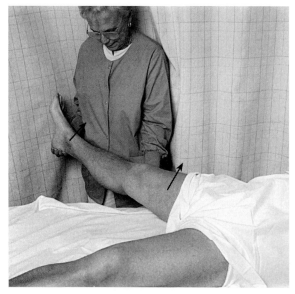

■ **FIGURE 5–27**
Hip abduction.

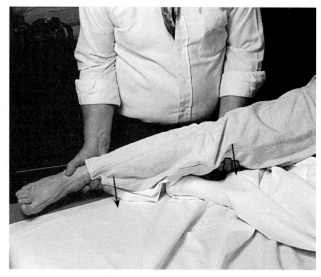

■ **FIGURE 5–28**
Hip adduction in the side-lying position.

Articulation: Acetabular-femoral.

Movement: Hip adduction–side lying (Fig. 5–28).

Hand placement and position: With the patient in a side-lying position and his/her uppermost hip and knee extended and the lowermost extremity flexed, use one hand to support the knee or distal thigh. With the other hand, grasp the ankle and lower the extremity toward the floor and keep the knee extended.

Articulation: Acetabular-femoral.

Movement: Hip internal and external rotation (Fig. 5–29).

Hand placement and motion: With the patient's hip and knee extended and resting on the treatment table, use one hand to grasp the distal thigh proximal to the knee, and use your other hand to grasp proximal to the ankle. Roll the extremity inward and outward, but do not abduct or adduct the hip. Be certain motion occurs in the hip.

For an alternative technique, flex the hip and knee to 90 degrees. Use one hand to support under the patient's knee, and use your other hand to grasp the ankle or cradle the leg. Move the leg inward and outward to cause the femur to rotate, but do not abduct or adduct the hip. Be cautious; avoid excessive stress to the medial or lateral aspects of the structures of the knee. Terminate the motion when you sense maximal tension in the muscle or joint or when the patient complains of discomfort in the groin or lateral hip (Fig. 5–30).

Articulation: Tibial-femoral.

Movement: Knee flexion with the hip extended (Fig. 5–31).

Hand placement and motion: With the patient supine and the thigh supported with the knee and leg at the edge of the support surface, use one hand to support the patient's ankle, and use your other hand or towel roll to protect the posterior thigh. Lower the leg to flex the knee over the edge of the table. You will need to stoop to attain

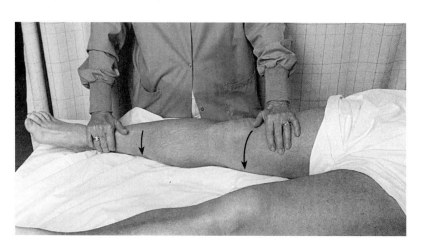

■ **FIGURE 5–29**
Internal (medial) hip rotation.

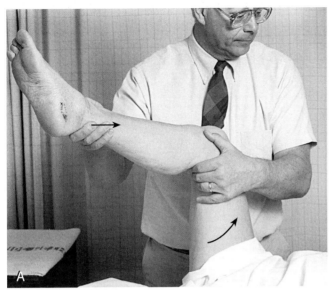
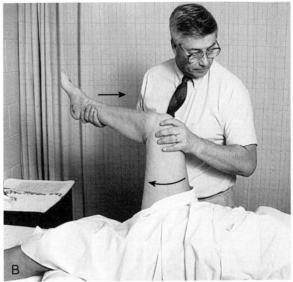

■ FIGURE 5–30
A, External (lateral) hip rotation (alternate method). *B,* Internal (medial) hip rotation (alternate method).

full range and to avoid unnecessary strain to the structures of your back.

You may also perform this motion with the patient prone. Use one hand to grasp the ankle, and use your other hand to rest on the buttock. Bend the knee by moving the heel toward the buttock. Terminate the motion when you sense maximal tension in the quadriceps muscle or when the patient complains of discomfort along the anterior thigh or hip flexion occurs. Hip flexion indicates that the rectus femoris has reached its fullest elongation and causes anterior pelvic rotation resulting in hip flexion. To elongate the rectus femoris, the hip is extended simultaneously with knee flexion.

Articulation: Crual-tibial.

Movement: Ankle dorsiflexion and plantar flexion (Fig. 5–32).

Hand placement and motion:

Dorsiflexion: Use one hand to grasp both sides of the calcaneus; place your forearm along the plantar surface of the foot, and use your other hand to stabilize the distal tibia. Pull downward on the calcaneus while pushing upward with the forearm against the metatarsal heads. It is important that the calcaneus move, and you should avoid pushing only against the metatarsal heads or the forefoot. The knee can be extended or flexed slightly.

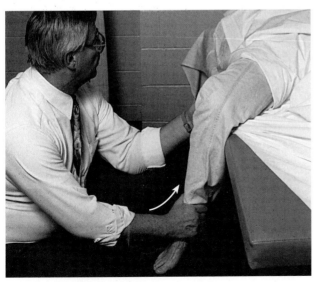

■ FIGURE 5–31
Knee flexion with the hip extended.

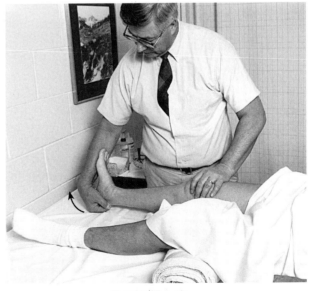

■ FIGURE 5–32
Ankle dorsiflexion.

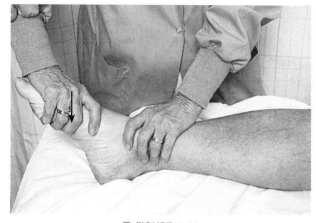

■ **FIGURE 5–33**
Plantar flexion.

When it is flexed, a more complete range of ankle motion will be possible, because the gastrocnemius, a multijoint muscle, is partially relaxed. When the knee is extended, the gastrocnemius will be elongated more and will limit the range of ankle dorsiflexion.

Plantar flexion: Use one hand to grasp the dorsum of the foot, and use your other hand to stabilize the distal tibia. Press down on the foot to produce plantar flexion (Fig. 5–33) but avoid pressure over the toes.

Articulation: Talo-crual.

Movement: Ankle inversion and eversion (Fig. 5–34).

Hand placement and motion: Use one hand to grasp the dorsum of the foot, and use your other hand to stabilize the distal tibia. Turn the foot inward and outward, avoiding hip rotation. All motion should occur at the lower ankle joint.

Articulation: Metatarsophalangeal (MTP) and IP.

Movement: Toe flexion and extension (Fig. 5–35).

Hand placement and motion: Use one hand to grasp and stabilize the foot or to stabilize each proximal bone, similar to the technique described for the fingers. Use the thumb and index finger of your other hand to grasp the phalanx immediately distal to the metatarsal being stabilized; flex and extend the phalanx. All of the MTP and IP joints may be moved simultaneously after the range of each joint has been evaluated. Avoid ankle dorsiflexion or plantar flexion by stabilizing the foot. The toes can be abducted using a technique similar to that described for the fingers.

Articulation: Metatarsal head joint play.

Movement: Elevation and depression of the metatarsal heads.

Hand placement and motion: Use the thumb and index finger of one hand to stabilize one metatarsal, and use the thumb and index finger of your other hand to grasp the adjacent metatarsal. The metatarsal that is not being stabilized is moved upward and downward; avoid simultaneous movement of two metatarsals.

Elongation of Multijoint Muscles

Hamstrings: Start with the patient supine and the knee extended; perform hip flexion while maintaining the knee in extension. Terminate the motion when you sense maximal tension in the hamstring muscles or when the patient complains of discomfort (see Fig. 5–26).

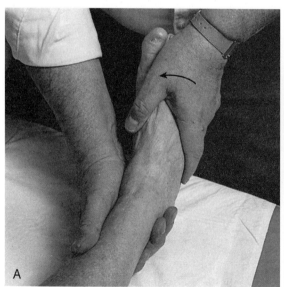
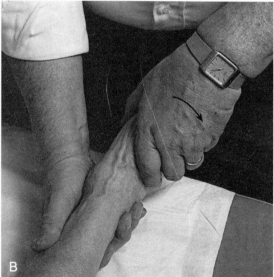

■ **FIGURE 5–34**
Inversion *(A)* and eversion *(B)* of the foot.

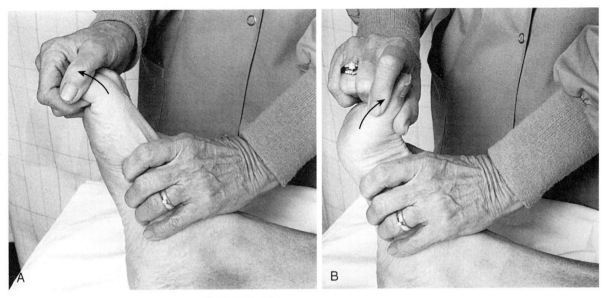

■ **FIGURE 5–35**
Flexion *(A)* and extension *(B)* of the toes.

Rectus femoris: Start with the patient prone, and perform simultaneous knee flexion and hip extension. This motion can also be performed with the patient in a side-lying position, providing he/she is secure and you can stabilize his/her pelvis to prevent an anterior pelvic tilt. Terminate the motion when you sense maximum tension in the quadriceps muscle, when lumbar lordosis increases, or when the patient complains of discomfort (Fig. 5–36).

Tensor fascia lata (iliotibial band): Start with the patient in a side-lying position and with the hip and knee of the uppermost extremity extended. Perform the motion described for hip adduction by lowering the uppermost extremity toward the floor or surface of the table. Terminate the motion when you sense maximum tension in the tensor fascia lata or when the extremity ceases to move downward (see Fig. 5–28).

Gastrocnemius: Start with the patient supine and with the hip and knee extended. Perform the motion described for ankle dorsiflexion by moving the dorsum of the foot toward the shin; be certain the calcaneus moves. This motion can also be combined with straight leg raising. Terminate the motion when maximal tension is sensed in the gastrocnemius or when the patient complains of discomfort (see Fig. 5–32).

Trunk Movements

Traditional Anatomic Planes Proper body mechanics must be used when you attempt some of these motions to prevent unnecessary strain to the structures of your back and to protect the patient from discomfort and injury.

Cervical spine: Stand at the head of the patient and facing him/her. With the patient's shoulders at the edge of the support surface, support the patient's head in your hands. Perform the motions slowly and cautiously (Fig. 5–37).

Forward bending (flexion): Support the patient's head with your hands placed firmly at the occiput. Lift the head so that the chin moves toward the chest. Encourage the patient to relax his/her posterior neck muscles (Fig. 5–38).

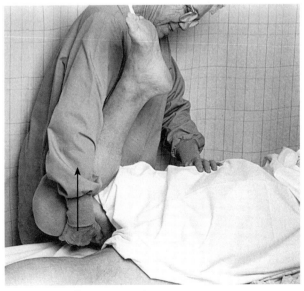

■ **FIGURE 5–36**
Elongation of the rectus femoris.

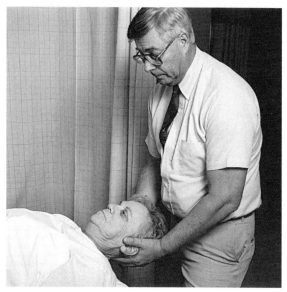

■ **FIGURE 5–37**
Hand positions for midposition of the cervical spine.

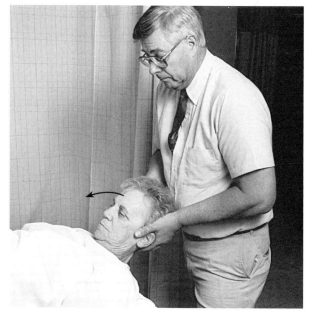

■ **FIGURE 5–38**
Forward bending (flexion) of the cervical spine.

Backward bending (extension or hyperextension): Support the patient's head with your hands at the occiput. Lower the head so that the occiput moves toward the floor. Encourage the patient to relax his/her anterior neck muscles (Fig. 5–39).

Side bending (lateral flexion): Support the patient's head at the occiput, and move the head so that one ear moves toward the acromion. Maintain the cervical spine in neutral flexion-extension, and do not allow the scapula to elevate toward the ear. Encourage the patient to relax his/her lateral neck muscles on the side of the neck opposite to the direction in which you move the head (Fig. 5–40).

Rotation: Support the patient's head at the occiput, and turn the head to the left and to the right. Maintain the cervical spine in neutral flexion-extension. Perform this motion slowly to avoid vertigo. Encourage the patient to relax the muscles of his/her neck (Fig. 5–41).

Lumbar spine: Stand on one side of the patient at the level of the pelvis with him/her close to the near edge of the support surface.

Lumbar flexion: With the patient supine, lift both of the thighs toward the chest by performing hip and knee flexion (i.e., a bilateral knee-to-chest maneuver). Elevate the distal portion of the sacrum from the support surface to produce full posterior pelvic rotation (Fig. 5–42). *Caution:* Do not attempt this maneuver when the patient's lower extremities are too heavy or too large for you to control and lift safely; be alert for indications of patient discomfort.

Lumbar extension: With the patient prone, flex both knees and lift both thighs to cause an anterior pelvic tilt and lumbar spine extension. *Caution:* Do not attempt this maneuver when the patient's lower extremities are too heavy or too large for you to control and lift safely; be alert for indications of patient discomfort. For small patients, the patient's chest can be lifted from the support surface by grasping the anterior surface of both shoulders, or the patient can perform a partial push-up to elevate the chest while maintaining the pelvis on the support surface (Fig. 5–43).

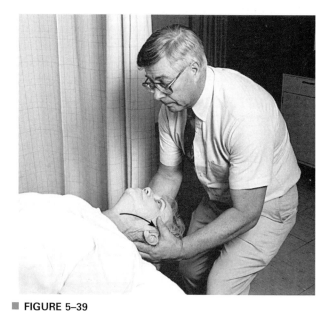

■ **FIGURE 5–39**
Backward bending (extension or hyperextension) of the cervical spine.

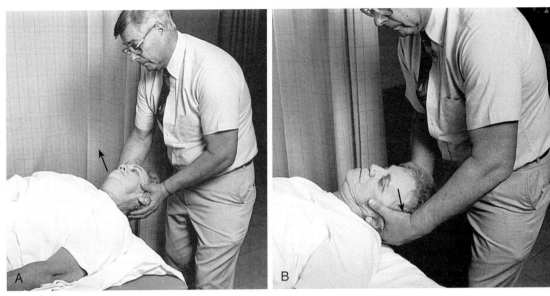

■ **FIGURE 5–40**
Side bending (lateral flexion) of the cervical spine.

Lumbar rotation: Position the patient supine with the hips and knees flexed and the feet on the support surface in a hook-lying position. Move the thighs to the left and to the right with one hand by applying a rotational force to the pelvis on the side opposite to the movement of the thighs, using your other hand to stabilize the chest. The right side of the pelvis should elevate when the thighs are moved to the left, and vice versa. Use caution if this technique is performed on a patient with a known hip abnormality or lumbar spine dysfunction, and avoid this exercise in a patient who has had a recent total hip replacement (Fig. 5–44).

Thoracic spine: Stand at the side of the patient at the level of the upper thorax. The patient's upper extremities should be folded over the chest, and he/she should be close to the near edge of the support surface.

Thoracic rotation: With the patient supine and with the hips and knees extended, grasp under the right scapula with one hand, and use your other hand to stabilize over the right anterior-superior iliac spine (ASIS). Lift and rotate the upper trunk to the left, and then perform the motion in the opposite direction with your hands positioned under the left scapula and over the left ASIS. Re-

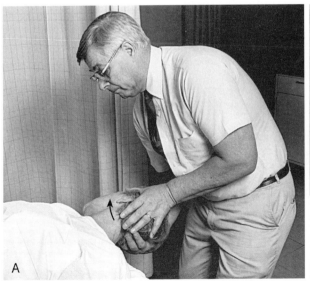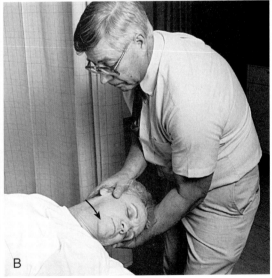

■ **FIGURE 5–41**
Rotation of the cervical spine.

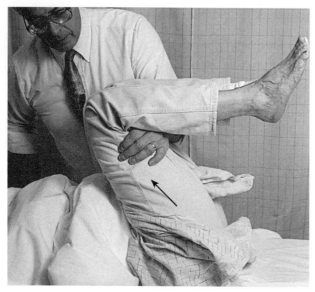

■ **FIGURE 5–42**
Lumbar flexion.

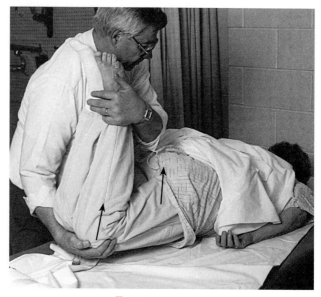

■ **FIGURE 5–43**
Lumbar extension.

quest the patient to lift and control his/her head while this motion is performed (Fig. 5–45).

DIAGONAL PATTERNS FOR PROM MOVEMENTS

Instead of using the traditional anatomic planes of motion, diagonal patterns can be used. Four of the stated and reported advantages of these patterns are

1. They incorporate rotation with all movements.
2. The midline of the body is crossed with many of the movements.
3. The movements tend to be more functional than traditional movements.

4. A combination of motions occurs within each pattern.

The patterns were developed as components of the therapeutic approach known as proprioceptive neuromuscular facilitation, or PNF, mentioned earlier. The patterns can be performed actively by the patient, passively by a caregiver, or resistively against some external force.

There are two basic diagonal patterns for the upper and lower extremity—diagonal 1 and diagonal 2—and each of them can be performed in flexion and extension, resulting in a total of four different movements. Thus, the patterns are identified as "diagonal 1 flexion," "diagonal 2 flexion," "diagonal 1 extension," and "diagonal 2 extension." Furthermore, each pat-

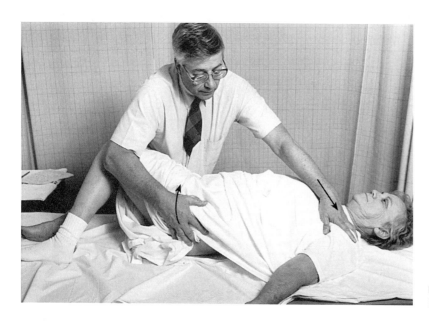

■ **FIGURE 5–44**
Lumbar rotation.

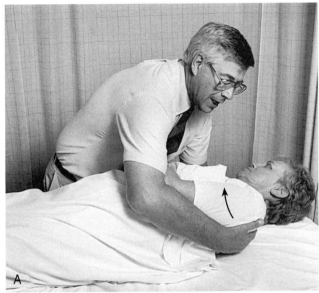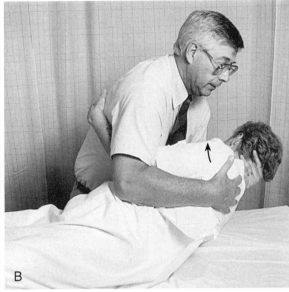

■ **FIGURE 5–45**
Thoracic rotation.

tern can be performed by the upper and lower extremity and so are termed "diagonal 1 flexion upper extremity" or "diagonal 1 flexion lower extremity," and so on. Common abbreviations of the patterns are D1 Fl UE, D2 Fl UE, D1 Ex UE, D2 Ex UE, D1 Fl LE, D2 Fl LE, D1 Ex LE, and D2 Ex LE.

The patterns are named according to the position of the proximal joint of the pattern—that is, the shoulder or the hip—at the *conclusion* of the pattern. Thus, the pattern is initiated with the proximal joint positioned opposite to its position at the conclusion of the pattern. Each pattern contains a flexion or extension component, an abduction or adduction component, and an internal or external rotation component for the proximal joint. All three motions must be per-

formed, especially the rotation component. Other extremity joints or components will also have a final position, but the patterns are described according to the final position of the proximal joint. Refer to Table 5–1 for a description of each pattern.

The caregiver should be positioned so he/she can move in a diagonal direction as the patterns are performed. It will be necessary to pivot on your feet to avoid improper and stress-producing body mechanics. Proper positioning and movement must be used consistently by the caregiver when diagonal patterns are performed passively to reduce stress and strain and to be able to complete each pattern.

Remember: These are the positions of the components at the *completion* of the pattern. To initiate a

Table 5–1
DIAGONAL PATTERNS: COMPONENT POSITIONS

	Diagonal 1		Diagonal 2	
	Flexion	*Extension*	*Flexion*	*Extension*
Upper extremity				
Scapula	Elevation, abduction, upward rotation	Depression, adduction, downward rotation	Elevation, adduction, upward rotation	Depression, abduction, downward rotation
Shoulder	Flexion, adduction, external rotation	Extension, abduction, internal rotation	Flexion, abduction, external rotation	Extension, adduction, internal rotation
Elbow	Flexion, extension	Flexion, extension	Flexion, extension	Flexion, extension
Forearm	Supination	Pronation	Supination	Pronation
Wrist	Flexion, radial deviation	Extension, ulnar deviation	Extension, radial deviation	Flexion, ulnar deviation
Fingers	Flexion, adduction	Extension, abduction	Extension, abduction	Flexion, adduction
Lower extremity				
Hip	Flexion, adduction, external rotation	Extension, abduction, internal rotation	Flexion, abduction, internal rotation	Extension, adduction, external rotation
Knee	Flexion, extension	Flexion, extension	Flexion, extension	Flexion, extension
Ankle	Dorsiflexion, inversion	Plantar flexion, eversion	Dorsiflexion, eversion	Plantar flexion, inversion
Toes	Extension	Flexion	Extension	Flexion

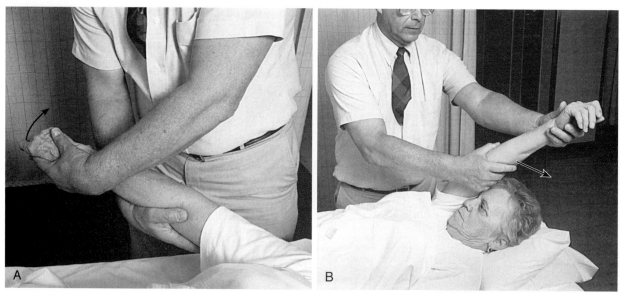

■ **FIGURE 5–46**
Diagonal 1, flexion with the elbow extended.

pattern, the proximal joint of the extremity is placed in the position that is the reciprocal of the completed pattern. For example, to initiate D1 Fl UE, the shoulder is positioned in D1 Ex UE. How would you position the extremity to initiate D1 Fl LE or D2 Fl UE?

Upper Extremity

Diagonal 1, Flexion With the Elbow Extended

Movement: Shoulder flexion, adduction, and external rotation. Start with the shoulder of the upper extremity slightly abducted, internally rotated, and extended. The elbow is extended, and the forearm is pronated with the wrist and fingers extended (Fig. 5–46).

Hand placement and motion: For the right upper extremity, use your left hand to support the patient's hand and wrist, and use your right hand to support the distal aspect of the upper arm. Lift the extremity diagonally across the chest and over the face; simultaneously, externally rotate the shoulder, supinate the forearm, and flex the wrist and fingers. Perform diagonal flexion within the width of the shoulder. Reverse your hand placement and grip for the left extremity.

Diagonal 1, Extension With the Elbow Extended

Movement: Shoulder extension, abduction, and internal rotation. Start with the shoulder of the upper extremity adducted, flexed, and externally rotated. The elbow is extended, the forearm is supinated, and the wrist and fingers are flexed (see Fig. 5–46).

Hand placement and motion: For the right upper extremity, use your left hand to grasp the patient's hand and wrist, and use your right hand to grasp the posterior distal upper arm. Move the extremity diagonally away from the face; simultaneously, internally rotate the shoulder, pronate the forearm, and extend the wrist and fingers. Perform the diagonal extension within the width of the shoulder. Reverse your hand placement and grip for the left extremity.

Diagonal 2, Flexion With the Elbow Extended

Movement: Shoulder flexion, abduction, and external rotation. Start with the shoulder of the upper extremity positioned diagonally across the patient's body and internally rotated. The elbow is extended, the forearm pronated, and the wrist and fingers flexed (Fig. 5–47).

Hand placement and motion: For the right upper extremity, use your left hand to grasp the dorsum of the patient's hand, and use your right hand to grasp the dorsal surface of the forearm or the lateral surface of the upper arm. Lift the extremity diagonally up from the body into flexion, abduction, and external rotation. Perform diagonal flexion within the width of the shoulder. Reverse your hand placement and grip for the left extremity.

Diagonal 2, Extension With the Elbow Extended

Movement: Shoulder extension, adduction, and internal rotation. Start with the shoulder of the upper extremity flexed, abducted, and externally rotated. The elbow is extended, the forearm supi-

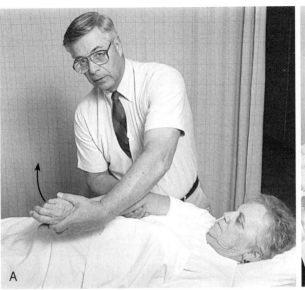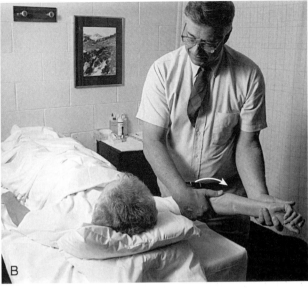

■ **FIGURE 5–47**
Diagonal 2, flexion with the elbow extended.

nated, and the wrist and fingers extended (see Fig. 5–47).

Hand placement and motion: Retain your grasp as described for the D2 Fl pattern, and move the upper extremity diagonally toward the body into extension, adduction, and internal rotation. Perform diagonal extension within the width of the shoulder.

These four patterns can be performed with the elbow flexed. Your hand placement will be similar to those described previously, and the motions will be the same as those described for the upper extremity patterns with the elbow extended.

Lower Extremity

Diagonal 1, Flexion With the Knee Flexed

Movement: Hip flexion, adduction, and external rotation. Start with the hip of the lower extremity slightly abducted, extended, and internally rotated and the knee extended (Fig. 5–48).

Hand placement and motion: Use one hand to grasp and support the patient's heel, and use your other hand to grasp and support the posterior distal thigh by reaching over the thigh. Lift the extremity diagonally toward the abdomen and the opposite shoulder; simultaneously, externally

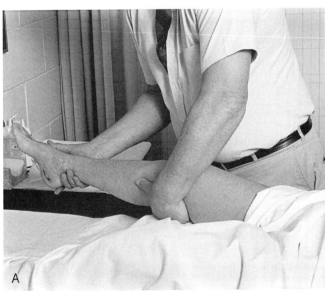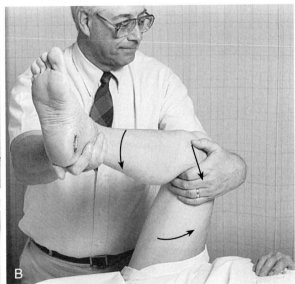

■ **FIGURE 5–48**
Diagonal 1, flexion with the knee flexed.

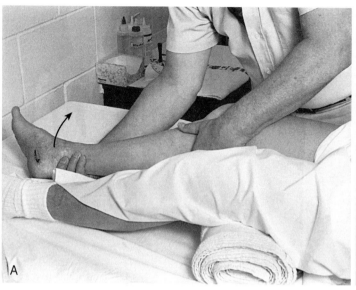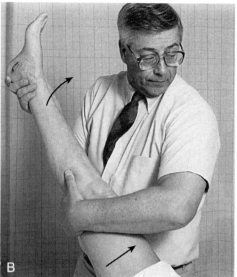

■ **FIGURE 5–49**
Diagonal 2, flexion with the knee extended.

rotate the hip and dorsiflex the foot. Perform diagonal flexion within the width of the hip. When this motion is performed with the knee extended, the full range of hip flexion will not be available.

Diagonal 1, Extension With the Knee Extended

Movement: Hip extension, abduction, and internal rotation. Start with the hip of the lower extremity flexed, adducted, and externally rotated and the knee extended (see Fig. 5–48).

Hand placement and motion: Maintain your hand placement as used for the D1 Fl pattern, and return the extremity diagonally so that the hip is extended, abducted, and internally rotated. Perform diagonal extension within the width of the hip.

Diagonal 2, Flexion With the Knee Extended

Movement: Hip flexion, abduction, and internal rotation. Start with the hip of the lower extremity slightly adducted, externally rotated, and extended and the knee extended (Fig. 5–49).

Hand placement and motion: Use one hand to grasp the lateral dorsal surface of the foot, and use your other hand to grasp the distal posterior thigh. Lift the extremity diagonally up and away from the body; simultaneously, internally rotate the hip. Perform diagonal flexion within the width of the hip.

Diagonal 2, Extension With the Knee Extended

Movement: Hip extension, adduction, and external rotation. Start with the hip of the lower extremity flexed, abducted, and internally rotated and the knee extended.

Hand placement and motion: Maintain the hand placement used for the D2 Fl pattern, and return the extremity diagonally toward the opposite lower extremity; simultaneously, externally rotate the hip. Perform diagonal extension within the width of the hip (see Fig. 5–49).

These four patterns can be performed with the knee flexed. Your hand placement will be similar to those described previously, and the motions will be the same as those described for the lower extremity patterns with the knee extended.

ACTIVE EXERCISE

Some of the advantages, uses, and goals associated with active exercise have been described previously in this chapter. For the patients who are capable, it is important for the exercise program to progress from passive to active, because normal function requires muscle strength and endurance. Numerous resources that provide detailed explanations of the effects of active exercise are available, and therefore, such explanations will not be given here.

Active exercise has been described previously as any exercise in which the movement of the body or body segment is accomplished by or in conjunction with an active, voluntary muscle contraction, with or without externally applied assistance or resistance. Many combinations or types of muscle contractions and assistance or resistance can be used in an active exercise program. The ingenuity and experience of the caregiver, the ability of the patient, and the goal of the exercise or program all affect the selection and application of techniques. This text will not describe or present information related to resistive exercise; sources of such information can be found in the Bibliography.

TYPES OF MUSCLE CONTRACTION AND EXERCISE

There are two basic types or forms of muscle contraction: *isotonic* and *isometric*. Isotonic contractions can be subdivided into *eccentric* and *concentric contractions*. There is visible joint motion when the muscle contracts isotonically, and the load, or *resistance*, against which the muscle contracts can remain constant or can vary. When the muscle contracts concentrically, its fibers produce a relative shortening of the muscle. When the muscle contracts eccentrically, its fibers allow a relative lengthening of the muscle. An example of a concentric contraction is contraction of the biceps to produce elbow flexion when the person is sitting or standing. An example of an eccentric contraction is contraction of the biceps to control elbow extension when returning the forearm from 90 degrees of flexion to a completely extended position when the person is sitting or standing.

The position of the patient, especially his/her relationship to gravity, will affect the type of contraction produced and the muscles that produce the contraction. For example, when a person is supine and performs active shoulder flexion through the shoulder's full normal range, the shoulder flexors function concentrically from 0 to 90 degrees of flexion, while the shoulder extensors function eccentrically from 90 to 180 degrees of flexion. When the extremity is returned to the patient's side, the shoulder extensors function concentrically from 180 to 90 degrees of extension, and the shoulder flexors function eccentrically from 90 to 0 degrees of extension. The concepts of concentric and eccentric muscle contractions can be applied to different muscles or muscle groups as you vary the position of the patient.

Isotonic exercise can be used to maintain or increase strength, power, and endurance; to promote local circulation; to enhance cardiovascular efficiency; to create *hypertrophy* of muscle fibers; to maintain the physiologic elasticity of a muscle; to maintain joint motion; and to maintain or enhance coordination. An eccentric muscle contraction develops more tension in the muscle than a concentric contraction and thus may develop strength more rapidly. External resistance or assistance can be applied manually or mechanically to either the eccentric or the concentric contraction (Box 5–3).

BOX 5–3

Benefits of Active Exercise

1. Maintain physiologic elasticity, strength, and contractile endurance of muscle.
2. Increase local circulation.
3. Increase awareness of joint motion and sensory awareness.
4. Maintain and improve cardiopulmonary functions, especially with aerobic exercise.
5. Can be used to prevent thrombus formation in lower extremities using ankle flexion–extension movements (i.e., "ankle pumping").
6. Maintain and promote structural integrity of tendon–bone interface.
7. Improve muscle strength with the use of external resistance.

In an isometric muscle contraction, there is little or no observable joint motion and no significant change in the length of the muscle. An isometric contraction can be performed with or without external resistance. When no resistance is applied, the contraction is frequently termed "muscle setting."

Isometric exercise can be used to maintain muscle tone or, when resistance is applied, to increase strength; to focus the muscle contraction at one or several specific portions of the total joint range; and to avoid the pain associated with joint motion. It may also economize the time spent to perform the exercise. This type of exercise does little to contribute to cardiovascular fitness or joint or muscle flexibility or to maintain coordinated movement. Resistance can be applied manually or mechanically; when resistance is applied, increased tension occurs in the muscle fibers, resulting in increased strength.

A third form of exercise, termed *isokinetic exercise*, is possible when specific equipment is used. Isokinetic exercise equipment controls the speed of the patient's contractions and produces a variable resistance to the muscle as it contracts through its arc or ROM. Some equipment provides resistance to only the concentric contractions, while other equipment resists both concentric and eccentric contractions. Published studies indicate that isokinetic exercise strengthens muscle more efficiently than other forms of resistive isotonic exercise.

Refer to the information presented previously in this chapter to review the possible benefits and uses of passive and active exercise. Several criteria or factors must be considered when performing passive or active exercise to obtain the greatest benefit from the exercise and to protect the patient from injury.

Maintain the exercise activities within the physiologic capabilities of the patient, keeping in mind the goals of therapy, while encouraging the patient to perform at maximally tolerated levels. The Valsalva maneuver should be avoided during exercise to prevent the possibility of serious complications that could lead to a cerebrovascular accident or even death. Therefore, instruct the patient to breathe normally during the exercise program, particularly when performing resisted isometric exercise. Use caution to avoid causing unnecessary or excessive trauma to a skeletal or soft tissue structure when resistance is applied. At the same time, you should protect unstable or vulnerable structures (e.g., the site of a recent fracture, a hypermobile joint, a recent muscle strain, or a recent surgical site) during exercise. Finally, you should carefully grade the severity and monitor the effects of exercise for the patient who has experienced a recent myocardial infarction or has a history of cardiac dysfunction.

During exercise with a patient who has an unprotected healing fracture, avoid applying resistance to the distal segment of the fracture. Isometric and eccentric exercise may be contraindicated for those persons who are in the immediate or subacute phase of recovery from a myocardial infarction, especially if resistance is applied. Exercise that produces pain during or after exercise for a period of 24 to 36 hours may be contraindicated, and this reaction should be considered a precaution for its future application. Exercise that produces abnormal results, such as an undesired or adverse change in the patient's symptoms or intensification of his/her condition, should be terminated and the program re-evaluated before it is continued. Finally, certain exercise movements may be contraindicated after selected surgical procedures; an example is excessive hip movement, especially hip adduction, flexion, and rotation, during the first several days after total hip replacement surgery (Box 5–4).

TYPES OF ACTIVE EXERCISE

There are three common forms of active exercise: active assistive, active or active free, and active resistive. Before performing any form of exercise, you should introduce yourself, explain the activity, inform the patient of the expected outcome or purpose of the activity, obtain his/her consent to participate in the program, and provide specific instructions. Once the exercise has been initiated the caregiver should observe the patient and correct improper performance (Procedure 5–3).

Isotonic Exercise Application

Active Assistive Exercise   As the term implies, active assistive exercise is exercise that requires the pa-

---

BOX 5–4

Precautions Related to Active Exercise

Revision or cessation of an exercise program should be considered when

1. Pain occurs during or persists after exercise.
2. Undesired cardiopulmonary stress occurs.
3. The breathing pattern of the patient becomes abnormal.
4. The patient exhibits an undesired, adverse response to exercise.
5. Stress occurs to an unstable area or segment.
6. Undesired movements or movement patterns occur.
7. Undesired tone of muscle develops or increases.
8. The patient's condition or functional ability regresses.

---

tient to actively contract the muscles involved in the exercise to the maximum extent he/she is capable while receiving assistance from another source to perform the exercise. The assistance may be provided manually or by a mechanical or gravitational force. It is important that the patient contract his/her muscles maximally during the exercise and that the caregiver alter the assistance according to the patient's performance. The greatest amount of assistance should be provided when the patient has the greatest difficulty performing the activity. Conversely, assistance should be reduced when the patient has the least difficulty performing the activity. An eventual goal for most patients is to progress from active assistive to active exercise.

Assistance or resistance to motion can be affected by the patient's position and his/her relationship to the effects of gravity. The effect of gravity as a resistance force can be eliminated by the use of external assistance or patient positioning. Although the patient may not be able to perform full hip flexion when supine, he/she may be able to perform the activity when graded assistance is provided manually or mechanically or when he/she is in a side-lying position and the lower extremity is supported on an elevated smooth surface. The resistance of gravity to the movement of hip flexion or extension or knee flexion or extension will be eliminated when the side-lying position is used. However, friction between the lower extremity and the surface will be created when the lower extremity is moved actively over the surface.

Before initiating the exercise, position the patient to provide stability and comfort. When you initiate the

PROCEDURE 5 – 3
Application of Active Exercise

1. Position the patient for support, stability, and type of active exercise to be performed; provide access to the area, or segment to be exercised, and drape as necessary.
2. Explain the purpose and goals of the exercise; obtain consent for treatment, and select equipment if necessary.
3. Position the patient to promote the use of proper body mechanics by patient and caregiver.
4. Grasp the part to be treated to provide support, stability, control, or resistance as necessary, or verbally instruct and guide the patient to perform the exercise. Refer to the photographs and instructions in this chapter for specific information.
5. The patient performs the exercises smoothly and slowly through the complete, unrestricted range of motion with a pause at the start and end positions of the exercise.
6. The patient performs the predetermined number of repetitions and frequency of exercises based on his/her abilities, needs, and goals.
7. At the conclusion of the treatment, the patient assumes or is assisted to assume proper alignment, support, and safety; drape or replace clothing for modesty and body temperature control.
8. Evaluate the patient's response to treatment; document important findings.

exercise, be certain to support, protect, stabilize, and control the segment being exercised, using the same hand placements described for passive exercise. Instruct the patient to actively contract the appropriate muscles through the available ROM, and establish an appropriate exercise velocity. Your instructions may include touching, tapping, or stroking the muscle to be contracted; having the person initially perform the contraction with the opposite uninvolved muscle; demonstrating the contraction yourself; and using terms such as "bend," "lift," or "straighten." Provide assistance only to the extent necessary to allow the patient to smoothly complete the movement through the available ROM and to avoid substitute motions. The external assistance you provide can be decreased gradually as the patient demonstrates an increase in strength. The patient should progress to active free exercise when he/she is able to smoothly complete the desired movement through the available ROM without substitute motions and without assistance. The exercises may be performed in traditional anatomic planes or in the diagonal patterns described previously.

Active Free Exercise   Active free exercise is performed by the patient without any assistance or resis-

tance other than gravity and the weight of the extremity or segment involved in the exercise. The patient should have sufficient strength to perform the activity against the resistance provided by gravity. The position of the patient will affect the resistance provided by gravity. You can demonstrate to yourself how the effect of gravity is altered by attempting the same exercise while supine, sitting, standing, or prone. The more exercises you attempt and the more positions you use, the better you will be able to determine how to position a patient to obtain maximal effort while avoiding substitutive or undesired motions.

Before initiating the exercise, position the patient depending on how you desire gravity to affect the exercise and the movement to be performed. For example, do you desire gravity to resist, assist, or be neutral during the exercise? Instruct the patient to perform the desired movement through the available ROM smoothly and without any substitute motions. If necessary, encourage or guide the patient as the activity is performed.

Establish an appropriate exercise speed to produce a smooth, controlled movement, and require that speed to be maintained. He/she should be encouraged to briefly pause ("hold") at the end and start positions during each repetition. A brief rest between each bout or series of repetitions will usually be necessary to reduce the effects of fatigue.

The exercises may be performed in traditional anatomic planes or in the diagonal patterns described previously.

Active Resistive Exercise *Active resistive exercise* requires the addition of a resistive force other than gravity; this can be done manually or mechanically. The resistance should require the patient to use a maximal contraction to perform the activity, but he/she should be able to complete the movement slowly, smoothly, and through the entire available ROM. Gravity will have a resistive effect, as described previously, so the position of the patient should be considered. Furthermore, the length of the lever arm and the amount of torque the patient can develop will both affect the location of the resistance. For example, greater resistance to the shoulder flexors will be required or need to be applied if the resistance is positioned above the elbow, while less resistance will be required or need to be applied if the resistance is located in the patient's hand. The shorter the lever arm, the greater the torque the patient can develop and the more resistance his/her muscles will be able to overcome. A goal for many patients is to progress from active free exercise to active resistive exercise, especially when a gain in muscle strength is desired.

When the patient performs an isotonic contraction, the maximal resistance he/she will be able to move is the resistance that can be overcome through the part of the range where the muscle has the poorest contractile capacity. Most muscles have the poorest contractile capacity at the beginning and the end of the ROM, and most muscles tend to develop their greatest tension during the midportion of the range. (These last two statements are general statements and may not be accurate for all body positions or exercise activities. However, they do explain the general concept of the *length-tension curve* of a muscle.) Although the load (resistance) remains constant, the effect of the resistance on the muscle will vary at different points within the range as the muscle lengthens and shortens as a result of a change in the lever arm relationships of the body segments involved.

Before initiating the exercise, position the patient depending on how you desire gravity to affect the exercise, the movement required, and the amount or type of support or stabilization the patient requires. Instruct the patient to perform the desired movement through the available range of motion smoothly and without any substitute motion as resistance is applied perpendicular to the extremity or segment. You will have to determine the most appropriate site or location for the resistance to be applied based on the patient's condition, ability, and exercise goals, with consideration of the concept of lever arm length.

The body segment to which the proximal component or origin of the muscle being exercised is attached should be stabilized. The patient's body weight or position may accomplish this, or an external strap or firm surface may be required. It may be necessary to vary or adjust the resistance during the exercise to allow the patient to complete the available range of motion smoothly and without substitute motions.

If manual resistance is used, the site of the application of the resistance and the amount of resistance applied can be revised during the exercise to provide maximal resistance while allowing the patient to complete the movement through the available ROM smoothly and without substitute motions. That is, the resistance lever arm can be lengthened or shortened, a new location can be used to avoid discomfort or to avoid an unstable area, or the applied resistance can be increased or decreased depending on the point in the range where the muscle is contracting.

The exercises may be performed in traditional anatomic planes or in the diagonal patterns described previously.

Isometric Exercise Application

Isometric Exercise Isometric exercise is used when a muscle is immobilized, when a joint or soft tissue is painful when moved through its range, or when inflammation is present in the area. No joint motion should occur when an isometric muscle contraction is performed. Gravity has less effect on the muscle contraction when this type of exercise is used, and the patient's position is not as important as it usually is for isometric exercise. The segment may be positioned at any point within the ROM depending on the patient's condition and the goal of the exercise. Manual or mechanical resistance can be applied, and the length of the lever arm can be varied. The benefits of resisted isometric exercise and the reasons to select it have already been presented.

Muscle setting is a form of isometric exercise that can be beneficial to maintain some muscle tone, to maintain contractile awareness, and to allow exercise to an immobilized, innervated, muscle. Before initiating the exercise, position the patient to provide a stable, comfortable position and to have access to the muscle that will contract. Instruct the patient to contract or tighten ("set") a specific muscle or muscle group without producing joint motion or changing the length of the muscle.

By describing the motion, you may assist the patient to use mental imaging to initiate the contraction. Tactile or verbal cueing may be used to initiate the contraction by touching the muscle or telling the patient the movement the muscle will perform. For example, you can instruct a supine or prone patient to squeeze or pinch the buttocks together to "set" (contract) the gluteus maximus. If the patient holds or squeezes his/her arms close to the side of the chest, as if trying to hold a newspaper or small purse, the pectoral muscles will contract. When a patient has a full-length cast on one lower extremity, you can instruct him/her to try to pull the kneecap of that extremity toward the hip by tightening the muscle on top of the thigh to isometrically contract the quadriceps. To facilitate this motion, have the patient perform it with the opposite, nonimmobilized quadriceps while you tactilely stroke upward on the quadriceps or gently push up on the patella. These are a few techniques that can be used to initiate an isometric contraction; you may need to consider other methods to teach a patient to contract the muscles isometrically.

Instruct the patient to maintain and "hold" the contraction for approximately 5 to 8 seconds and then relax. He/she should be instructed to breathe normally to avoid the Valsalva phenomenon.

Isometric Resistive Exercise Isometric resistive exercise can be used to increase muscle strength through the addition of manual or mechanical resistance. The segment can be positioned at any point in the range depending on the patient's condition and the goal of the exercise. The amount of resistance and the length of the lever arm can be varied. It is particularly important that the patient be instructed to breathe normally and to avoid the Valsalva phenomenon when he/she performs isometric resistive exercise.

Before initiating the exercise, position the patient to provide stability, comfort, and access to the muscle that will contract. Determine where you desire to apply the resistance on the segment, and position the segment within the available joint ROM. Be certain resistance is applied perpendicular to the segment, and instruct the patient to maintain and "hold" the position selected. Joint motion should not occur or be permitted. Instruct the patient to maintain the contraction for approximately 5 to 8 seconds while breathing normally and then to relax for 5 to 8 seconds before repeating the contraction. Additional information about the concept, use, and application of active exercise is contained in many of the references listed in the Bibliography.

SUMMARY

Exercise is used in the management of a variety of conditions or problems. There are several forms or types of exercise, including passive, active assistive, active, and active resistive. The caregiver must be knowledgeable and competent to be able to select the exercise type that will most benefit the patient.

There are two primary types of muscle contraction: isotonic (which can be subdivided into concentric and eccentric) and isometric. Exercise can affect the person's strength, endurance, joint flexibility, coordination, and cardiopulmonary system.

Exercises can be performed with the patient positioned supine, sitting, prone, in a side-lying position, or standing. The position selected is based on the purpose of the exercise, the condition of the patient, the patient's ability to assume and maintain a specific position, and the equipment to be used.

The patient's response to exercise during and after each treatment session should be monitored and should include the observation of changes in the appearance of the segment exercised, evaluation of vital signs, and assessment of any changes in ROM or movement (coordination, strength, quality, or control), complaint, or indication of pain. Provide specific support and stabilization to any unstable or pain-producing segments, such as a recent fracture site, areas of hypermobility or paralysis, or a wound or incision site. The extremity or segment should be moved through the entire, unrestricted, pain-free, normal range of the associated joint or joints. Forceful movement into a restricted component of the range constitutes stretching and should be avoided when performing PROM exercise. A description of stretching techniques is beyond the scope of this textbook and will not be presented.

All exercises should be performed smoothly and slowly throughout the unrestricted range. A brief rest at the ending and starting position of the exercise should also be incorporated into the exercise.

The number of repetitions required to accomplish the goals of treatment will vary, as will the frequency of the exercises. Some patients may benefit from or require the exercises to be performed two or more times per day for 10 or more repetitions. Other patients may benefit from or require one exercise session per day and fewer than 10 repetitions per joint or area. The patient's response to treatment, any change in the patient's condition, and the judgment of the caregiver are the factors used to determine the parameters of the exercise program.

The exercises may be applied using traditional anatomic planes or using diagonal or a combination of planes, by using functional movement patterns, or by combining two or more of these techniques. At the termination of the treatment, the patient should be repositioned with proper support, security, and alignment. Any equipment or assistive devices that were used should be stored and the treatment area prepared for other patients. Information about the patient's response to treatment or his/her condition should be documented.

■ SELF-STUDY/DISCUSSION ACTIVITIES

1. Describe some factors you would consider when determining the type of active exercise to select for a patient.
2. How would you determine whether a patient had performed active exercise maximally?
3. Describe how you would determine whether a patient performs active exercise properly.
4. Describe the actions you would use to enhance proper active exercise motions.
5. Explain what happens when you lengthen or shorten the lever arm used to apply manual resistance.

6. List at least one body position you would use to place each of the following muscles in a maximal gravity-resisted position; in a maximal gravity-assisted position; and in a gravity-neutral position: middle deltoid, biceps, triceps, pectoralis major, upper trapezius, quadriceps, hamstrings, gluteus maximus, erector spinae, and abdominals.
7. Explain how you would decide that a patient is ready to progress from passive to active exercise.
8. What are some reasons or patient conditions for which you would perform passive exercise?
9. Demonstrate the positions and motions you would use to perform concentric and eccentric contractions of the quadriceps, hamstrings, anterior deltoid, triceps, and abdominal muscles.

Chapter 6

Transfer
Activities

After studying this chapter, the reader will be able to:

1 Instruct and assist another person to perform various transfer techniques.

2 Instruct one or more assistants to perform a safe lift transfer.

3 Adjust the position of a person who is recumbent with or without the assistance of another person in preparation for the transfer.

4 Teach a person independent bed mobility and functional activities preparatory to performing a transfer.

5 Properly guard and protect a person during the performance of a transfer.

Exacerbation: An increase in the severity of disease or any of its symptoms.

Graft: Any tissue or organ for transplantation or implantation.

Hemiplegia: Paralysis of one side of the body.

Ipsilateral: Homolateral; on the same side.

Mobility: The ability to move in one's environment with ease and without restriction.

Osteoporosis: A decreased mass per unit volume of normally mineralized bone when compared with that in age- and sex-matched controls; loss of bone mass.

Paralysis: Loss of power of voluntary movement in a muscle through injury or disease of its nerve supply.

Paresis: Partial or incomplete paralysis.

Plinth: A padded table for a patient to sit on or lie on while performing exercises, receiving a massage, or undergoing other physical therapy treatment.

Safety belt: An adjustable belt or strap that is secured around a person's waist; used to protect and control the person; also referred to as a guard, transfer, ambulation, or gait belt.

Syncope: A temporary suspension of consciousness as a result of cerebral anemia; fainting.

Transfer: The moving of a patient from one surface to another surface.

Vertigo: A sensation of rotation or movement of one's self or of one's surroundings.

INTRODUCTION

A *transfer* is the safe movement of a person from one surface or location to another or from one position to another. Depending on the mental and physical ability of the patient, a transfer may be performed independently by the patient, with the direct assistance of one or more persons (i.e., dependently) or with the indirect assistance of one person (i.e., standby assistance or verbal cueing). Adjusting the patient's position or bed mobility activities are included in the broad definition of a transfer. The ability to move upward, downward, or from side to side; to roll, to turn over, and to move to sitting from a recumbent position are important activities for a patient to accomplish for independence. Often these movements are preliminary to the actual transfer from a bed or mat table to a wheelchair. They are also necessary to permit the patient to alter his/her position for comfort and avoid the

development of contractures or skin breakdown. The caregiver should not overlook teaching the patient to perform these movements and should emphasize their importance to the patient and his/her family. Preparatory activities may include muscle strengthening, development of joint and muscle flexibility (range of motion), and development of endurance.

Equipment such as a sliding board, a hydraulic or pneumatic lift, an electric hoist or a lift, a rope, a bed rail, and an over-the-bed frame or bar ("trapeze") may be required or used to assist with a transfer. These devices can perpetuate dependence in a patient, and therefore they are recommended only for those patients who are unable to perform a safe transfer without using them or when the caregiver is unable to safely assist the patient without one or more of them.

ORGANIZATION OF PATIENT TRANSFERS

A transfer requires planning and organization before the patient attempts to perform it. The patient should be informed about the transfer and instructed on how to assist with or perform it before attempting it. A demonstration of the activity by another patient or by the caregiver may be necessary. Careful attention to the safety factors associated with each transfer will enhance the patient's confidence and lead to a more effective transfer.

Be certain to obtain and use sufficient assistance or equipment to ensure a safe procedure. When the patient is able to assist more fully with the procedure, the external assistance can be reduced, leading to increased patient independence. Although patient independence is a frequent goal associated with transfer activities, your primary responsibility is to guard and protect the patient to avoid injury to him/her or to yourself.

PREPARATION

You will have to prepare the patient, the environment, yourself, and possibly other persons before performing the transfer activity. Initially you should review the medical record and interview the patient for information to assist you in planning the activity. For example, what has the patient accomplished previously? How does he/she transfer now? What are his/her limitations and abilities? How much assistance does he/she require to move in bed or to transfer? Are there specific precautions that must be used to protect the patient or to avoid further injury or trauma? Your assessment or evaluation of the patient will help you to determine his/her abilities and limitations. Physical abilities that should be considered are muscle strength, joint and soft tissue flexibility, sitting and standing balance, endurance, tolerance to sitting and standing positions, and motor control. A decision will have to be made, based on your evaluation, the written information available, and the goals of treatment, regarding the appropriate transfer or activity to be used. As you mentally plan and organize the activity, you can consider whether mechanical or human assistance will be needed. If equipment will be needed, you should obtain, position, and stabilize it before beginning the transfer.

Introduce yourself to the patient and prepare him/her for the transfer by explaining the activity and, in many instances, by demonstrating it. You should inform and instruct the patient about his/her role and how to assist with or perform the activity. The patient should be properly dressed for the transfer. Excessively loose clothing; excessively long trousers, slacks, or pajamas; and slippery, loose, or ill-fitting footwear should be avoided. A *safety belt* should be applied if the patient will move from one surface to another, especially during the early treatment sessions. Even though you may expect that the patient has consented to the proposed treatment, you should obtain his/her consent after you have explained the activity and the possible risks, if any, associated with it.

PRINCIPLES

After these planning activities have been completed, you will have to apply certain concepts or principles to better ensure a safe and successful outcome. You must analyze the transfer into its component parts, such as the position of the equipment, operation of the equipment by the patient, the position of the patient's body, and the movements the patient will have to perform. You may find that it is necessary for the patient to practice and accomplish the component activities before he/she attempts the total transfer. After you have instructed the patient, ask him/her to describe your instructions in his/her own words. Avoid asking the patient, "Do you understand the instructions?" Most patients will answer "yes" when asked such a question, even when they may not have comprehended everything you have explained. Instead, require him/her to explain the procedure to you to verify what he/she really understands.

Once the transfer is initiated, you should remain close to the patient to guard him/her. Use the safety belt and the patient's knees, pelvis, or upper thorax for stabilization or control. Do not use the patient's upper extremity for guidance or stability because you will not be able to control the trunk and you may injure the extremity. Your instructions to the patient and to any persons who assist you should be brief, concise, and action oriented. You might instruct the patient like this: "First, lock your chair; now lift the footrests; move your hips forward; place your right foot closer to the chair and your left foot farther from the chair," and so on. Try to avoid "Now the first thing I want you to do is. . . ." Many patients will still be processing these nondirective words when you are beginning to state the actual instructions. Any persons who are to assist you must be informed of and understand their roles and must be instructed how to assist with the transfer. Instructions and guidance to the patient and to those who are assisting may be necessary as the transfer is performed. It may be possible to incorporate some patient teaching while the activity is performed. Encourage the patient to participate mentally and physically in the transfer to his/her maximal ability and within the limits of safety. Be certain to use proper body mechanics as you assist the patient to protect and control his/her movements and to avoid self-injury.

PRECAUTIONS

There are several precautions you should consider when assisting a patient with a transfer, especially a standing transfer, regardless of the patient's condition. The patient should wear proper shoes to perform a standing transfer. Slippers, sandals, shoes with smooth leather soles, or socks without shoes are likely to decrease safety. These items usually do not provide adequate support and security and should not be used by the patient. A safety belt provides a secure object to grasp and decreases the need to use the patient's clothing. You should anticipate and be alert for unusual patient actions or equipment that may create unexpected risks. Any bandages or equipment attached to or used by the patient should be protected, including casts, drainage tubes, intravenous tubes, and dressing sites (Box 6–1).

You must determine the best position to use to protect the patient. To prevent injury to the patient due to a fall, it is usually best to be in front of and slightly to one side of the patient when he/she stands. Your body mechanics may be compromised when you are in this protective position, but it will enable you to provide maximal protection for the patient. At the conclusion of the transfer, the patient may be protected by applying a lap belt, engaging the bed rails, being positioned in the center of the bed, or using other similar methods. Do not leave him/her unattended unless there is adequate support, stabilization, and protection to prevent injury.

General Precautions During Transfers

1. Predetermine the patient's mental and physical capabilities to perform the transfer.
2. The patient's clothing and footwear should be suitable for the transfer.
3. Mentally preplan the activities and sequence associated with the transfer.
4. Select, position, and secure equipment before the transfer; put a safety belt on the patient.
5. Be alert for unusual events that may occur.
6. Do not guard the patient by using his/her clothing or grasping his/her arm.
7. Position yourself to guard and protect the patient throughout the transfer.

Whenever a patient performs a transfer, it is important that the environment be free of unneeded equipment and other hazards and that the area needed for the transfer be clearly visible to the caregivers and assistants. When transfers are performed in an area protected by curtains or drapes, you should know what is on the other side of the curtain when it is closed.

PRECAUTIONS FOR SPECIAL PATIENT CONDITIONS

When assisting patients with certain conditions to alter their positions in bed or on a mat or to transfer, special care and precautions must be used to avoid additional trauma or *exacerbation* of their condition. Examples of some of these patient conditions are shown in Box 6-2.

TYPES OF TRANSFERS

Transfers are designated by a variety of terms. Some transfers are described according to the number of persons required to assist the patient (e.g., Plus 1, Plus 2), and most descriptions indicate whether the patient is dependent on assistance or can function independently. The designation of the transfer is important because it is part of the documentation to which other caregivers will refer. All persons involved with the care and management of the patient should use the same terminology when describing the transfer, and there must be a consensus regarding the termi-

nology that will be used by all caregivers. Once the transfer method or type has been selected, it is important for all caregivers to perform each transfer the same way with a particular patient to enhance learning and competence by the patient. If modifications are made to the transfer, each caregiver should be aware of them. The patient's family should observe the transfer and practice providing assistance while being guided by the appropriate caregiver (Procedure 6-1).

Standing, Dependent Pivot The standing, dependent pivot requires at least one other person to assist the patient. The patient is assisted to a standing position, usually from a bed, *plinth*, toilet seat, or wheelchair, and pivoted so that his/her back is toward another object to which he/she is lowered. You may be required to lift the patient to a standing position, to stabilize the knees and hips for the pivot, and to assist him/her to sit. Some patients may be able to assist with the transfer by using their extremities, whereas others may be totally dependent on another person.

Standing, Semi-independent Pivot The standing, semi-independent pivot may require the physical or standby assistance of another person. Some patients using this transfer may be able to stand, pivot, and sit, transferring from one object to a second object with minimal assistance. The assistance required may vary, from verbal cueing to close or casual guarding, or to actual stabilization or support. Safety is still a concern with this type of transfer, and you must be alert for the patient's need for your assistance.

Standing, Independent Pivot The patient is able to perform the entire transfer safely and efficiently without any physical or verbal assistance from another person.

Sitting, Dependent Transfer The patient is able to move from one surface to a second surface while in a sitting position with the assistance of at least one other person. This transfer may require the use of a transfer or sliding board, an overhead bar or frame, overhead straps, or other equipment. These items are used to bridge the space between the two objects or to permit the patient to use the upper extremities for assistance. The patient may be able to physically assist with the transfer but requires physical assistance, and he/she must be guarded and protected throughout the transfer.

Sitting, Independent Transfer The patient is able to safely and efficiently move from one surface to a second surface while in a sitting position, without assistance from another person. It still may be necessary for the patient to use a transfer or sliding board, an

Conditions Requiring Special Precautions During Transfers

1. *Total hip replacement, especially within the initial 2 weeks after surgery.* The surgically replaced hip should not be adducted or rotated, flexed more than 60 degrees, or extended beyond neutral flexion-extension. This means you must not cross the ankle of the surgically affected extremity over the opposite extremity, pull on the surgically affected extremity, or allow the patient to lie on the surgically replaced hip. However, you must maintain the surgical extremity in abduction when moving to and during side lying, you must require the patient to sit in a semireclining position, and you must require the patient to maintain the surgically affected extremity in abduction when moving from side to side.

    These precautions can also be used for the patient with a recent hip fracture or dislocation to decrease the possibility of dislocation or trauma to the fracture site.

2. *Low back trauma or discomfort.* These patients should avoid excessive lumbar rotation, trunk side bending, and trunk flexion. When turning, they may experience less discomfort if they "logroll" (i.e., rolling the entire body simultaneously) rather than roll segmentally (i.e., rolling the shoulders and upper trunk first, then the pelvis, and then the lower extremities). They may be more comfortable with the hips and knees partially flexed when they are in a supine or side-lying position.

3. *Spinal cord injury.* For the patient with a recent spinal cord injury, the injury site may be protected by some type of external appliance (e.g., a brace or a plaster or plastic body jacket), internal fixation (e.g., bone graft, metal rods, or wires), or a combination of the two methods. Distracting and rotational forces should be avoided, so you should not pull downward on the lower extremities and the person should be logrolled. Protective positioning or restraints will be required when this patient is in a side-lying position or sits without a back support. For the person with an injury that occurred several months or years earlier, you should be aware that *osteoporosis*, especially in the long bones of the lower extremities and the vertebral bodies, may be present. Even mild to moderate stress or strain to these bones may lead to a fracture. Some patients could experience a fracture when turning over or transferring from a wheelchair to the floor or to other objects.

4. *Burns.* The primary precaution is to avoid sliding or dragging the patient across the surface of the burn wound, *graft* site, or area from which the graft was taken. Sliding creates a shear force, which causes friction, which in turn disrupts the healing process. The patient should be instructed to elevate the body when moving to avoid the effect of shear forces.

5. *Hemiplegia.* Pulling on the involved or weakened extremities should not be used to control or move the patient. This is particularly important for the shoulder because the muscles will not provide adequate support to the joint due to the effects of paralysis. Many patients will experience pain or discomfort when they lie on or roll over the involved shoulder.

overhead bar or frame, overhead straps, or other equipment.

Sitting, Dependent Lift One, two, or three persons may be required to lift the patient and move him/her from one surface to a second surface. A mechanical lift may be used instead of multiple persons. If a lift is used, only one caregiver is usually needed to perform the transfer. This transfer is used when the patient is totally unable to physically assist with the transfer and other persons or equipment are required.

Recumbent, Dependent Transfer The recumbent, dependent transfer is used when the patient is physically unable to assist with the transfer and is unable to be placed in a sitting position. One, two, or three persons or special equipment are required to lift and move the patient from one surface to a second surface.

PROCEDURE 6 – 1
General Transfer Principles

1. Evaluate the patient to determine his/her mental and physical capacities to perform the transfer.
2. Select, position, and secure needed equipment; apply a safety belt on the patient.
3. Instruct the patient how to perform the transfer; demonstrate the transfer as necessary.
4. Practice components of the transfer as necessary before attempting the entire transfer.
5. Position yourself to guard and protect the patient throughout the transfer.
6. Request the patient to initiate and perform the transfer; assist him/her as necessary.
7. Guide and direct the patient throughout the transfer and closely guard him/her.
8. At the conclusion of the transfer, position the patient for comfort, stability, and safety.

The equipment may be a mechanical lift, mechanical transfer stretcher, mattress pad, bed liner (e.g., a draw sheet), or plastic transfer board.

MOBILITY ACTIVITIES FOR A BED OR MAT

Mobility activities are used to adjust the patient's body position while he/she is recumbent. They may be performed independently by the patient, with assistance from another person, or by using various types of equipment. The most common movements are turning from a supine to a side-lying position and returning; from a supine to a prone position and returning; moving upward, downward, or from side to side and returning to the center; and moving from a lying to a sitting position and returning. The equipment may include bed rails; an overhead bar or frame; loops attached to the bed, mat, or mattress; or linen items such as a draw sheet.

These activities should be taught to a patient to improve independence and assist in preventing the development of skin problems or contractures as a result of lying in one position too long. The patient must become independent in all phases of bed/mat mobility, to become independent in sitting or standing transfers. Remember to use proper body mechanics as you

assist the patient and to guard the patient when his/her safety is threatened.

The patient should mentally and physically participate in these activities even when he/she is being assisted. You can begin to initiate patient involvement by asking the patient to control his/her head, position the upper or lower extremities, or use the upper and lower extremities to help with the activity within his/her functional capacity. The patient should perform these assistive movements to promote independent movement as his/her condition improves. You and the patient may need to problem solve together to determine the most effective way to use his/her abilities to lead to independent movement and decrease the amount of assistance required.

To perform mobility activities with greater ease, you should attempt to reduce friction between the patient's body and the surface of the bed/mat, centralize the weight of the patient, reduce the effects of gravity, and use gravity as an assistive force. Each of these techniques will reduce the patient's and your energy expenditure and will enhance the patient's ability to move. There are many "tricks of the trade" that you can discover and apply by using your problem-solving skills and ability. Some are presented later in this chapter.

Knowledge of many of the basic principles of physics and body mechanics will assist you in developing innovative and safe methods to adjust a patient's position or to transfer him/her. Role playing with a friend, classmate, or coworker and simulating specific patient conditions or limitations are excellent methods to initiate the problem-solving process. The better you mimic a patient's condition, the better you will be able to devise techniques to alter your position on the bed/mat.

DEPENDENT OR ASSISTED MOBILITY ACTIVITIES

To move a supine or prone patient, you should move individual body segments to reduce the effort required and to provide greater control. Begin by positioning yourself close to the side of the patient or the bed or mat table. This will allow you to use your upper extremities with short lever arms to reduce strain and increase the mechanical advantage of your muscles. By kneeling on the mat or flexing your hips and knees as you treat the patient who is in bed, you will minimize strain to your back. If it is possible to adjust the height of the bed, position it at the most comfortable

and most beneficial level for you to function. Remember to apply the principles of body mechanics to reduce stress and strain to your muscles, joints, and ligaments.

Be certain to explain the activity to the patient and encourage him/her to assist with each of the movements. You should continue to guide and encourage the patient throughout the activity to promote his/her motivation and independence.

Side-to-Side Movement, Patient Supine Position one forearm under the patient's neck or upper back and one forearm under the middle of the back, and gently slide the upper body and head toward you (Fig. 6–1). Do not lift the upper body; slide it on your forearms. It may be necessary to support the patient's head with your upper arm as you move him/her. Next, position your forearms under the patient's lower trunk and just distal to the pelvis, and gently slide that body segment toward you. Finally, position your forearms under the thighs and legs, and gently slide them toward you. When you slide rather than lift the patient toward you, the amount of energy required and the

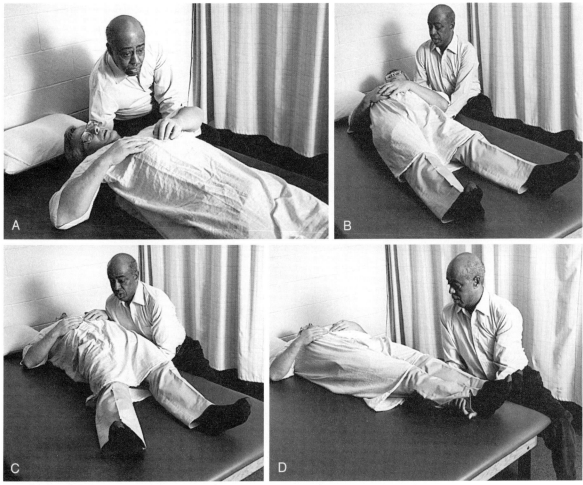

■ **FIGURE 6–1**
Moving a supine patient sideward.

stress to your upper extremity and back muscles will be reduced. The force you use to pull and slide the patient should be applied parallel to the surface of the bed/mat to further reduce the energy required. Remember to lower your trunk by flexing your hips and knees or raising the bed before moving the patient. This will position your center of gravity as close to the patient's center of gravity as possible. Position your feet to widen your base of support by placing one foot in front of the other. These actions allow you to control the patient better, to reduce stress and strain to your arms and back and to reduce the energy required to move the patient. When it is necessary to move the patient sideward over a large distance, such a transfer will be easier if each body segment is moved several times. Moving the patient closer to one side of the bed/mat is important prior to performing exercise or a transfer. Having the patient close to you allows you to take advantage of the use of proper body mechanics.

Upward Movement, Patient Supine Before attempting to move the patient upward, bring him/her closer to the near edge of the bed/mat, especially if the patient is lying in the center of the bed/mat. This position will allow you to use the muscles of your upper extremities more effectively by using short lever arms. Short lever arms can develop greater force than long lever arms, with less energy expenditure and better patient control.

To initiate the move, flex the patient's hips and knees so the feet rest flat on the bed or mat. This will reduce friction between the extremities and the bed/mat surface and will position the patient so he/she can assist by lifting the pelvis or pushing with the extremities.

It may be necessary to support the thighs with one or more pillows if the patient is unable to maintain the proper position. You should face toward the patient's head and stand approximately opposite the patient's mid chest with the foot that is farthest from the bed in front of your other foot (i.e., in stride in an anterior-posterior position). Support the patient's head and upper trunk with your arms, and lift until the inferior angles of the scapulae clear the bed/mat; your chest should be close to the patient's chest so that you will use short lever arms with your arms (Fig. 6–2). This position will reduce the friction of the patient's trunk on the bed/mat but should not place excessive strain or stress on the structures of your back.

If you are unable to lift the patient's trunk or if the lift creates excessive strain or stress to your back, it may be necessary to ask another person for assistance. Slide the lower trunk and pelvis upward approximately 6 to 10 inches; do not attempt to move the patient over a long distance unless the patient is able to assist. To move the patient farther, you will have to re-

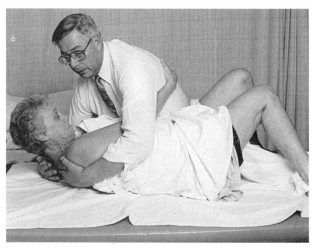

■ FIGURE 6–2
Moving a supine patient upward.

position both yourself and the patient's lower extremities and then repeat the process. Some patients may be able to grasp your trunk to help elevate their trunk. However, this may increase stress or strain to your back, and you must determine whether it is a safe technique. After you have moved the patient upward to the final position, reposition him/her in the center of the bed/mat to reduce the possibility of him/her rolling off the bed/mat.

Downward Movement, Patient Supine Initially, move the patient closer to the near edge of the bed/mat and partially flex the hips and knees. If necessary, use a pillow to support the thighs. Position yourself approximately opposite to the patient's waist or hips or at the patient's feet (Fig. 6–3A,B). Cradle and lift the pelvis slightly before you slide the patient's upper body and head downward. Move the patient approximately 6 to 10 inches, and then reposition yourself and the patient's lower extremities if further movement is required. Reposition the patient in the center of the bed/mat.

Note: Movement of a recumbent patient upward, downward, or sideward can be accomplished more easily if a small sheet or linen pad is placed beneath the patient. This item is frequently called a "draw" sheet/pad; it usually extends from the upper back to the buttocks or midthighs. Two persons, one on either side of the bed or mat, grasp the sheet/pad and, on command from one of them, simultaneously move the patient by sliding him/her. Some lifting may be required, but the primary force used is sliding. The patient should be encouraged to assist by using his/her upper or lower extremities to partially elevate his/her trunk or pelvis. When the patient is moved upward or sideward, the upper portion of the bed should be lowered; if he/she is moved downward, the upper portion of the bed can be raised.

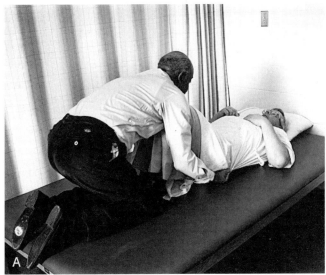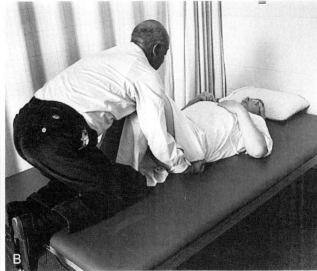

■ **FIGURE 6–3**
Moving a supine patient downward.

Move to a Side-Lying Position, Patient Supine To have sufficient space on the bed/mat, it may be necessary to initially position the patient close to the far edge of the bed/mat. This is a potentially dangerous position, and you, another person, a bed rail, or a wall must protect the patient so he/she does not roll off the bed/mat.

Stand facing the patient so you can roll (turn) him/her toward you to a side-lying position. If you plan to roll the patient toward the right extremities, place the left lower extremity over the right lower extremity, place the left upper extremity on the chest, and place the right upper extremity in straight abduction. Roll the patient toward you by pulling gently on the left posterior scapula (shoulder) and the left posterior pelvis. Do not use the upper or lower extremity to initiate the roll because you will not be able to properly control or initiate movement of the trunk, and you may injure the extremity. When the patient is in a side-lying position, flex the hips and knees and place a pillow under the head, between the knees and ankles, and along the front and back of the trunk. The downmost upper and lower extremities should be positioned for comfort. Refer to the description of the side-lying position in Chapter 3 for more complete information about this position. If the patient is to remain in this position unattended, it may be necessary to apply trunk restraints or engage the bed rails. *Caution:* Be careful when readjusting the patient's position while he/she is in a side-lying position. This is an unstable position, and the patient can easily roll forward or backward. Inform the patient when you move from one side of the bed/mat to the other side, and it is recommended that you maintain manual contact with the patient as you move. You should roll the patient toward you and guard the edge of the bed/mat to pre-

vent him/her from rolling too far. This will require you to stand close to the side of the bed/mat toward which you roll the patient, with at least one thigh against the edge of the bed/mat. These precautions must be followed when moving the patient from a supine to a prone position or from a prone to a supine position to protect and maintain control of him/her.

Move to a Prone Position, Patient Supine Move the patient closer to one side of the bed or mat, and prepare to roll him/her to a side-lying position as described previously, with one modification. The arm over which the patient will roll should be positioned either close along his/her side with the shoulder externally rotated, elbow straight, palm up, and the hand tucked under the pelvis; or with the shoulder flexed so the arm rests next to the ear with the elbow straight. The other upper extremity remains by the side (Fig. 6–4*A–C*).

Stand facing the patient and roll him/her to a side-lying position. Determine whether there is sufficient space to allow the roll to a prone position to be completed. If the space is insufficient, move him/her backward, while side lying, until there is sufficient space to complete the roll to prone. *Caution:* The patient is very insecure while in a side-lying position, so you must guard him/her closely.

Be certain to roll the patient toward you, and protect the near edge of the bed/mat by placing one of your thighs against it. This will prevent the patient from rolling off the bed/mat if he/she rolls too far.

Move to a Supine Position, Patient Prone Move the patient close to one edge of the bed/mat. If he/she is going to roll toward the right side, cross the left leg over the right leg. Position the right upper extremity

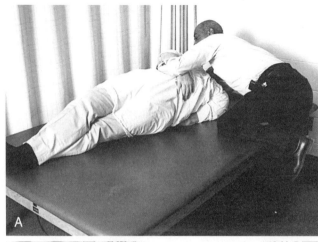

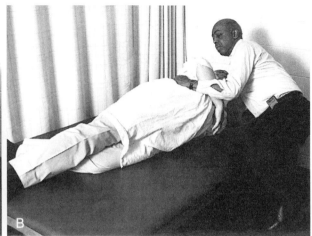

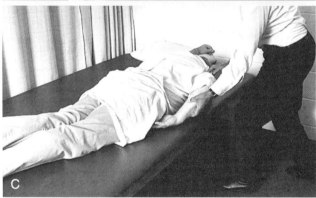

■ **FIGURE 6–4**
Moving a supine patient to a prone position.

close to the side with the elbow straight, palm up, and hand tucked under the pelvis, or the right shoulder can be flexed and the arm positioned close to the patient's ear; place the other upper extremity next to the side. Stand on the far side of the table, and roll the patient toward you to a side-lying position. Determine whether there is sufficient space to allow the roll to a supine position to be completed. If the space is insufficient, move the patient forward, while side lying, until there is sufficient space to complete the roll to a supine position.

Guide the patient from a side-lying to a supine position by resisting against the posterior left shoulder and pelvis to retard the movement to a supine position. Reposition him/her in the center of the bed/mat.

Be certain to roll the patient toward you and to protect the near edge of the bed/mat by placing one of your thighs against it.

Move to a Sitting Position, Patient Supine Move the patient close to one edge of the bed or mat, and flex the hips and knees with the feet flat on the bed/mat (see Fig. 6–2). Fold the arms across the chest unless they will be used to elevate the trunk or to hold onto your upper back. Place one or both of your arms under the patient's upper back and head, and elevate the trunk until a sitting position is attained.

Pivot the patient by supporting under the thighs and behind the back to a short sitting or dangling position. *Caution:* Do not allow the patient to sit unattended or without support, even briefly. Some patients may experience *vertigo* or syncope (i.e., become faint) when they are moved quickly from a supine to a sitting position. Other patients may lack sufficient strength or balance to remain sitting without some form of support.

Alternative Method Move the patient close to one edge of the bed/mat, and roll him/her to a side-lying position with the lower extremities partially flexed. Elevate the trunk by lifting under the shoulders or by instructing the patient to push up using either or both upper extremities (Fig. 6–5).

Pivot the lower extremities over the side of the bed or mat as the trunk is raised. Do not allow the patient to sit unattended or unsupported.

This alternative method is recommended for the patient who has a lower back condition that might be aggravated by trunk flexion or for the patient who has functional use of only one upper and lower extremity. This method concentrates the patient's body weight closer to his/her center of gravity (COG), which will make it easier for you to lift the trunk. Position your feet in an anterior-posterior position to widen your base of support (BOS) and to avoid twisting your back as you lift the patient.

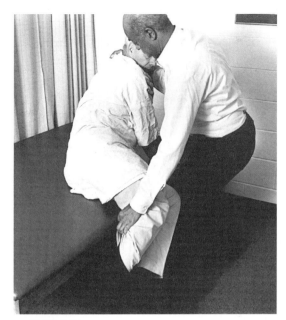

■ **FIGURE 6–5**
Assisting a supine patient to a sitting position.

Move to Supine Position, Patient Sitting   Reverse the sequence of activities described in the preceding section to move from a supine to a sitting position. Reposition the patient in the center of the bed/mat after he/she is supine.

INDEPENDENT MOBILITY ACTIVITIES

Each patient should be taught and encouraged to independently perform or assist with all bed/mat mobility activities within his/her abilities. Initially, these activities can be used while practicing dependent or assisted bed/mat mobility activities. The patient will have to be instructed and guided in the activities to be performed. Assistive equipment such as bed rails or overhead bars should not be used unless the patient is unable to safely perform the activity without equipment. *Remember:* These activities are necessary for the patient to be able to perform transfers and avoid soft tissue pressure and the development of contractures as a result of prolonged immobilization.

Side-to-Side Movement, Patient Supine   Instruct the patient to flex his/her hips and knees and place the feet flat on the bed/mat. He/she positions one upper extremity next to the trunk and abducts the other upper extremity approximately 4 inches from the trunk.
Instruct the patient to push down with the lower extremities to lift the pelvis and move it toward the abducted upper extremity. He/she elevates the upper trunk by pushing into the mat with the elbows and the back of the head and moves toward the abducted el-

bow. Then he/she repositions the lower and upper extremities to move again or for comfort.
An alternative method for some patients is to elevate the pelvis and upper trunk by simultaneously pushing down with the legs and the back of the head. He/she then shifts the body toward the abducted upper extremity. The patient should be taught to move to the left and to the right.

Upward Movement, Patient Supine   Instruct the patient to fully flex his/her hips and knees, position the feet flat on the bed/mat with the heels close to the buttocks, and position the upper extremities with the elbows flexed, next to the trunk with the shoulders (scapulae) pulled up toward his/her ears (Fig. 6–6).
The patient elevates the pelvis using the lower extremities and elevates the upper trunk by simultaneously pushing into the bed/mat with the elbows and the back of the head. He/she moves upward by pushing with the lower extremities and depressing the shoulders (scapulae). He/she then repositions the lower and upper extremities for successive movements.

Downward Movement, Patient Supine   Instruct the patient to partially flex his/her hips and knees to position the feet flat on the bed/mat; the heels should be 8 to 12 inches distal to the buttocks. The upper extremities should be positioned next to the trunk with the elbows flexed and the shoulders (scapulae) depressed (Fig. 6–7).
The patient elevates the pelvis using the lower extremities and elevates the upper trunk by simultaneously pushing into the bed/mat with the elbows and the back of the head. He/she moves downward by pulling with the lower extremities and by simultaneously pushing up with the shoulders (scapulae) and pulling downward with the elbows or forearms. He/

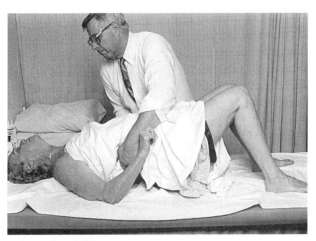

■ **FIGURE 6–6**
Assisting a supine patient to move upward.

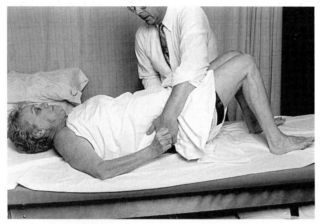

■ **FIGURE 6–7**
Assisting a supine patient to move downward.

she then repositions the lower and upper extremities for successive movements.

Move to a Side-Lying Position, Patient Supine Instruct the patient to move to the far side of the bed or mat. To roll toward the right, he/she simultaneously reaches across the chest with the left upper extremity and lifts the left lower extremity diagonally over the right lower extremity; the patient then uses head flexion and his/her abdominal muscles to roll onto the side.

Instruct the patient to maintain the side-lying position by using the left hand on the bed/mat and by flexing the lower extremities. A pillow may be needed for the head.

To roll to the left, the patient performs the same process with the opposite extremities.

Alternative Method An alternative method is to instruct the patient to move to the far side of the bed/mat. To roll to the right, he/she pushes with the left upper extremity and the left lower extremity before reaching across the body. Some patients may prefer to reach with their upper extremity and push with their lower extremity to initiate the roll. To roll to the left, the patient performs the same process with the opposite extremities.

Caution: You must inform the patient about the relative insecurity of the side-lying position. Be certain you instruct the patient to flex the hips and knees and to place the uppermost hand in front of the chest on the bed/mat to increase stability. In addition, you may need to teach the patient to reposition his/her body in the center of the bed/mat to provide as much surface as possible in front and behind him/her.

Move to a Prone Position, Patient Supine Instruct the patient to move to one side of the bed or mat. To roll to the right, he/she positions the right upper extremity under the right side of the body or flexes the shoulder so that it is positioned next to the right ear.

He/she moves to a side-lying position; if the space is insufficient to roll to prone, he/she repositions the body away from the near edge of the bed/mat. As the patient rolls to prone, he/she uses the left upper extremity for protection and then adjusts the position as desired for comfort.

Move to a Supine Position, Patient Prone Instruct the patient to move to one side of the bed/mat. To roll to the right, he/she positions the right upper extremity under the right side or flexes the right shoulder so it is positioned next to the right ear. The left hand is placed flat on the bed/mat near the anterior left shoulder; the left hip and knee can be partially flexed or extended.

The patient pushes with the left upper extremity, lifts the left lower extremity over the right lower extremity, and moves to a side-lying position. If space on the bed/mat is insufficient to roll to a supine position, he/she repositions the body away from the near edge of the bed/mat, then rolls to a supine position, and adjusts his/her position as desired for comfort.

Caution: You must instruct the patient to determine his/her position on the bed/mat before any rolling activities are attempted. Depending on the width of the bed/mat, it may be necessary for the patient to adjust his/her position by moving forward or backward while in a side-lying position.

Move to a Sitting Position, Patient Supine Instruct the patient to move to the near edge of the bed/mat. Start with the hips and knees flexed and the feet flat on the bed/mat; the upper extremities are slightly abducted, with the shoulders internally rotated and the forearms resting on the bed or mat (Fig. 6–8*A*).

He/she lifts his/her head and pushes with the upper extremities to elevate the trunk using a tripod support, with the hands placed on the bed/mat behind the hips with the elbows extended. By alternately moving his/her hands forward, the patient attains a sitting position (Fig. 6–8*B*). He/she can pivot the lower extremities over the edge of the bed/mat in preparation for standing.

Alternative Method Instruct the patient to move toward one edge of the bed/mat but leave sufficient space to roll to a side-lying position. He/she rolls to a side-lying position and flexes the hips and knees to maintain the side-lying position briefly; he/she positions the hand of the uppermost upper extremity on the bed/mat opposite to the mid chest.

The patient pushes with the upper extremity to raise the trunk and maintains this position by resting on the elbow and forearm of the lowermost upper extremity; then the trunk is elevated fully by pushing with both upper extremities to a side-sitting position. The lower extremities can be pivoted simultaneously

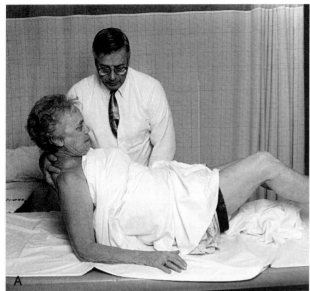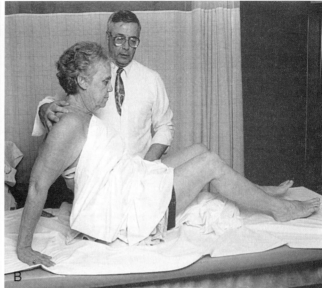

■ FIGURE 6–8
Assisting a supine patient to a sitting position.

over the edge of the bed/mat in preparation for standing. This technique is beneficial for the patient with low back dysfunction or pain because less stress is directed to the lumbar spine through the avoidance of rotation and flexion. The patient can return to a supine position by performing the movements in reverse sequence. Occasionally a patient with low back dysfunction may desire to move to the floor and return to standing. Procedure 6–2 presents techniques designed to accomplish the movements safely and with reduced stress and discomfort.

It may be necessary to alter or modify these activities for the patient who has reduced strength or reduced function of one or more of the extremities. For example, the *paralysis* or *paresis* of the *ipsilateral* upper and lower extremity that results from a cerebrovascular accident (i.e., stroke) will require the patient to use the remaining functional extremities to adjust his/her position and to be mobile in bed or on a mat. The patient who has limited function as a result of joint disease or trauma will need to rely on the noninvolved or least involved joints to adjust his/her position. Finally, the patient with paralysis of the lower extremities and lower trunk (i.e., a paraplegic) or with paralysis of all four extremities and trunk (i.e., a quadriplegic) will require a longer period of training and practice to learn how to safely and efficiently adjust his/her position. The quadriplegic patient may require aids such as loops attached to the mattress or to an overhead bed frame, bed rails, an overhead trapeze, or loops of cloth sewn to clothing to assist him/her to alter his/her position. The techniques or procedures that must be learned and practiced by the patient with multiple or severe paralyzing injuries are beyond the scope of this text. The reader is referred to the Bibliography for

sources of information about these types of patient conditions.

STANDING, SITTING, LIFTING TRANSFERS

Standing Transfer, Dependent Pivot A safety belt should be applied before attempting any sitting or standing transfer, particularly during the early treatment sessions. The patient should be instructed in the procedures required to maneuver, position, and operate the wheelchair and its components. These procedures are described in Chapter 7.

Movement From a Wheelchair to a Bed, Mat, or Low Plinth Position the wheelchair parallel or at a 45- to 60-degree angle to the bed midway between the head and foot of the bed, mat, or plinth (Fig. 6–9A). Apply a safety belt, and lock the wheelchair with the caster wheels positioned forward to increase the BOS of the wheelchair. *Note:* The caster wheels may pivot or turn to one side when the patient performs the transfer. That movement does not cause a safety problem, and the patient can continue to perform the transfer. However, the caster wheels should not be permitted to be directed backward because that position reduces the stability of the chair, particularly when the patient moves to the front portion of the seat. Remove the patient's feet from the footrests, and elevate the footrests; remove or swing away the front rigging, and place the patient's feet flat on the floor. Remove the armrest nearest to the bed, mat, or low plinth if the top surface of the bed, mat, or low plinth is lower than

---

PROCEDURE 6 - 2
Protective Transfer to and From the Floor for a Person With Low Back Dysfunction

The patient should be encouraged to use a firm, stable object for support and to reduce stress to the back as these activities are performed.

1. Movement to the floor
   a. The patient places one hand on a firm object and moves to a single knee (half-kneeling) position, keeping the trunk erect.
   b. He/she moves to kneeling on both knees (high kneeling) position and then moves to an "all fours" (hands and knees) position.
   c. He/she "walks" his/her hands forward until in a prone position or he/she gently side sits from the hands and knees position; he/she then lowers onto one elbow to a side-lying position.
   d. He/she can adjust his/her position as desired.

2. From the floor to standing
   a. He/she starts from a prone position and pushes to a hands and knees position, or he/she may "logroll" to side lying.
   b. If on "all fours," he/she pushes to a high kneeling position and then moves to a half-kneeling position and then to standing; he/she may desire to use a firm object for assistance.
   c. If side lying, he/she pushes to side sitting and then moves to a hands and knees position and performs the movements listed in step b.

---

the armrest. Move the patient forward in the chair by grasping the posterior pelvis and pulling on it so the buttocks slide forward (see Fig. 6–8B) and position his/her feet parallel to each other. Partially stoop and position your knees and feet outside and touching the patient's knees and feet. If he/she is able, he/she can hold your middle or upper back with the upper extremities. *Caution:* Do not allow the patient to hold around your neck. You must use proper body mechanics to prevent undue strain to your back.

Grasp the safety belt at the sides of the patient's waist and inform him/her when and how the move to standing is performed. If necessary, you may rock the patient to develop momentum before standing the patient (Fig. 6–9C).

Instruct the patient using terms such as "Ready, stand" or "One, two, three, stand." As you lift on the safety belt, simultaneously straighten your lower extremities and stabilize the patient's knees by pushing in and forward with your knees as he/she stands. Elevate the body high enough to clear the wheelchair wheel and stand the patient to the height necessary to elevate the pelvis above the level of the surface of the bed, mat, or plinth. Pivot yourself and the patient toward the bed, mat, or plinth and lower him/her onto the surface when his/her buttocks are turned so that they are directed toward the bed, mat, or plinth. Set

the patient on the edge of the bed, mat, or plinth, and then assist him/her to a supine position (see Fig. 6–9D–G). *Caution:* Do not leave the patient sitting unattended or without sufficient support to prevent a fall.

The return to the wheelchair is performed using the same procedures in reverse. The patient should be transferred to his/her left and right side and requested to assist with the transfer. As the patient gains strength, the assisted standing transfer should be attempted.

If a safety belt or strap is not used, the assistant may lift the patient by grasping under the buttocks. However, this procedure may be difficult to perform on large patients, and some patients may prefer that you not use this method. Your hands may slip or slide over the patient's clothing, and it may not be as easy to control him/her as it would be with a safety belt. *Caution:* You should not use patient clothing, including his/her belt, to lift or protect the patient. You could soil and tear the clothing or unbuckle the belt or cause patient discomfort if you use them as a means of control.

Standing Transfer, Assisted Pivot When performing this transfer with a patient who has greater strength in one upper and lower extremity than in the other upper and lower extremity, a decision should be made as to the direction in which the patient will trans-

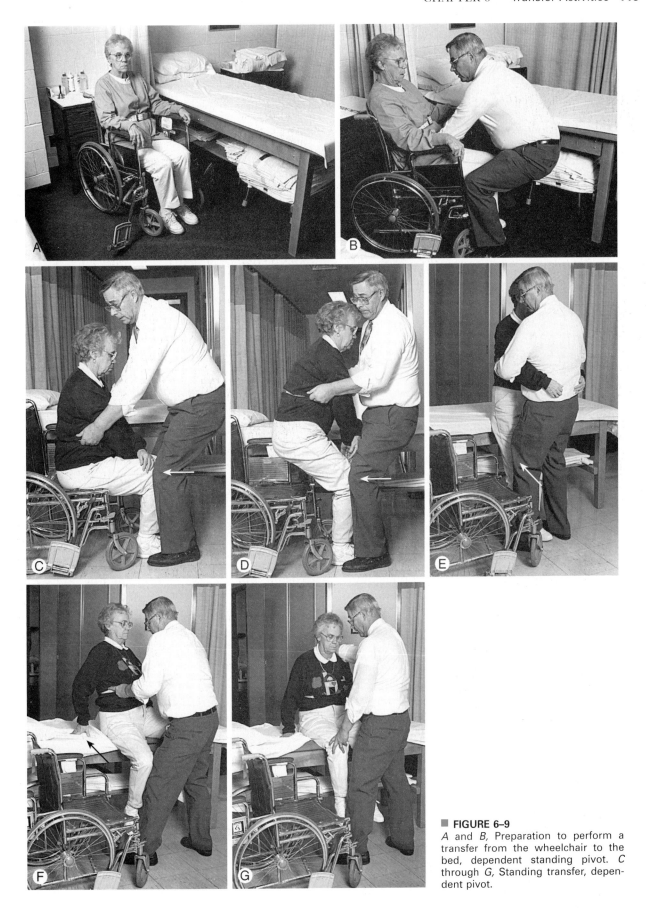

PROCEDURE 6 – 3
Procedures Associated With a Standing Transfer

1. Evaluate the patient to determine whether he/she has the mental and physical capacities to perform or assist with the transfer.

2. Position, secure, and stabilize the wheelchair and other items involved with the transfer; swing away front rigging or elevate foot plates, and apply safety belt on the patient.

3. Instruct the patient in the steps of the transfer; indicate the activities he/she will be expected to perform, and demonstrate the transfer as necessary.

4. Instruct the patient to move forward in the chair, or provide assistance; position the patient's feet flat on the floor parallel or anterior-posterior to each other.

5. The patient initiates standing with trunk momentum or by inclining the trunk forward ("nose over toes"); the caregiver is positioned in front and slightly to one side of the patient to protect and guard him/her.

6. The patient uses his/her upper and lower extremity or extremities to rise to stand; assistance is provided by the caregiver as needed using his/her knees and the safety belt.

7. The patient stands briefly to establish his/her balance and to acclimate to the upright position before turning or pivoting toward the object to which he/she is transferring.

8. As he/she turns or pivots or after the turn or pivot has been completed, the patient reaches for the object (i.e., armrest, grab bar, edge of bed mattress, automobile seat) and uses his/her upper and lower extremity or extremities to lower himself/herself onto the object; assistance is provided by the caregiver as needed.

9. The patient's position is adjusted for proper support, stability, and safety; his/her reaction and physiologic response to the activity are evaluated by the caregiver. Documentation of the performance of the patient is provided as needed, and the safety belt is removed.

---

fer. Initially, it will be easier and safer for most patients to transfer by leading with the stronger extremities. However, there are reasons to have the patient learn to lead with the weaker extremities. When the patient leads with the weaker extremity and uses the weaker upper extremity to assist with the transfer, this may begin to improve proprioception and kinesthesia in those extremities, and the patient is more likely to "sense" or "feel" them in a functional way. In addition, if the patient learns to transfer using both the left and the right extremities, he/she will be better prepared to move in either direction at home depending on the location of objects such as the bed, toilet, or bathtub. Thus the patient should learn to transfer by leading with both the weaker and the stronger extremities to increase his/her

independence and to encourage use of the weaker extremities (Procedure 6–3).

Initially the patient may feel more secure if the stronger knee is blocked, which ensures that one lower extremity will be stable throughout the transfer. When the patient transfers by leading with the left (stronger) extremities, you should stabilize the left knee by placing your left foot next to the *medial* side of the left foot and placing your left knee on the *lateral* side of the knee. Grasp the safety belt with your right hand and place your left hand on the right shoulder or on the posterior-lateral thorax by reaching under the right upper extremity. *Caution:* Do not use the right upper extremity or clothing as a point of control because both are insecure and you

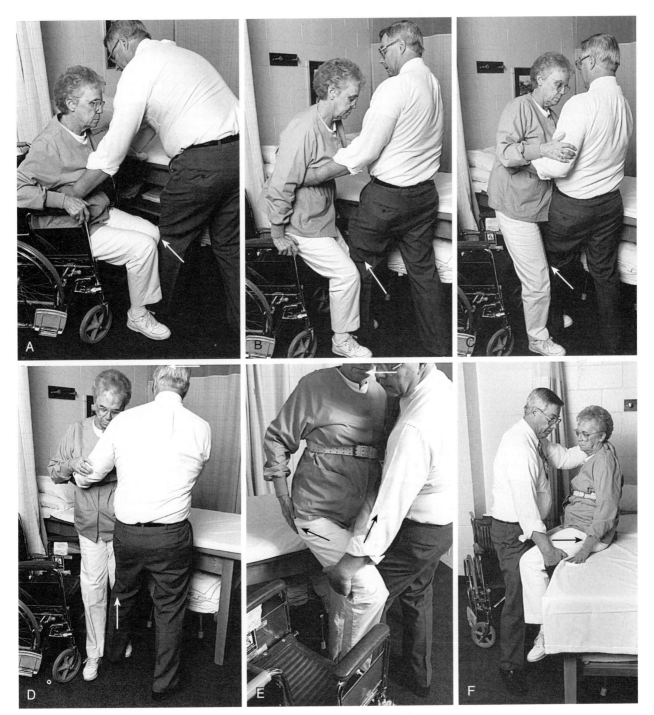

■ **FIGURE 6–10**
Standing transfer, assisted pivot, with the patient leading with the stronger (left) extremities.

will not be able to guard the patient satisfactorily (Fig. 6–10).

When you determine the patient is able to safely and independently support his/her weight on the stronger lower extremity, you may choose to stabilize the weaker extremity. This will allow the patient to increase the use of the lower extremities and improve his/her independence. When the patient transfers leading with the left (stronger) extremities, you

should stabilize the weaker (right) knee by placing your left foot next to the lateral side of the right foot and placing your left knee on the medial side of the right knee. You can control the patient's trunk by grasping the safety belt with your left hand and by placing your right hand on the left shoulder or on the posterior-lateral thorax by reaching under the left upper extremity (Fig. 6–11). *Caution:* Do not use the patient's right upper extremity or clothing

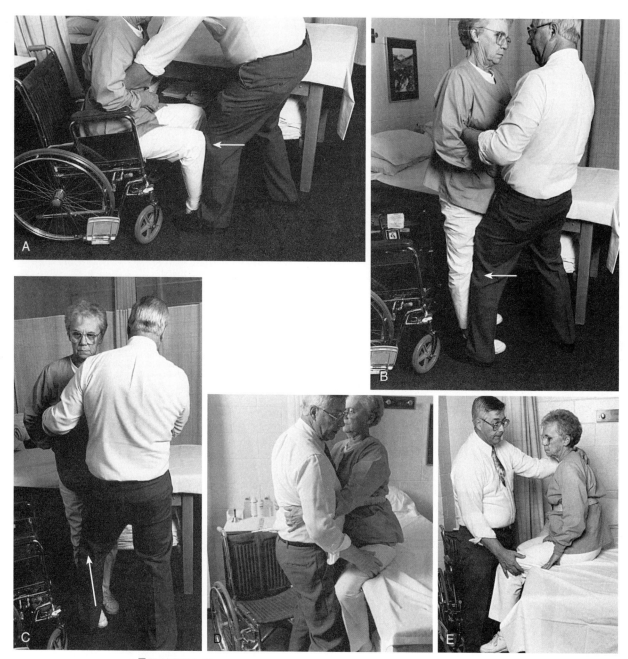

■ **FIGURE 6–11**
Standing transfer, assisted pivot, with the weaker (right) knee stabilized.

as a point of control, for the reasons stated previously.

Movement From the Wheelchair to the Bed, Mat, or Low Plinth Instruct the patient to position the wheelchair parallel or at a 45- to 60-degree angle to the bed, with the stronger extremities nearest the bed. The chair should be at the midpoint between the head and foot of the bed or mat (see Fig. 6–11).

Instruct the patient to lock the wheelchair with the caster wheels directed forward; remove his/her feet from the footrests, and remove or swing away the front rigging. Desk type armrests should be reversed so that the highest part is forward. Instruct the patient to move forward to the center or forward part of the seat either by shifting his/her weight off one buttock and elevating the pelvis on that side and moving it forward to the desired position in the chair or by leaning against the chair back and pushing the pelvis forward to the desired position in the chair and then moving the trunk to an erect or forward-inclined position to place the COG over the feet.

The patient positions the feet with the stronger/least affected foot posterior to the weaker/most affected foot. (*Note:* An elderly patient may perform better with the feet positioned parallel to each other rather than anterior-posterior to each other.) He/she places his/her hands forward on the armrests and simultaneously pushes down with the upper and lower extremities while inclining the trunk forward slightly ("nose over toes") to stand. He/she may initiate some trunk motion by rocking the trunk forward and back to develop momentum before attempting to stand. You may need to stabilize one or both of the knees as described previously when the patient initiates the stand while you maintain control using the safety belt and the shoulder or the posterior neck. *Caution:* Do not use the patient's upper extremity or clothing for control, for the reasons stated previously.

Allow the patient to stand briefly to establish balance and to determine whether he/she experiences lightheadedness or a dizzy sensation. He/she pivots toward the bed so that his/her back is nearest to the bed, reaches with the nearest upper extremity to the surface of the bed, and lowers to sitting on the bed. The patient places his/her lower extremities onto the bed and then lies down; if necessary, you may need to lift the lower extremities onto the bed and assist him/her to recline.

Movement From the Bed, Mat, or Low Plinth to the Wheelchair   The wheelchair should be positioned and locked as previously described. The patient should position it prior to lying down, or it will have to be positioned after he/she is sitting on the edge of the bed or by another person before the transfer. Instruct the patient to rise to a sitting position using one of the methods described previously. Assistance should be provided as necessary for safety and to complete the change in position. Instruct him/her to move the hips to the edge of the bed and place the feet on the floor in the position described previously. Again, an elderly patient may perform best with his/her feet parallel to each other. You may need to stabilize one or both knees as he/she stands.

Instruct the patient to push to a standing position and to reach for the near armrest of the wheelchair. He/she then starts to pivot, reaches to the far armrest, and continues to pivot so his/her back is toward the chair. He/she then lowers into the chair, repositions the front rigging and the footrests, places his/her feet on the footrests, and moves the hips (pelvis) back into the chair seat.

Caution: For patients with a recent total hip replacement, care must be taken to avoid (1) adduction of the surgically replaced hip beyond a midline position, (2) excessive internal or external hip rotation, and (3) excessive hip flexion, which is usually restricted to 60 to 90 degrees. Thus the patient *must not* pivot on that extremity when standing, flex the surgically replaced hip or his/her trunk excessively, or adduct the hip at any time during the transfer.

Standing Transfer, Assisted Pivot Using a Footstool

Occasionally it may be necessary for the person with short stature to use a footstool to elevate his/her hips to the height of a nonadjustable bed or plinth. The important principle to remember is that the person should step onto the stool with the stronger lower extremity, and it may be necessary to guard the opposite knee during the transfer. The footstool should have four legs, and the feet of the legs should be located beyond the edges of the top. The feet should have rubber tips, and the top should have a nonslip surface. The footstool should be between 8 and 12 inches high.

As with other transfers, the chair must be positioned properly, and the patient should initiate the transfer with the stronger extremities nearest to the bed or plinth. The preliminary steps are the same as those listed for a standing transfer, assisted pivot. The caregiver guards the weaker knee as the patient steps onto the footstool with the stronger lower extremity. That extremity is used to lift the body high enough to position the buttocks slightly above the surface of the bed or plinth. The caregiver assists the patient to pivot so the buttocks are turned toward the bed or plinth. He/she sits on the edge of the bed or plinth and establishes balance (Fig. 6–12). The caregiver can assist the patient to lie down by controlling the trunk and the lower extremities.

Another method is to instruct the patient to place the stronger foot on the footstool and to stand with assistance (Fig. 6–12*E–G*). *Caution:* The patient must be instructed to push down with the foot and to not push forward to avoid sliding or tipping the footstool.

Usually it is not necessary to use a footstool to transfer from the bed or plinth to a wheelchair. The caregiver can assist the patient to sit on the edge of the bed or plinth and turn so the stronger lower extremity is directed outward. With assistance, he/she slides forward gradually and reaches toward the floor with the stronger lower extremity. When that foot is secure on the floor, the other lower extremity is lowered to the floor. Then he/she pivots on the stronger lower extremity, reaches for the chair armrest, completes the pivot, and is assisted to sit in the chair.

Remember to apply and use a safety belt for these transfers. Transferring a patient from a wheelchair to a motor vehicle will also require a safety belt (Fig. 6–13*A–D*).

Sitting Transfer Assisted With a Sliding Board

Movement From the Wheelchair to a Bed, Mat, or Low Plinth   Instruct the patient to position the wheelchair at an angle to the bed and midway between the head and foot of the bed, mat, or low plinth; apply a safety belt to the patient. Instruct him/her to lock the wheelchair, remove his/her feet from the footrests,

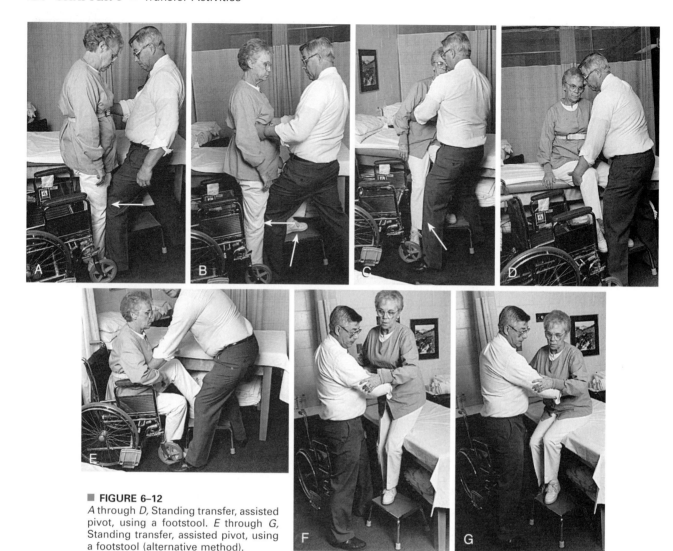

■ **FIGURE 6–12**
A through *D,* Standing transfer, assisted pivot, using a footstool. *E* through *G,* Standing transfer, assisted pivot, using a footstool (alternative method).

swing away or remove the front rigging, and place his/her feet on the floor. Instruct or assist him/her to move forward in the chair and to remove the armrest nearest to the bed. The sliding board is positioned under the patient's thigh, in front of the drivewheel, so it rests on the seat and bed, mat, or low plinth (Fig. 6–14*A–F*).

If the patient is going to move to the right, the right hand is placed on the board 4 to 6 inches from the right thigh, and the left hand is placed next to the left thigh. He/she performs a push-up with the upper extremities to elevate the body and begins to move toward the bed by quickly moving the head to the left and pushing toward the right with the left arm. This procedure is repeated until the hips are on the bed. To move to the left, the position of the patient's hands is reversed. (*Note:* Some patients will be able to totally elevate the pelvis and move across the board without assistance. However, some patients will not be able to totally elevate the pelvis and must slide their buttocks, using a series of small movements, to progress across the board.) You should guard the patient's knees and

use the safety belt to assist in elevating the body or moving the buttocks across the board. You can prevent the patient's loss of balance by placing your hand on the upper trunk. The sliding board is removed when he/she is seated securely on the bed, mat, or low plinth. He/she then lies down independently or is assisted to a lying position. Do not leave the patient sitting unattended.

The return to the wheelchair is performed using the same techniques in reverse order. The patient should learn to transfer to his/her left and right to maximize his/her independence.

This transfer is most commonly used for the patient who is unable to stand but has functional upper extremities. A similar transfer can be performed by a patient with weakness in one upper and lower extremity and normal strength in the other extremities but who is unable to stand safely. Some patients will require the use of a sliding board at all times, whereas other patients will develop the balance, strength, and skill to permit them to perform the transfer without the board. This type of transfer is frequently referred

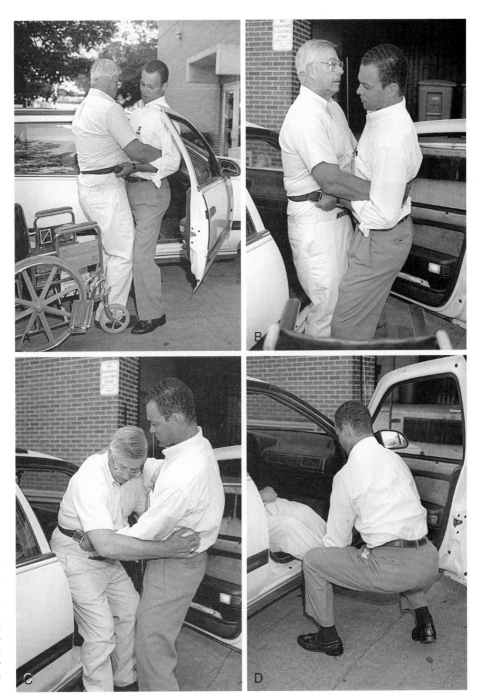

■ **FIGURE 6–13**
Assisted transfer into a motor vehicle. *A,* The caregiver protects the person's knees and assists him in standing; chair is prepositioned and locked. *B,* The knees are protected as the person pivots. *C,* The caregiver uses the safety belt to assist the person in sitting. *D,* The lower extremities are placed in the car.

to as a "lateral" or "swinging sitting transfer" (Procedure 6–4).

Sitting Transfer, Independent Lateral/Swinging
Movement From the Wheelchair to a Bed, Mat, or
Low Plinth Instruct the patient to position the wheelchair at an angle to the bed and midway between the head and the foot of the bed, mat, or low plinth. The caster wheels should be positioned forward to expand the BOS of the chair. Instruct him/her to remove his/her feet from the footrests, remove or swing away the front rigging, and place his/her feet on the floor.

Instruct the patient to move forward in the chair to clear the buttocks past the drivewheel and to remove the armrest nearest to the bed. He/she moves the buttocks to partially pivot his/her body so his/her back is toward the bed. If he/she is going to move to the right, the right hand is placed on the edge of the bed and the left hand is placed on the armrest, on the seat of the chair, or on the back of the chair, depending on the patient's strength, size, and skills. Instruct the patient to push with the upper extremities to elevate the body and to swing the buttocks onto the edge of the bed by moving his/her head quickly to the left and pushing toward the right with the left arm.

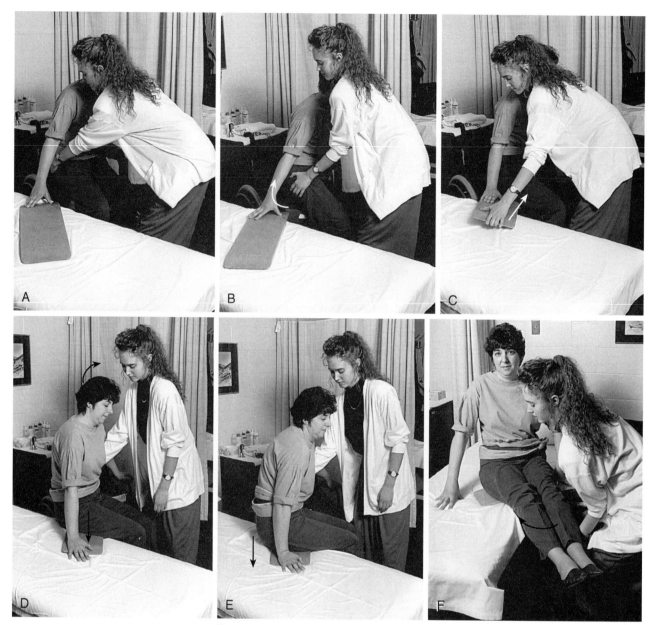

■ **FIGURE 6–14**
Sitting transfer assisted with a sliding board.

He/she repositions the hands and moves farther onto the bed. The patient then stabilizes himself/herself on the edge of the bed, places the lower extremities onto the bed, and lies on the bed. It may be necessary to assist some patients in placing their lower extremities onto the bed and lying on the bed (Fig. 6–15).

The return to the wheelchair is performed using the same techniques in reverse order. The patient should learn to transfer to his/her left and right to maximize his/her independence.

One-Person Lift Transfer The one-person lift transfer can be used when a patient is unable to stand or is unable to perform any type of sliding board

transfer and when the assistant is sufficiently strong and skilled to perform the lift. The caregiver must use proper body mechanics and perform the lift over the shortest possible distance (Fig. 6–16).

Movement From the Wheelchair to a Low Bed, Mat, Plinth, or Toilet *Caution:* If you have not been taught how to perform this transfer or have not practiced it with an able-bodied person, do not attempt it with a patient. Position the wheelchair at an angle to and touching the other surface, and apply a safety belt to the patient. Position the caster wheels forward, lock the chair, and remove the patient's feet from the footrests. Elevate the footrests or remove or swing away

PROCEDURE 6 – 4
Sliding Board Transfer

If the bed height can be adjusted, it should be positioned as near the height of the wheelchair seat as possible before the transfer is attempted.

1. Bed to wheelchair
   a. Position the wheelchair at an angle next to the bed, facing the foot of the bed and opposite the patient's hips; lock the chair, remove the armrest nearest the bed, and swing away the front rigging.
   b. Assist the patient to long sit; apply a safety belt, and assist him/her in moving to the edge of the mattress. The lower extremities may be positioned over the edge of the mattress or remain parallel to the edge of the mattress.
   c. Position one end of the sliding board under the patient's upper thighs and buttocks; the other end should rest on the chair seat. Position yourself slightly in front and to the near side of the patient to guard and protect him/her throughout the transfer.
   d. Assist him/her in moving across the board and onto the chair seat. Guard and protect him/her if the lower extremities need to be lowered from the mattress and when the board is removed.
   e. Place his/her feet on the footrests; position him/her for safety and comfort, and remove the safety belt.

2. Wheelchair to bed
   a. Position the chair at an angle next to the bed, facing the foot of the bed and midway between the head and foot of the bed. Lock the chair, and remove the armrest nearest the bed. Swing away the front rigging.
   b. Assist the patient in moving forward in the chair. Place one end of the board under his/her thighs and buttocks; the other end should rest on the mattress. Position yourself slightly in front and to one side of him/her to guard and protect him/her.
   c. Assist him/her in moving across the board onto the mattress; his/her legs may dangle over the edge of the mattress, or they may be lifted onto the mattress. Guard and protect him/her when the lower extremities are placed onto the mattress.
   d. Remove the board; assist him/her to move toward the center of the mattress and to lie down.
   e. Position him/her for safety and comfort, and remove the safety belt.

the front rigging, and place the feet on the floor. Remove the armrest nearest to the object to which the patient is to be transferred and move him/her forward to the front of the chair.

Stand in front of the patient, flex your hips and knees, and position your knees and feet on the outside but next to the patient's knees and feet. Lift his/her thighs and hold them between your knees or lower thighs so his/her feet are off the floor. Flex the patient's trunk with his/her head positioned on the side of your hip that is on the side opposite to the di-

rection of the transfer; the arms should be folded in the lap or across the chest (see Fig. 6–16*A,B*).

Grasp the safety belt on each side of the patient, and lift him/her from the chair. Pivot your body, and turn the patient's buttocks toward the transfer object (see Fig. 6–16*C,D*). Lower the patient onto the transfer object, place the feet on the floor, and straighten him/her to an upright, sitting position. Be certain to protect him/her while sitting and then reposition as necessary.

The return to the wheelchair is performed using the same techniques in reverse order. *Caution:* Do not

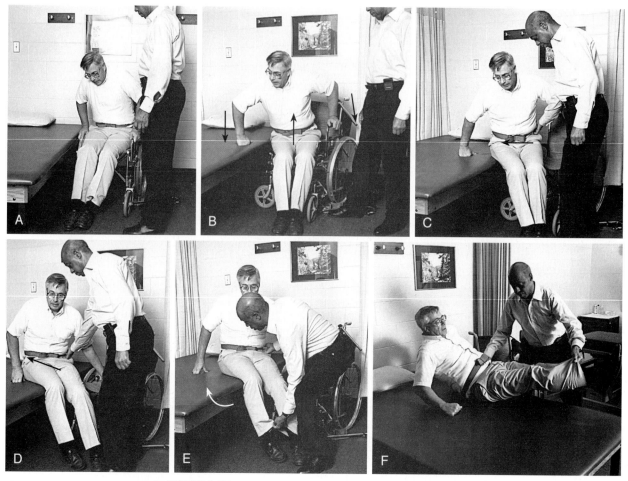

■ **FIGURE 6–15**
Sitting transfer with an independent lateral/swinging movement.

leave the patient sitting unattended on the edge of the bed, mat, or plinth. If you have returned the patient into the wheelchair, be certain the hips are repositioned back on the seat so he/she will be supported by the chair back.

Two-Person Lift Transfer The two-person lift transfer can be used when the patient is unable to stand, when the transfer is performed from two surfaces of unequal height, or when the patient is unable to assist with the transfer. The use of proper body mechanics for the persons performing the lift is extremely important. Each person should mentally review and plan how he/she will perform the lift, and one person must assume the role of the leader. The leader will instruct the patient and the other person so all three can work together. The transfer procedure should be explained to the patient, and he/she should understand what is planned and what to expect. This information should be provided before performing any of the lifting transfers to reduce possible fears or apprehensions the patient may have.

Movement From the Wheelchair to a Bed or Mat
Position and lock the wheelchair as described previ-

ously. The armrest nearest to the bed/mat should be removed only if it is higher than the surface of the bed/mat. The taller and stronger person stands behind the chair, and the other person removes the patient's lower extremities from the footrests and swings away or removes the front rigging. The person standing behind the patient reaches through the patient's axillae, grasps the patient's opposite forearms with his/her hands, and folds the patient's forearms over the abdomen (Fig. 6–17). (*Note:* A safety belt can be used instead of the patient's forearms, but it must be secured tightly and firmly below the flair of the rib cage so it will not slip upward when the lift occurs.) The other person stands facing the outer side of the patient's lower extremities. He/she stoops and places one forearm under the patient's distal thigh and the other forearm under the patient's lower leg and extends the patient's knees.

The person standing behind the patient instructs him/her to push down and hold the position with the shoulder muscles. The other person is instructed when to lift (e.g., "One, two, three, lift"; "Ready, lift"; "Prepare to lift"; "Lift"), and the two persons lift at the same time and place the patient onto the near side of

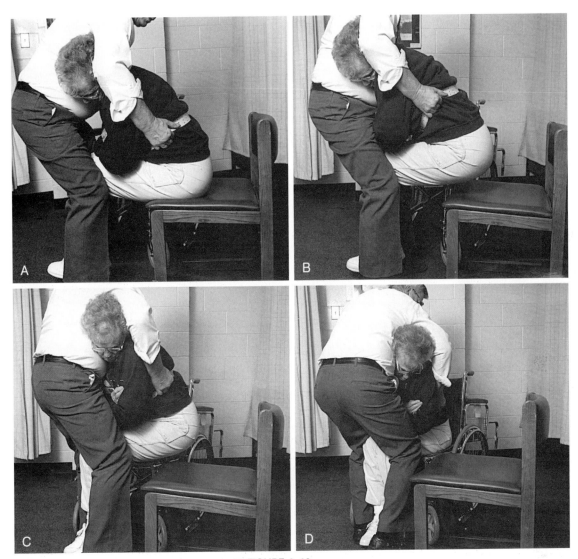

■ FIGURE 6–16
One-person lift transfer.

the bed/mat. The patient is maintained in an upright position (long sitting position) by the person at the patient's back while the other person moves the wheelchair. The patient is positioned in the center of the bed/mat by both persons and is assisted to recline onto the bed/mat (Procedure 6–5).

Alternative Method There are several other two-person lifts that can be used depending on the size of the patient and the strength of the persons who will perform the lift. This alternative method distributes the patient's weight more equally but requires the patient to be lifted and carried over a longer distance than the previous lift. It also requires the assistants to step and turn while carrying the patient. The wheelchair is positioned and locked either parallel to and approximately 2 feet from the head of the bed or facing the center of the bed approximately three feet from the side of the bed, with both armrests and the front rigging removed (Fig. 6–18).

The persons doing the lift approach the patient

from each side. Each lifter uses one forearm to cradle the patient's thighs while the other upper extremity crosses the patient's posterior upper trunk and grasps the other lifter's forearm. The patient's upper extremities are placed over each lifter's upper back or shoulders. One person gives the command to lift, and the lifters walk forward, away from the chair, carrying the patient. They then turn so that the patient's back is toward the bed and move backward toward the bed. The patient is seated on the edge of the bed, assisted to a supine position, and centered in the bed. *Caution:* Do not allow the patient to sit unattended or unsupported.

Movement From the Bed or Mat to the Wheelchair
The patient is moved toward the near edge of the bed/mat, and the wheelchair is positioned and locked as described previously.

One person elevates the patient's trunk so that he/she is in a long sitting position, and the patient's forearms are grasped as described previously. The

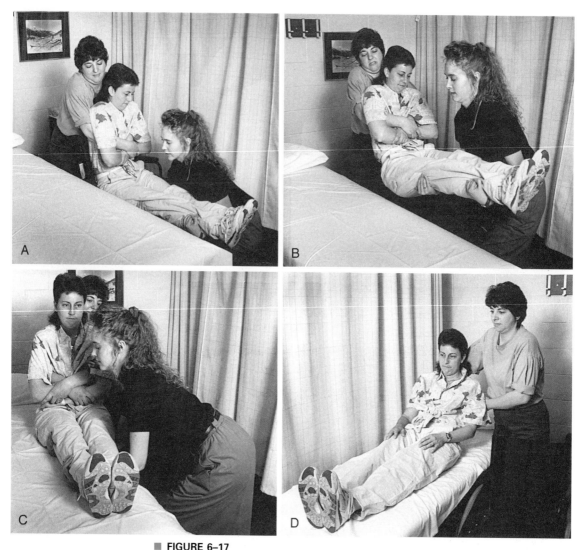

■ **FIGURE 6–17**
Two-person lift transfer from the wheelchair to the bed.

other person cradles the patient's lower extremities as described previously, keeping the patient's knees straight. One person gives the command to lift, and the patient is transferred to the wheelchair. *Caution:* Both persons performing the transfer must use proper body mechanics to lower the patient into the chair by flexing at the hips and knees and avoiding excessive trunk flexion. Some trunk rotation may be required by the person who stands behind the patient during the lift, so this person must be prepared to pivot using his/her hips and feet to avoid lower back strain. The patient's body is moved to the rear of the chair seat, and his/her feet are repositioned on the footrests. If necessary, a lap or chest belt is applied to protect or stabilize the patient.

Alternative Method The wheelchair is positioned as described previously, and the patient is positioned sitting on the edge of the bed with the lifters positioned on each side of the patient.

The patient is supported by the lifters as described previously. One lifter gives the command to

lift, and the patient is lifted and carried to the wheelchair. The patient is lowered into the chair and positioned as described previously. The lifters must use proper body mechanics to lower the patient into the chair. The armrests and front rigging are replaced, and a lap or chest strap is applied, if necessary, to protect or stabilize the patient.

Movement From the Chair to the Floor Position the wheelchair parallel to the area on the floor to which the patient is to be transferred. One person stands behind the patient, and other person stands at the near side of the lower extremities. The patient is lifted from the chair as described previously, and the lifters move sideward away from the chair. On command, both lifters stoop to lower the patient to the floor (Fig. 6–19A–D). *Caution:* The lifters must flex their hips and knees and avoid trunk flexion as the patient is lowered to the floor. The patient is assisted to a lying position or maintains a sitting position, using the upper extremities to form a tripod with the hips.

PROCEDURE 6 – 5
Two-Person Lift Transfer

1. Wheelchair to bed
   a. Position the wheelchair parallel to the side and midway between the head and foot of the bed, and lock the chair. Lift the foot plates or swing away front rigging; remove the armrest nearest the bed.
   b. One person stands behind the wheelchair, the patient crosses his/her arms over his/her abdomen, and the person reaches through the axillae and grasps the patient's lower forearms near the wrists.
   c. A second person stoops/squats at the side of the patient's lower extremities, facing the bed; he/she places one forearm under the thighs and one forearm under the lower legs to cradle the lower extremities.
   d. On command from the person standing behind the patient, the two persons simultaneously lift and place the patient on the near side of the mattress; the patient's knees should be straight during the lift.
   e. The two persons partially lift the patient and place him/her in the center of the mattress; the person holding the patient's forearms assists him/her to lie back.

Note: If the bed height can be adjusted, it should be lowered as near the height of the wheelchair seat as possible before the transfer is attempted.

2. Bed to wheelchair
   a. Move the patient to the near edge of the bed. Position the wheelchair parallel to the bed and opposite the patient's hips, lock the chair, lift the foot plates or swing away the front rigging, and remove the armrest nearest the bed.
   b. Elevate the patient's trunk so he/she is long sitting; guard and protect him/her.
   c. One person stands behind the patient; the patient crosses his/her arms over his/her abdomen, and the person reaches through the axillae and grasps the patient's lower forearms near the wrists.
   d. A second person stands at the side of the patient's lower extremities, facing the bed; he/she places one forearm under the thighs and one forearm under the lower legs to cradle the lower extremities.
   e. On command from the person standing behind the patient, the two persons simultaneously lift and lower the patient into the wheelchair; the patient's knees should be straight during the transfer. The person holding the lower extremities must stoop/squat to lower the patient.
   f. The front rigging is replaced or the front plates are lowered, and the patient's feet are placed on the footrests.
   g. The patient's position is adjusted for safety and comfort as necessary.

Note: If the bed height can be adjusted, it should be lowered to as near the height of the wheelchair seat as possible before the transfer is attempted.

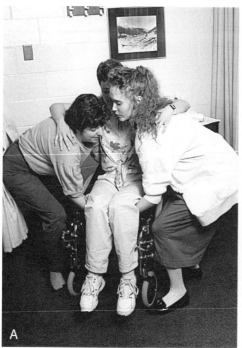
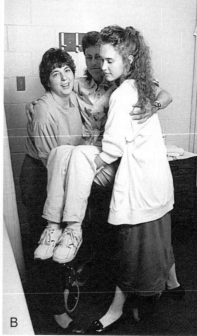
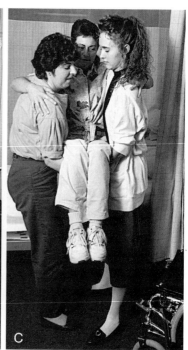

■ **FIGURE 6–18**
Two-person lift transfer (alternative method).

To return the patient to the chair, he/she is placed in a long sitting position. The two lifters stoop and grasp the patient as described previously. On command, the lifters stand simultaneously to lift the patient; then they step toward the chair. The patient is lowered into the chair and properly positioned.

Three-Person Lift Transfer The three-person lift transfer can be used to transfer a patient from one flat surface to another (e.g., from a wheeled stretcher to a bed, or vice versa) while leaving the patient supine. The two stronger and taller of the three persons should be positioned at the patient's head, shoulders, and pelvis. The third person is positioned to control the lower extremities. One person becomes the leader to instruct and give commands to the lifters.

Proper body mechanics must be used to prevent possible injury to the lifters. They should flex their hips and knees before lifting, and when lowering the patient, they should be close to the patient and cradle the patient's body in their arms by flexing their elbows to use short lever arms when lifting or lowering the patient.

Movement From the Bed to the Stretcher The stretcher is positioned and locked at a right angle to the bed with either the foot of the stretcher nearest to the head of the bed or the head of the stretcher nearest to the foot of the bed.

The lifters place their upper extremities under the patient's head and upper trunk, just above and below the pelvis and under the upper thigh and lower leg to maintain the knees straight (Fig. 6–20*A*). The patient is moved to the near edge of the bed with his/her upper extremities positioned along the sides of the body. Moving the patient close to the near edge of the bed will allow the lifters to use their upper extremities as short lever arms and will position the patient's COG closer to their COGs. The leader commands the lifters to roll the patient so he/she is in a side-lying position and cradled in their flexed elbows (Fig. 6–20*B*). Next, the leader commands the lifters to lift the patient, keeping him/her on one side; to step back from the bed; to pivot so the patient's back is toward the other surface onto which he/she is to be placed; and to sidestep to carry the patient to the stretcher (Fig. 6–20*C*). The lifters should use short steps and should sidestep rather than use a crossover step to avoid stepping on another person's foot. Once the patient is positioned over the stretcher, the leader commands the lifters to lower the patient by flexing their hips and knees until their elbows contact the stretcher top (Fig. 6–20*D*). The patient should remain in a side-lying position until the lifters' elbows contact the top of the stretcher (Fig. 6–20*E*). The leader commands the lifters to slowly release their elbows to position the patient supine onto the stretcher. The patient is properly positioned toward the center of the stretcher, and side rails or body straps are applied, if necessary, to protect or stabilize the patient.

Movement From the Stretcher to the Bed The process described previously is performed in reverse sequence. It is important to properly position the stretcher in relation to the bed or item to which

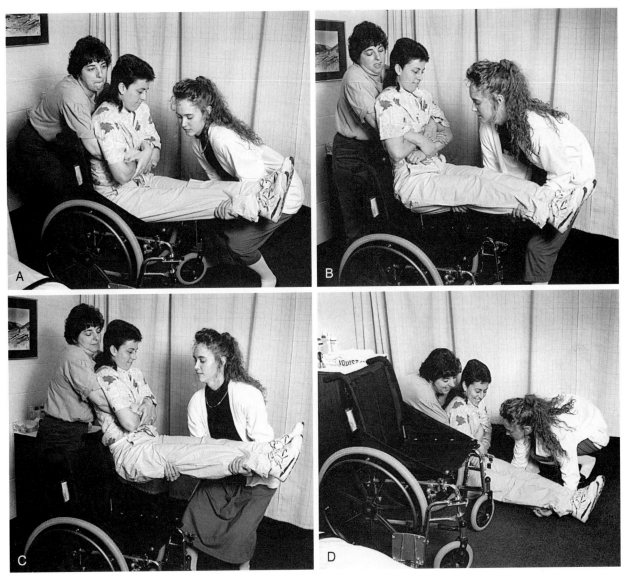

■ **FIGURE 6–19**
Two-person lift transfer from the wheelchair to the floor.

the patient is to be transferred before lifting the patient (Procedure 6–6).

MECHANICAL EQUIPMENT

When a large or very dependent patient needs to be lifted and transported, a hydraulic or pneumatic lift may be the safest and most effective device to use. This device has a "U"-shaped base supported by four caster wheels, at least two of which usually can be locked. A tubular metal support column is attached to the base, which contains the controls for the adjustable lift column with its attached overhead spreader bar (Fig. 6–21A). A body seat or wide support slings can be attached to the adjustable overhead bar by chains or web straps, which are sewn directly or attached to the

seat or slings by metal "S"-shaped hooks. The base can be narrowed for storage or widened to increase its support or to allow it to be positioned around a wheelchair or the end of a bathtub. A long control lever attached to the base of the lift is used to widen or narrow the base (Fig. 6–21B).

A valve on the tubular support column controls the release or containment of air or fluid from a closed chamber (cylinder). When the valve is closed (tightened), the adjustable bar is raised by using a handle to compress the air or hydraulic fluid in the chamber (Fig. 6–21C). This raises the adjustable bar and elevates the patient. When the valve is opened (loosened), the adjustable bar will descend to lower the patient as the air or fluid pressure is released. The amount the valve is opened will affect the rate of descent of the patient and will be dependent on the weight of the patient. It is important to remember to

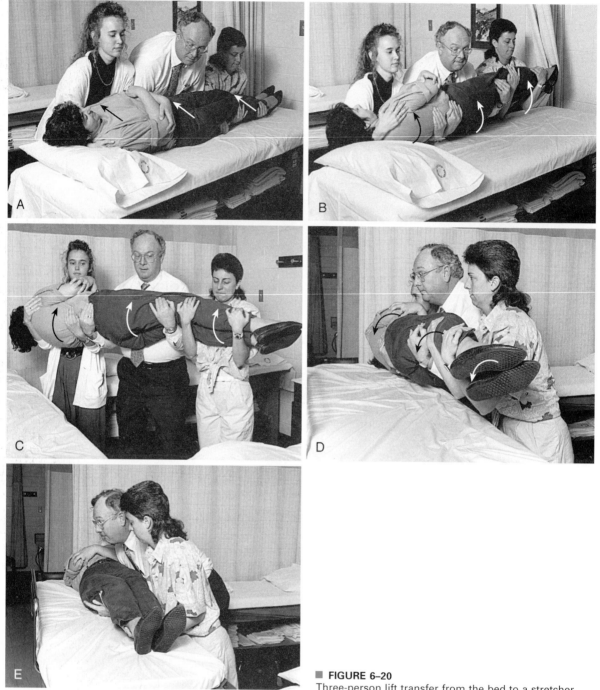

■ **FIGURE 6–20**
Three-person lift transfer from the bed to a stretcher.

close the valve whenever the patient is elevated and when the unit is not in use. *Caution:* When the patient has been lowered to the proper level, the valve must be closed to prevent the adjustable bar from continuing to descend and striking the patient's head.

This device is very safe for one person to use to lift and transfer a very large (up to 250- to 300-pound) patient or a patient who is extremely dependent, providing the device is operated correctly.

Transfer From the Bed to the Wheelchair Roll the patient onto one side and slide the slings under the upper trunk and thighs. Next, roll the patient onto his/her other side, and pull the slings completely under the body so that the sling attachments are exposed, with the seams of the sling on the outside of the sling, directed away from the patient (Fig. 6–22*A*–*C*).

Position the base of the lift perpendicular to the patient and the edge of the bed and with the spreader bar directed across the patient's upper body. *Caution:* Be certain the valve that controls the adjustable arm is closed as you position the lift. Open the valve and carefully lower the adjustable arm so that the spreader

P R O C E D U R E   6 – 6
Three-Person Lift Transfer

1. Bed to a new support surface (e.g., stretcher, cart, tilt table)
   a. Position the head of the new support surface perpendicular (i.e., at a right angle) to the foot of the bed; move the patient close to the near edge of the bed.
   b. One of the stronger lifters slides his/her forearms under the patient's head and upper trunk; another strong lifter slides his/her forearms under the patient just below the pelvis; and the third lifter slides his/her forearms under the thighs and lower legs near the ankles.
   c. On command from the lifter at the head of the patient, roll the patient to a side-lying position.
   d. On command from the lifter at the patient's head lift the patient; cradle his/her body between your forearms and upper arms.
   e. Carry the patient to the stretcher, treatment table, or tilt table using short side steps.
   f. On command from the lifter at the patient's head, lower the patient to the new support surface by bending your knees and hips; keep the body cradled until your elbows rest on the support surface.
   g. On command, lower your forearms to the support surface to place the patient flat.
   h. Move the patient toward the center of the support surface; position him/her for comfort and safety, and apply security straps, pillows, towel rolls, and so on as necessary.

2. Return to bed
   a. Reverse the sequence of the transfer from bed to a new support surface to return the patient to the bed.

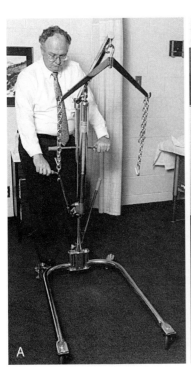
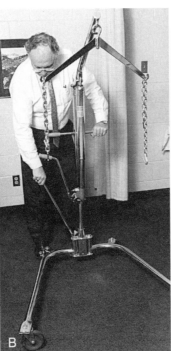
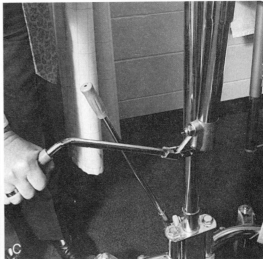

■ **FIGURE 6–21**
Mechanical lift to transfer large or very dependent patients.

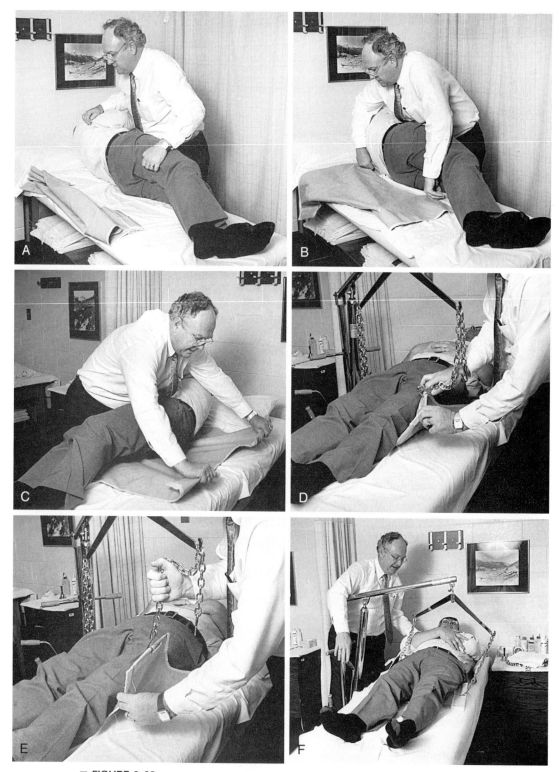

■ **FIGURE 6–22**

A through K, Transfer from the bed to the wheelchair using a hydraulic lift device.

bar is close enough to the patient to attach the sling (Fig. 6–22D). *Be certain to close the valve when the proper position of the adjustable arm is attained.*

Apply the rings of the web strap or the "S" hook of the chain to the sling. The shortest segment of the chain or web strap should be attached to the upper part of the sling, and the longest segment should be attached to the lower part of the sling. These positions will ensure that the patient will be lifted into a sitting position. The open end of the "S" hook should be directed away from the patient to prevent injury to the skin (Fig. 6–22E).

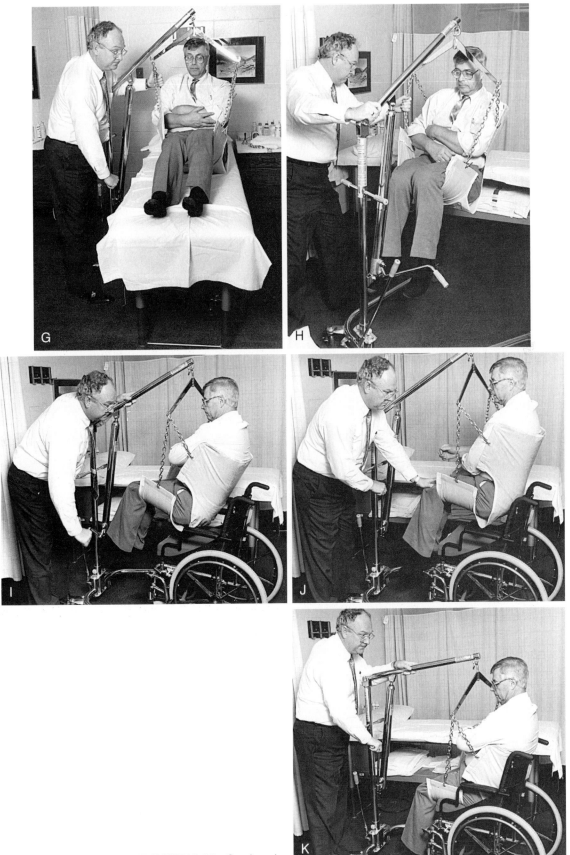

■ **FIGURE 6–22** *Continued*

PROCEDURE 6 – 7
Mechanical Lift Transfer

1. Bed to wheelchair

   a. Explain the activity to the patient the first time it is performed.

   b. Place the sling or slings under the upper trunk and buttocks and upper thighs by rolling him/her onto one side and then onto the other side.

   c. Position the lift perpendicular and close to the bed with the spreader bar over the chest; attach the chains or web straps to the spreader bar.

   d. Partially open the control valve to slowly lower the spreader bar until the chains or web straps can be attached to the sling or slings. *Close the valve* so the spreader bar does not continue to lower.

   e. Attach the chains or web straps to the sling or slings; attach the shorter segment of the chains or web straps to the trunk sling. When "S" hooks are used, they should be directed away from the body.

   f. Adjust the sling or slings and attachments as necessary; fold his/her arms onto the chest, and elevate him/her using the pump handle.

   g. Check all attachments and the position of the sling or slings; continue to elevate him/her until the buttocks are off the mattress.

   h. Move the lift away from the bed using the cross handles on the center post. The knees can be allowed to flex or be supported by the caregiver; maintain the patient within the base of the lift.

   i. Transport the patient to the wheelchair. Turn him/her so his/her back is toward the front of the chair; position the buttocks over the center of the chair seat.

   j. Partially open the control valve to slowly lower him/her into the chair; move his/her body toward the back of the seat by pushing on the knees before the buttocks contact the seat. *Close the valve* as soon as he/she is seated.

   k. Remove the chains or web straps from the sling or slings, but leave the sling or slings in place so he/she can be transferred back to the bed at a later time.

2. Wheelchair to bed

   a. Reverse the sequence of the activities of the transfer from the bed to chair. Position patient on mattress; remove sling(s).

   b. Be certain to check the position of the sling or slings and security of the chains or web straps before lifting the patient from the chair.

   c. Remember to close the valve after the spreader bar has been positioned to attach or remove the chains or web straps.

Before you attempt to lift the patient, check all the attachments, fold his/her arms over the abdomen, and check the position of the slings (Fig. 6–22F). Caution the patient not to reach for or grasp the spreader bar as he/she is raised. Elevate the patient until the buttocks clear the surface of the bed; re-evaluate his/her position, the location of the slings, and the security of the attachments before you move him/her away from the bed (Fig. 6–22G). Continue to elevate the patient and assist him/her by moving the lower extremities from the bed so he/she is sitting properly in the slings. The knees can be allowed to flex or can be kept extended as you carefully move the lift away from the side of the bed; then turn the patient to face the support column (Fig. 6–22H). Transport the patient to the wheelchair by using the cross handles on the support column. *Caution:* Be certain the floor is free of objects and there is sufficient space to maneuver the lift. Objects that could interfere with or block the caster wheels from moving smoothly, such as a throw rug, a door threshold, or a line cord, should be avoided. Maneuver the patient so that his/her buttocks are over the front or the middle of the seat of the locked wheelchair and open the valve to lower him/her into the chair (Fig. 6–22I). As the patient is lowered, you may need to push against the knees to position the hips back into the chair (Fig. 6–22K). *Caution:* Be certain to close the valve as soon as the patient is properly positioned in the chair so the adjustable bar does not continue to lower and strike the patient's head.

Remove the sling attachments and move the lift away from the chair; however, the slings remain under the patient so that he/she can be transferred back to bed at a later time. If the slings are removed, they will be difficult to reposition under the patient while he/she is sitting. Position his/her feet on the footrests, and apply a lap or chest strap, if necessary, to protect or stabilize the patient (Procedure 6–7).

Movement From the Wheelchair to the Bed Transfer from the wheelchair to the bed is accomplished by reversing the sequence described for transferring the patient from the bed to the wheelchair. After the patient has returned to his/her bed, the slings are removed.

It will be helpful to have multiple slings available if this equipment is to be used for several patients. In addition, it will be necessary to launder the slings periodically, and therefore, more than one sling should be available to use when one of them is being laundered.

Patients are apt to be apprehensive the first few times this device is used. To help overcome any fear or apprehension, explain the procedure to the patient and provide information about the safety of the unit prior to using it. It may be helpful to allow the patient to observe the unit being used for another person before it is used for him/her.

OTHER TYPES OF TRANSFERS

Movement From Stretcher to Bed or Bed to Stretcher, Totally Dependent Patient When the two surfaces are approximately the same height, position the stretcher parallel to and touching one edge of the bed. *Caution:* Be certain the stretcher and the bed are locked or secured so they will not separate during the transfer.

If the stretcher has a loose pad, slide it and the patient onto the bed and then remove the pad; if a draw sheet is available, use it to slide the patient from the stretcher onto the bed.

The patient can be rolled from the stretcher toward you onto the bed, or you can segmentally slide the patient from the stretcher to the bed, as you kneel on the bed using your forearms to support under the patient to avoid skin irritation.

Caution: Extreme care must be used when any of these techniques are attempted, as the stretcher and bed could separate and the patient could fall. Another person may be needed to hold the two objects together or to assist with the transfer.

Caution: You are advised not to use bed linen to lift and carry a patient from one object to another because the linen could tear and the patient could fall. This technique should be used only in an emergency when no other technique is possible or when the situation requires a rapid transfer. It is relatively safe to use a sheet to transfer a patient by sliding because even if the sheet tears, the patient remains supported by a firm surface. Do not use this technique if there are contraindications to sliding the patient or when the shear forces associated with sliding are apt to cause skin irritation.

Standing Transfer, Assisted, for a Total Hip Replacement Patient There are special precautions or considerations that should be used with a patient after surgery for a total hip replacement. Each surgeon will have instructions or preferences for the amount of weight bearing and the movement activities to be permitted and the alignment of the trunk in relation to the surgically replaced hip. The person who assists the patient must be aware of these specific precautions, instructions, and preferences. Most of the precautions or contraindications are designed to reduce the possibility of hip dislocation during the first 10 to 14 days of postoperative care. Some of the generally and widely accepted precautions or contraindications for this patient condition are listed in Box 6–3.

Precautions for Patients With a Total Hip Replacement

1. Maintain the surgically replaced hip slightly abducted from the midline of the body and in neutral rotation (patella and toes positioned toward ceiling) when the patient is supine. The hip should not be adducted beyond the midline of the body when the patient lies, sits, or stands.

2. Maintain the surgically replaced hip in neutral extension. The hip should not be extended beyond a midposition of flexion and extension.

3. Maintain hip abduction and neutral rotation while the patient is in a side-lying position by supporting the affected lower extremity on pillows, powder board, or a bolster. The affected extremity should be in the uppermost position.

4. Avoid external hip rotation when an anterior or anterior-lateral surgical approach was used.

5. Avoid internal hip rotation when a posterior or posterior-lateral surgical approach was used.

6. Avoid rotating or twisting the upper body with the lower extremity fixed or immobile (e.g., as when reaching for an object on a bedside stand while lying in bed) because such activity indirectly causes hip rotation.

7. Avoid hip flexion beyond 60 to 90 degrees when a posterior or posterior-lateral surgical approach was used. This means the patient should not sit erect in a wheelchair or in bed, because bringing the trunk closer to the thigh, rather than bringing the thigh toward the trunk, creates hip flexion.

8. Avoid excessive trunk flexion while the patient is sitting, because this indirectly causes hip flexion. An elevated toilet seat and an elevated chair seat should be used for most patients.

Movement From the Bed to a Walker A walker is frequently used initially for hip replacement patients to improve stability and support, although bilateral axillary crutches may also be used. Before allowing the patient to stand, measure and adjust the walker for the patient, apply a safety belt, apply footwear, lock the bed, adjust the height of the bed slightly higher than its lowest position, and partially elevate the head of the bed to assist the patient to come to sitting before standing. Instruct the patient to move to the edge of the bed by using the upper extremities and the normal lower extremity to elevate the body. He/she can move toward the normal lower extremity to maintain the surgically replaced hip in abduction. He/she should maintain the trunk in no more than 60 degrees of flexion by semireclining on his/her arms, which are positioned behind the body. You should help to control the surgically replaced hip and its lower extremity and the trunk as the patient pivots and positions the lower extremities over the edge of bed. Instruct the patient to place the normal foot on the floor as you assist in lowering the surgically affected lower extremity to the floor. The patient maintains a semireclining position of the trunk by resting on the extended upper extremities, which are placed posterior to his/her hips. *Caution:* The patient may need to sit on the edge of the bed for a short time to avoid dizziness or syncope and to accommodate to being upright before standing. Do not allow the patient to sit unattended or unprotected.

Instruct the patient to push up from the bed, stand, and grasp the hand grips on the walker while you maintain control on the safety belt and shoulder. You may guard or stabilize the patient's normal foot so that it does not slide as he/she stands. The patient maintains his/her balance and takes time to accommodate to standing before ambulating. Monitor the pulse rate and ask the patient about his/her reaction to standing.

Instruct the patient to ambulate using a three-one pattern; instruct him/her to turn by pivoting on the normal lower extremity and stepping around the normal lower extremity with the surgically affected lower extremity. (For example, a patient with a right hip replacement will be taught to turn toward the left.) These procedures are explained in Chapter 8. *Caution:* The patient must not pivot or twist while standing on the surgically affected lower extremity.

Return to Bed Be certain the bed is locked and will not roll; elevate the bed so that it is slightly below the patient's buttocks. Instruct the patient to back toward the bed until the posterior thigh of the normal lower extremity touches the edge of the mattress; the surgically affected lower extremity should remain slightly forward of the opposite lower extremity.

Instruct the patient to reach back with his/her hands to the mattress and shift his/her weight onto the normal lower extremity while allowing the surgically affected lower extremity to slide forward. The patient sits on the edge of the bed in a semireclining position as you control the surgically affected lower extremity.

Instruct the patient to pivot toward the center of the bed, leading with the normal lower extremity and keeping the surgically replaced hip abducted. Assist in controlling the surgically affected lower extremity to maintain abduction and to limit flexion of the hip.

PROCEDURE 6–8
Standing Transfer; One NWB Lower Extremity

Note: NWB = non–weight bearing; FWB = full weight bearing.

1. Bed to wheelchair
   a. Position wheelchair at an angle on the side next to the hip of the FWB lower extremity, facing the foot of the bed; lock the chair, and swing away the front rigging or elevate the foot plates.
   b. Assist the patient in moving to the edge of the mattress and sitting up; apply a safety belt.
   c. Position yourself in front of the patient to guard and protect him/her; assist in moving the NWB extremity to the edge of the mattress. *Caution:* Avoid excessive hip flexion and adduction if the patient has had a total hip replacement.
   d. Assist him/her in standing on the FWB lower extremity; assist in controlling or supporting the NWB lower extremity.
   e. Instruct him/her to reach for and grasp the far armrest of the wheelchair and pivot on the FWB foot to position his/her hips in preparation to sit. Instruct him/her to use the upper extremities and FWB lower extremity to slowly lower his/her body into the chair; maintain control and support of the NWB lower extremity.
   f. Position the NWB lower extremity on an elevated legrest as necessary; place the other foot on the foot plate.
   g. Position him/her for safety and comfort, and remove the safety belt.

2. Wheelchair to bed
   a. Position the wheelchair at an angle next to the bed, facing the foot of the bed and midway between the head and foot of the bed; either lower extremity can be nearest the bed. Lock the chair, swing away the front rigging, and apply a safety belt.
   b. Assist the patient in moving forward in the chair; maintain control and support the NWB lower extremity. Position yourself in front of him/her to guard and protect him/her throughout the transfer.
   c. Instruct him/her to stand by pushing with the upper extremities and FWB lower extremity.
   d. Instruct him/her to pivot so his/her buttocks are toward the bed. Control and support the NWB lower extremity as he/she sits on the edge of the mattress.
   e. Assist in lifting the NWB lower extremity onto the mattress as he/she lifts the FWB lower extremity. *Caution:* Avoid excessive hip flexion and adduction if the patient has had a total hip replacement.
   f. Instruct him/her to move toward the center of the mattress and lie down.
   g. Position him/her for safety and comfort, and remove the safety belt.

The patient uses the normal lower extremity and the upper extremities to shift his/her body toward the center of the bed, while you guide the surgically affected lower extremity, until he/she is properly positioned.

(*Note:* Some patients may return to the center of the bed leading with the surgically affected lower extremity so it moves in abduction. The position of the bed and the ability to have access to either side of the bed may dictate how the return-to-bed transfer is accomplished. If this technique is used, care must be applied to avoid a relative position of adduction of the surgically replaced hip as the normal lower extremity is placed on the bed) (Procedure 6–8).

TRANSFER FROM THE WHEELCHAIR TO THE FLOOR AND RETURN

Initially the patient will need to be protected or guarded by another person using the general guarding principles and techniques described previously. The activity should be practiced in an area free of hazards, and mats may be placed on the floor to protect the patient. Some patients may benefit from the use of incremental steps or small platforms when they initially perform and practice this transfer. Eventually, the patient should be taught how to move down to the floor and return to the chair without any additional equipment, to maximize his/her independence.

Wheelchair to Floor: Strong Right Upper and Lower Extremities and Weak Left Upper and Lower Extremities Instruct the patient to position the caster wheels forward, lock the chair, remove his/her feet from the footrests, and remove or swing away the front rigging or elevate the footrests. The patient moves forward in the chair with the body pivoted or turned slightly so the right extremities are most forward (Fig. 6–23*A*).

Instruct the patient to shift his/her weight onto the right lower extremity and to reach toward the floor with the right upper extremity (Fig. 6–23*B*). When the right hand is on the floor, the patient uses the right upper and lower extremity to lower his/her body to the floor and sit on the right buttock (Fig. 6–23*C*). He/she can adjust the body position as desired.

Floor to Wheelchair: Strong Right Upper and Lower Extremities and Weak Left Upper and Lower Extremities Instruct the patient to sit on the right hip facing the locked wheelchair with its caster wheels forward. The

lower extremities should be flexed at the hips and knees (Fig. 6–24*A*).

Instruct the patient to reach to the back of the seat or the armrest and to pull himself/herself to a kneeling position. The patient moves to a half-kneeling position with the right foot forward and flat on the floor and kneeling on the left knee (Fig. 6–24*B*, *C*). Instruct the patient to place the right upper extremity on the near armrest or on the seat of the chair. The patient uses the right extremities to push to a partial or full standing position facing the wheelchair (Fig. 6–24*D*). *Note:* The caster wheels may pivot or turn to one side when the patient uses the chair for support. That movement does not cause a safety problem, and the patient can continue to perform the transfer. However, the caster wheels should not be permitted to be directed backward during these transfers because that position reduces the stability of the chair. The patient should be informed and taught not to allow the caster wheels to be directed backward or a chair with caster wheel locks may be recommended.

Instruct the patient to reach for the far armrest with the right upper extremity and to pivot on the right lower extremity so his/her back is toward the chair. Then the patient lowers himself/herself into the chair using the right extremities.

Wheelchair to Floor, Forward or Sideward: Strong Upper Extremities and Weak or Paralyzed Lower Extremities Instruct the patient to position the chair with the caster wheels forward, lock the chair, remove his/her feet from the footrests, and remove or swing away the front rigging. The patient moves to the front of the chair, and the lower extremities are positioned to one side with the knees extended or flexed and positioned under the chair.

Instruct the patient to maintain one hand on the

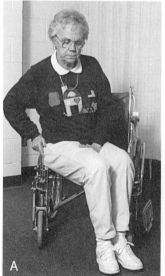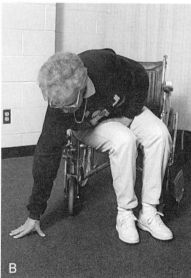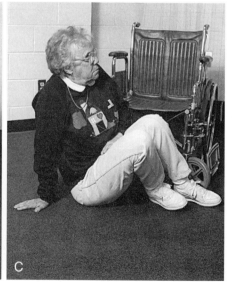

■ **FIGURE 6–23**
Transfer from the wheelchair to the floor for a patient with strong right upper and lower extremities.

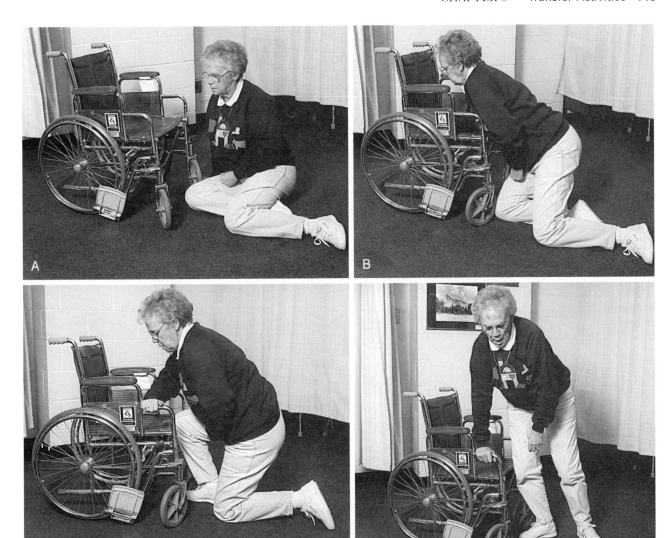

■ **FIGURE 6–24**
A through *D*, Transfer from the floor to the wheelchair for a patient with strong right upper and lower extremities. *Note:* For transfers from the chair to the floor and return to the chair, the caster wheels will probably pivot or turn to one side when the patient uses the chair for support unless the wheels can be locked in the forward position. If the caster wheels pivot, there is no safety problem, and the patient can continue to perform the transfer. However, the patient should not allow the caster wheels to be directed backward because that position reduces the stability of the chair.

armrest or chair seat rail and to reach toward the floor with the other upper extremity while flexing his/her head and trunk (Fig. 6–25*A*). After the hand has contacted the floor, the patient lowers himself/herself onto the floor and releases his/her grasp on the wheelchair (Fig. 6–25*B*). The patient repositions himself/herself as desired.

Floor to Wheelchair Forward: Push-Up, Strong Upper Extremities, Weak or Paralyzed Lower Extremities Instruct the patient to sit on one hip close to and facing the wheelchair with the hips and knees flexed (Fig. 6–26*A–F*). The chair must be locked, the front rigging swung away, and the caster wheels positioned forward or turned to one side. Some patients may prefer to initiate this transfer from an all-fours position (i.e., on hands and knees). Instruct the patient to move to the

front of the chair and to place one hand on the armrest or on the seat (Fig. 6–26*B*). The patient grasps the armrest or the seat of the chair and pulls to a high kneeling position, maintaining his/her balance (Fig. 6–26*C*). Instruct the patient to grasp both armrests or to place one hand on the seat of the chair and one hand on the armrest and then to perform a push-up to elevate the hips above the seat level (Fig. 6–26*D*). At the peak of the lift, he/she pivots so that one hip is over the seat and releases the innermost hand to lower one hip into the chair (Fig. 6–26*E*). The patient repositions the hands on the armrests and performs a push-up to position himself/herself in the chair (Fig. 6–26*F*).

This method requires exceptional upper extremity strength and trunk control, and the patient must

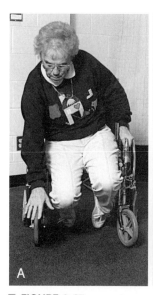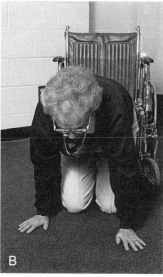

■ **FIGURE 6–25**
Transfer from the wheelchair to the floor, forward, for a patient with strong upper extremities.

have the ability to maintain his/her balance while in a high kneeling and push-up position. However, this is a safe and secure method, and many patients will be able to perform it very efficiently.

Wheelchair to Floor Backward: Strong Upper Extremities, Weak or Paralyzed Lower Extremities Instruct the patient to position and prepare the wheelchair as described previously. Instruct the patient to move to the front of the chair, pivot onto the right or left hip, and grasp the armrests. If he/she is sitting on the right hip, the right hand grasps the left armrest and the left hand grasps the right armrest to rotate the upper body so that he/she now partially faces the back of chair.

Instruct the patient to perform a partial push-up to clear the pelvis from the seat and then to use the upper extremities to lower onto his/her knees in a high kneeling position facing the front of the chair. Then instruct the patient to lower himself/herself to a side-sitting position or onto all fours and then onto one hip.

This method is the reverse of moving from the floor to the chair forward. It requires exceptional upper extremity strength, trunk control, and balance, and the patient must be flexible and agile. Some patients will be able to lift their buttocks onto the front edge of the chair seat using an initial push-up with one hand on the chair seat and one hand on the front rigging. The patient can reverse this method to move from the wheelchair to the floor.

Wheelchair to Floor Forward: Strong Upper Extremities, Weak or Paralyzed Lower Extremities Instruct the patient to position and prepare the wheelchair as described previously. The patient moves forward in the chair and positions his/her feet under the wheelchair by flexing the knees. The front rigging must be swung away or removed before the patient continues.

Instruct the patient to lean forward and to reach toward the floor with both upper extremities so that the hands will contact the floor as he/she falls toward the floor onto all fours (see Fig. 6–25*A*). Alternatively, the patient can reach forward with one hand and grasp the armrest with the other hand; when the first hand is on or close to the floor, he/she releases the armrest, with that hand reaching the floor so that the patient is on all fours. The patient can side sit or alter his/her position as desired.

Alternative Method Instruct the patient to position and prepare the wheelchair as described previously, except that one or both front riggings remain in place with the footrests elevated (Fig. 6–27*A*). The patient moves forward in the chair and positions the lower extremities away from the chair with the knees extended. Instruct the patient to place one hand on the front rigging and one hand on the chair seat; he/she performs a push-up with the upper extremities to elevate the buttocks from the chair seat while extending the head and upper trunk (Fig. 6–27*B*). The patient lowers the body to the floor with the buttocks between the footrests of the front rigging (Fig. 6–27*C*). A patient with wide hips will need to swing away, but not remove, one front rigging to have sufficient space for the hips when they descend to the floor. (*Note:* This method is the reverse of moving from the floor to the wheelchair backward.) The patient must have excellent flexibility in the shoulders and good strength in the upper extremities to perform this technique.

Caution: Many inactive or paralyzed patients may have osteoporosis in their lower extremities and vertebral bodies. Some of these transfer methods may be unsafe for these patients because of the floor reaction force that the patient may experience when he/she drops onto the knees or hip. This force may be sufficient to cause a fracture in weakened bone. Therefore, the patient may need to be assisted down to the floor to avoid injury.

The wheelchair-to-floor-and-return transfer methods described may be interchanged to meet the needs, strength, preference, flexibility, agility, balance, size, and skill of a given patient. For example, a patient may prefer or find it easier to transfer to the floor forward and return to the chair backward, or to transfer to the floor backward and return to the chair forward. The patient should be given the opportunity to attempt any of the methods to determine which is most suitable, safe, and efficient for him/her. Guard and assist the patient during practice sessions and until the patient is able to perform the transfer independently with safety. A safety belt should be used, and

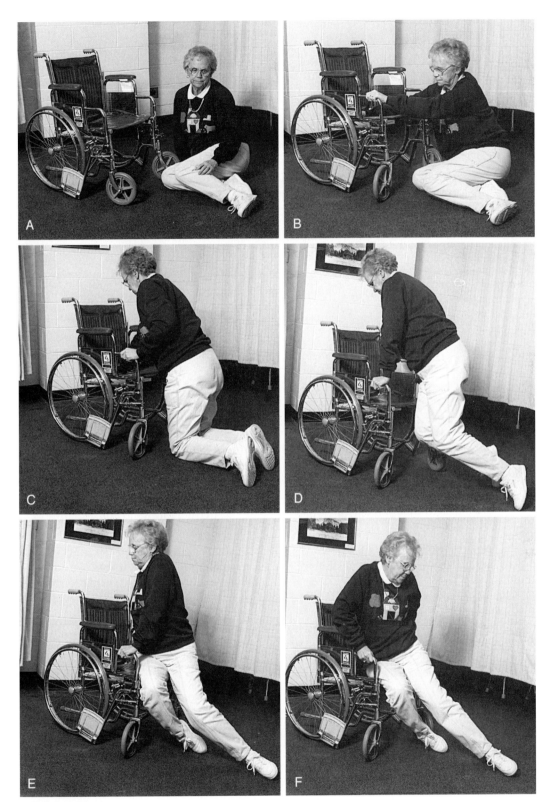

■ **FIGURE 6–26**
Transfer from the floor to the wheelchair, forward push-up, for a patient with strong upper extremities.
The procedure is reversed to move from the wheelchair to the floor. Note: The caster wheels may pivot
during this transfer if they cannot be locked in a forward position. The transfer can be performed safely
provided that the caster wheels do not pivot completely rearward.

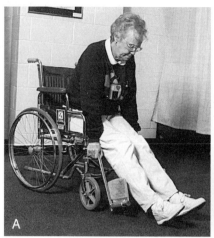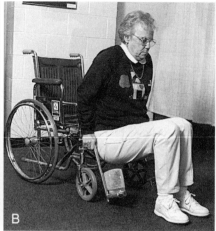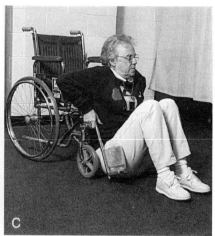

▪ FIGURE 6–27
Transfer from the wheelchair to the floor (alternative method). The procedure is reversed to move from the floor to the wheelchair.

you should not use the patient's clothing or upper extremities to control or guard him/her as these transfers are performed, for the reasons cited elsewhere in this text.

SUMMARY

Transfer activities are necessary to alter a patient's position, move a patient from one surface to another, and promote independent functional activities. Some patients require maximal assistance and will be dependent on other persons or mechanical equipment to perform or complete a transfer. Other patients are able to accomplish their transfers without assistance or with only minimal assistance. Transfers can be performed with the patient lying, standing, or sitting; some patients may need to be lifted by other persons or mechanical equipment. Regardless of the technique used, the caregiver must guard and protect the patient as he/she performs the transfer. A safety belt should be used with all patients when they transfer until they can perform the transfer safely and independently.

The procedures or techniques used to assist or teach the patient will vary depending on his/her condition, abilities, and needs. The philosophy and preferences of the caregiver may also affect the way the transfer is taught or performed. The caregiver and patient may need to problem solve together to develop the most efficient and safest technique for the patient to use. Observing other patients as they perform a specific transfer may assist the patient in understanding how to perform the transfer. Practicing the transfer, using the same technique consistently, should improve the patient's skill and efficiency.

▪ SELF-STUDY/DISCUSSION ACTIVITIES

1. Describe five different types of transfers.
2. Explain the rationale for teaching a patient bed mobility activities.
3. Describe at least five specific precautions that should be followed when transferring a patient who has recently undergone a total hip replacement.
4. Explain the wheelchair positions you might use for a standing and a sliding board transfer and indicate why these positions are necessary and important for the transfer.
5. Demonstrate two different methods to move from a wheelchair to the floor and return for a person with lower extremity paralysis.
6. Describe how you would reduce friction between a patient's body and the surface of the bed/mat; center the patient's weight; reduce the effects of gravity; and use gravity as an assistive force.

Wheelchair Features and Activities

After studying this chapter, the reader will be able to:

1 List the standard measurements for an adult wheelchair.

2 Measure a patient for a wheelchair and confirm the fit of the chair.

3 Teach a person to propel a wheelchair using both upper extremities or one upper extremity and one lower extremity.

4 Name the components of a standard wheelchair and describe the purpose of each.

5 Teach a wheelchair user various functional activities.

6 Perform various wheelchair functional activities with a person in the chair by providing plus-one assistance.

■ ■ ■ ■ K E Y   T E R M S

Condyle: A rounded projection on a bone.

Crash bar: The metal bar on a door that disengages the door latch when it is pushed.

Dependent: Requiring some level or type of assistance, which may be human or mechanical.

Descend: To go down; proceed from a higher to a lower level.

Femoral: Pertaining to the femur (thigh bone).

Independent: Able to function or perform without assistance from another.

Locomotion: The ability to move from one place to another.

Pedal: Pertaining to the foot or feet.

Pneumatic: Of or containing air or gases.

Popliteal: Pertaining to the area behind the knee.

Propulsion: The act of propelling; movement of a wheelchair by the person in the chair or by another person.

Restraint: The forcible confinement or restriction of movement of a person through the use of belts, straps, or other similar items.

Self-closing device: A device attached to a door that closes the door through the use of compressed fluid or air.

Semipneumatic: Partially containing air or gases.

INTRODUCTION

Persons who use a wheelchair as their primary mode of mobility should have a chair that fits properly to provide maximum function, comfort, stability, safety, and protection of body structures. The initial measurement and subsequent confirmation of fit must be done carefully. Information about special seating needs, chairs designed for special activities (e.g., chairs for recreation or sports participation), or chairs designed to fulfill special patient needs is not presented. However, it may be important to consider whether the person will require a cushion, a reclining back, an elevating or swing-away front rigging (leg rests), adjustable armrests, or other similar adaptations.

The type of wheelchair selected and its components will depend on the patient's disability, functional ability, size, weight, and functional needs or activities; the expected use of the chair; and the prognosis for change in the patient's condition. Proper fit of the chair becomes more important if the patient has decreased sensory awareness; limited ability to alter his/her position; decreased subcutaneous soft tissue, espe-

Table 7–1 TYPES OF WHEELCHAIRS	
Type	**Description**
Standard adult	Designed for persons who weigh less than 200 pounds and for limited use on rough surfaces or for vigorous functional activities.
Heavy-duty adult	Constructed for persons weighing more than 200 pounds or those who perform vigorous functional activities.
Intermediate or junior	Designed for persons with a body build smaller than an adult but larger than a child.
Growing	Designed to permit adjustments in the frame to accommodate the growth of the user.
Child or youth	Designed for persons up to the approximate age of 6 years.
Indoor	Constructed for use indoors, with the larger drive wheels placed at the front of the chair and the caster wheels at the rear. It functions better in confined areas but is more difficult to propel or for the user to perform many functional activities.
"Hemiplegic"	The seat is lowered approximately 2 inches to allow better use of the user's lower extremities to propel the chair; however, the lower seat may make it more difficult for the user to perform a standing transfer.
Amputee	The rear wheel axles are positioned approximately 2 inches posterior to their normal position to widen the base of support of the chair and compensate for the loss of the weight of the user's lower extremities.
One-hand drive	Two handrims are fabricated on one drive wheel, and the two drive wheels are connected by a linkage bar. The smaller handrim propels the near drive wheel; the large handrim propels the far drive wheel; and when both rims are moved simultaneously, both wheels are propelled.
Externally powered	The chair is propelled by a deep-cycle battery system, and there are various types of controls to operate the chair (e.g., joystick, chin piece, or mouth stick).
Sports	A low-profile chair with features such as a low back, canted rear wheels, small handrims, and adjustable axles. It can be used for various sports activities, and some users prefer this type of chair for day-to-day activities.
Reclining	Used for persons who need to partially or fully recline at some time when they are in the chair. The chair may be a semireclining or fully reclining chair. Semireclining chairs recline to approximately 30 degrees from vertical, and fully reclining chairs can recline to a horizontal position. Elevating leg rests and headrest extensions are necessary components for these chairs.

Factors Associated With the Selection of a Wheelchair Type and Components

1. Patient's disability and functional ability.
2. Patient's age, size, stature, and weight.
3. Expected use or patient needs of the wheelchair (e.g., indoors, outdoors, recreation, transfer needs, ability to transport the chair).
4. Temporary versus permanent use of the wheelchair.
5. Potential or prognosis for change in the patient's condition, especially as it affects his/her mobility.
6. Mental and physical condition or capacity of the patient.

cially over bony prominences; impaired peripheral circulation in the lower extremities; or abnormal skin integrity or condition, or if the chair is required for use for extended periods of time. Any of these factors individually or in combination could cause a serious secondary problem or complication for the patient (Box 7–1).

There are several wheelchair types and designs (Table 7–1). The more common or frequently prescribed types are described briefly. Product and accessory catalogs can be obtained from the manufacturers of wheelchairs. These catalogs will contain information about the styles and types of wheelchairs each company manufactures.

STANDARD WHEELCHAIR MEASUREMENTS

The initial measurements should be made with the user seated on a firm, flat surface such as a wood chair or on a piece of plywood placed on a mat platform. The user should wear clothing similar to the clothing he/she will usually wear. The person should sit with the trunk erect in a comfortable position and posture. If a seat cushion or back rest (e.g., a cushion or posture panel) is going to be used, it should be in place when the measurements are made. A tape measure that can be read easily is recommended to measure the person (Table 7–2).

The patient's age, weight, disability, or condition; the expected use of the chair; the functional and recreational activities to be performed; and specific fea-

Table 7–2 STANDARD WHEELCHAIR MEASUREMENTS FOR PROPER FIT

Measurement	Instructions	Average Adult Size
Seat height/leg length	Measure from the user's heel to the popliteal fold and add 2 inches to allow clearance of the footrest.	19.5 to 20.5 inches
Seat depth	Measure from the user's posterior buttock, along the lateral thigh, to the popliteal fold; then subtract approximately 2 inches to avoid pressure from the front edge of the seat against the popliteal space.	16 inches
Seat width	Measure the widest aspect of the user's buttocks, hips, or thighs and add approximately 2 inches. This will provide space for bulky clothing, orthoses, or clearance of the trochanters from the armrest side panel.	18 inches
Back height	Measure from the seat of the chair to the floor of the axilla with the user's shoulder flexed to 90 degrees and then subtract approximately 4 inches. This will allow the final back height to be below the inferior angles of the scapulae. (*Note:* This measurement will be affected if a seat cushion is to be used. The person should be measured while seated on the cushion or the thickness of the cushion must be considered by adding that value to the actual measurement.)	16 to 16.5 inches
Armrest height	Measure from the seat of the chair to the olecranon process with the user's elbow flexed to 90 degrees and then add approximately 1 inch. (*Note:* This measurement will be affected if a seat cushion is to be used. The person should be measured while seated on the cushion or the thickness of the cushion must be considered by adding that value to the actual measurement.)	9 inches above the chair seat

tures such as adjustable armrests, desk arms, reclining back, swing-away front rigging, elevating leg rests, and caster wheel locks should be specified when the chair is ordered.

CONFIRMATION OF FIT

The fit of a wheelchair should be determined with the user seated in the wheelchair and wearing his/her usual clothing, including shoes. Any cushions or other components that would affect the fit should be in place. The importance of proper fit of the chair must be reemphasized, because without it, the user will not be able to attain maximal comfort, stability, function, and safety. You should be able to confirm the fit of the wheelchair within approximately 1 to 2 minutes.

METHODS TO EVALUATE THE FIT

Seat Height/Leg Length Proper fit will allow you to place two or three fingers easily under the thigh from the front edge of the seat to a depth of approximately 2 inches (Fig. 7–1). The bottom of the footrest

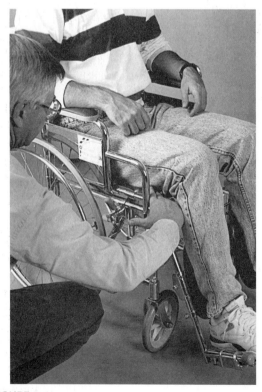

■ **FIGURE 7–1**
Proper fit allows two or three fingers to be placed under the thigh from the front seat edge.

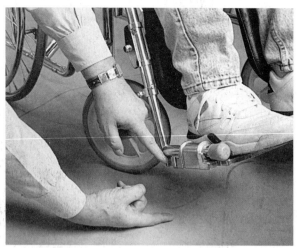

■ **FIGURE 7–2**
The footrest must be at least 2 inches from the floor.

must be at least 2 inches from the floor with the chair on a level surface when this evaluation is performed (Fig. 7–2). The 2 inches provide adequate distance from the bottom of the foot plate to the floor so the chair can be maneuvered easily and safely on most surfaces. The foot plate can be adjusted to the proper position using the adjusting bolt or nut located at the bottom of the shaft of the front rigging (Fig. 7–3).

Seat Depth Proper fit will allow three or four fingers to be placed between the front edge of the seat and the user's *popliteal* fold with your palm horizontal to the seat. It is important that the user is seated well back in the chair with the posterior pelvis in contact with the seat back when this component is evaluated. If he/she is not positioned back in the chair, the seat will appear to be too short, and the user may not have sufficient support for the thighs (Fig. 7–4).

Seat Width Proper fit will allow the placement of your hand between the user's trochanter, hip, or thigh and the armrest panels with your hand positioned vertically to the seat. Your hand should be in slight contact with the user and the armrest panel when the user is seated in the center of the seat. Both hands should be used, one hand on the side of each hip, to be certain there is sufficient space between each hip and each armrest panel when the user is in the center of the seat (Fig. 7–5).

Back Height Proper traditional fit will allow you to place four fingers, with your hand held vertically, between the top of the back upholstery and the floor of the user's axilla. The inferior angles of the scapulae should be positioned approximately one fingerbreadth above the back upholstery when the user sits with an erect posture (Fig. 7–6).

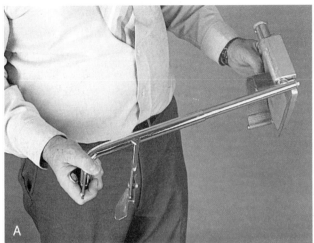

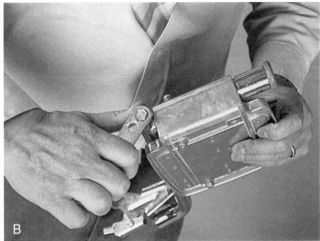

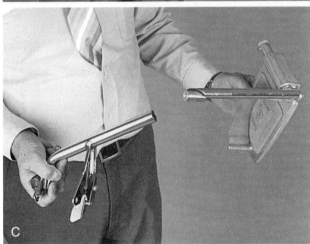

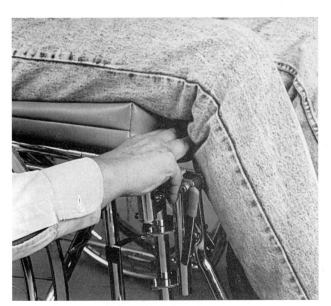

■ **FIGURE 7–3**
The footrest can be adjusted for proper fit.

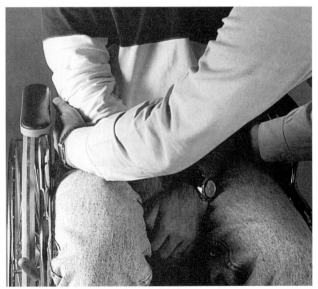

■ **FIGURE 7–4**
Proper fit of seat depth.

■ **FIGURE 7–5**
Proper fit of seat width.

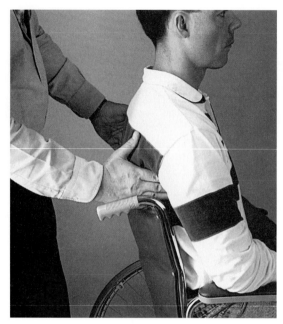

■ FIGURE 7–6
Proper fit of back height.

Armrest Height The user should be able to sit with the trunk erect and his/her shoulders level when bearing weight on the forearms as they rest on the armrest (Fig. 7–7). While in this position, a triangle should be formed by the user's posterior humerus, the top of the armrest, and the frame of the chair back (Procedure 7–1).

POTENTIAL ADVERSE EFFECTS OF IMPROPER FIT

Although there may be deviations in the proper fit that do not cause a problem for the patient, some deviations may cause or create serious problems. Thus each component of the fit must be evaluated to ensure that comfort, security, stability, and safety are maintained for the user. By observing the user when he/she maneuvers the wheelchair or performs functional activities, you may be able to detect problems associated with the fit of the chair.

Seat Height If the seat is too high, the user may experience (1) insufficient trunk support because the back upholstery will be too low, (2) difficulty positioning the knees beneath a table or desk because they are too high, or (3) difficulty propelling the wheelchair because he/she has difficulty reaching the handrims on the drive wheels.

If the seat is too low, the user may experience (1) difficulty performing a standing or lateral swing-type transfer because his/her center of gravity (COG) is lowered, making it difficult for him/her to elevate the

body; and (2) improper weight distribution. (3) If the foot plates are lowered to compensate for the low seat, they may contact objects on the floor or ground, leading to decreased mobility and unsafe use of the chair.

Seat Depth If the seat is too short from the front to the back, the user may experience (1) decreased trunk stability because he/she will have less support under the thighs, (2) increased weight bearing on the ischial tuberosities because his/her weight will be shifted posteriorly as a result of the lack of support to the thighs, or (3) poor balance because his/her base of support has been reduced.

If the seat is too long from the front to the back, the user may experience increased pressure in the popliteal area, leading to skin discomfort or compromise of circulation because the seat upholstery is longer than the thighs.

Seat Width If the seat is too wide, the user may experience (1) difficulty propelling the chair when using the upper extremities because the distance to the handrims is increased, (2) difficulty performing a standing or lateral swing-type transfer because the distance between the armrests is increased and the user will have to move his/her body over a greater distance, (3) difficulty moving through narrow hallways or doorways or using public restroom facilities because the overall width of the chair is increased, or (4) postural deviations because he/she may need to lean to one side of the chair for support.

If the seat is too narrow, the person may experience (1) difficulty changing position because there is

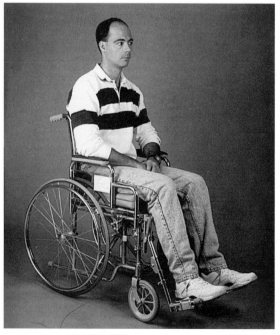

■ FIGURE 7–7
Proper fit of armrest height.

PROCEDURE 7 – 1
Wheelchair Fit Confirmation

The chair should be on a level, smooth surface, and the patient must sit erect with his/her pelvis in contact with the back upholstery.

1. **Seat height/leg length**
   a. With your hand parallel to the floor, you should be able to insert two or three fingers lengthwise between the patient's posterior thigh and the seat upholstery to a depth of approximately 2 inches.
   b. The bottom of the foot plate must be at least 2 inches above the floor.

2. **Seat depth**
   a. With your hand parallel to the floor, you should be able to place the width of three or four fingers between the front edge of the seat and the popliteal fold.

3. **Seat width**
   a. With your hands vertical to the floor, you should be able to slide each hand between the patient's hips and the clothing guard of the chair with minimal contact.

4. **Back height**
   a. With your hand vertical to the floor, you should be able to place the width of four fingers between the top of the back upholstery and the floor of the axilla.

5. **Armrest height**
   a. Observe the angle made by the posterior aspect of the upper arm and the back post when the elbows rest on the armrest approximately 4 inches in front of the back post.
   b. Observe the position of the shoulders; they should be level.
   c. Observe the position of the trunk; it should be erect.

---

not sufficient space to adjust his/her position, (2) excessive pressure to the greater trochanters because they are likely to contact the armrest panel, and (3) difficulty wearing bulky outer garments or orthoses because there will not be sufficient space for the object to fit between the user's hip or thigh and the armrest panel.

Back Height If the back is too high, the user may experience (1) difficulty propelling the chair because it will be more difficult to use his/her arms comfortably, (2) excessive irritation to the skin over the inferior angles of the scapulae as they rub against the upholstery, or (3) difficulty with balance because the trunk may be inclined forward by the high back.

If the back is too low, the user may experience decreased trunk stability or postural deviations, because he/she will have less support from the chair back. (*Note:* The current trend in many wheelchair styles is to have a low back to maximize function. However, many patients may require and desire the traditional higher back for safety, stability, and support.)

Armrest Height If the armrest is too high, the user may experience (1) difficulty propelling the chair because it will be difficult to reach over the high armrest to grasp the handrims, (2) difficulty performing a standing transfer because the armrest height will require his/her arms to be positioned in a poor mechanical position to push to stand, (3) postural deviation as a result of elevated shoulders when resting the forearms on the armrest, or (4) limited use of the armrests due to discomfort when trying to use them, leading to decreased trunk stability and fatigue.

If the armrest is too low, the user may experience (1) poor posture or back discomfort as a result of excessive forward trunk inclination when leaning forward to place the forearms on the armrest, (2) less efficient respiration because of the decreased function of the diaphragm when leaning forward, (3) inadequate balance, or (4) difficulty rising to stand from the chair because the armrests are too low to offer support as he/she pushes to a standing position.

Leg Length If the foot plates are too low, the user may experience (1) increased pressure to the distal posterior thigh and (2) decreased function and unsafe mobility because of lack of sufficient clearance of the foot plate from the floor or ground surface.

If the foot plates are too high, the user may experience (1) increased pressure to the ischial tuberosities, (2) difficulty positioning the chair beneath a table or desk, or (3) decreased trunk stability due to lack of support by the posterior thighs.

PATIENT AND FAMILY EDUCATION

The wheelchair user and his/her family should be educated to inspect the skin after periods of prolonged sitting. Inspection of the skin that overlies bony prominences such as the vertebral spinous processes, inferior angles of the scapulae, ischial tuberosities, greater trochanters, lateral *femoral condyles*, sacrum, and medial humeral epicondyles is particularly important. Instructions should be given to the patient, family, or personal care attendant so each person will know how to relieve weight bearing and how frequently to relieve it. The importance of pressure relief must be emphasized, and compliance with a relief schedule or program should be encouraged. Some users will have to perform several sitting push-ups each hour they are in the wheelchair, and some will need to elevate one buttock at a time by leaning to one side several times each hour they are in the wheelchair to relieve pressure to the ischial tuberosities. Other patients will have to adjust their position by shifting their trunk forward, backward, or to each side several times each hour they are in the chair. Some users may have to be removed from the chair after sitting for 1 to 4 hours or lifted briefly up from the seat by another person several times per hour. The user and the family member should be informed that sitting on a cushion or pillow does not eliminate the need to relieve pressure on the buttocks frequently by the methods described.

The patient and his/her family should be instructed to observe signs or symptoms of decreased circulation in the lower extremities. Ankle edema; color changes in the toes, feet, or legs; decreased sensory response to surface stimuli; loss of hair follicles; or other similar complaints that cannot be explained or are not associated with the person's disease or condition should be reported to a physician. If any of these signs or symptoms occur, it may be necessary to

reduce the amount of time the person sits in the wheelchair. Prevention of a severe secondary problem must be considered to be extremely important and should supersede the user's desire to sit in the wheelchair. Evaluation of the femoral, popliteal, and *pedal* pulses and observation of the legs should be performed frequently. Evidence of venous stasis or ischemic skin (e.g., dark skin over the malleolus) and soft tissue ulcers should also be reported to a physician. These activities are particularly important to perform for the person whose disease or condition predisposes him/her to circulatory changes, such as the person with a spinal cord injury, diabetes mellitus, or a kidney disorder or who uses nicotine or alcohol excessively.

WHEELCHAIR COMPONENTS AND FEATURES

There are several styles and types of wheelchairs with similar features, but the mechanical operation of these features may vary. The more common features and their operation are described and some of them are illustrated in this section. The components or features that are appropriate and necessary for one patient may be unnecessary or inappropriate for another patient. Decisions about the components and features selected for a patient's chair will depend on the criteria described previously. (See also Fig. 7–26, which illustrates the major components of a standard wheelchair and provides the nomenclature of these components.)

WHEEL LOCKS

Toggle Lock Forward movement of the lever engages the lock, and backward movement of the lever disengages it (Fig. 7–8). The lock should be engaged before any transfer to stabilize the chair and add to patient safety, but persons who become very proficient with the performance of a transfer may not opt to engage the locks before a transfer. The device should not be used as a brake to stop the chair or to retard the motion of the chair, such as when *descending* an incline. A special device can be added to the wheelchair to slow the chair's motion when the user ascends or descends an incline.

Lever or Ratchet Lock A lever lock requires the patient to push the lever in toward the chair arm to disengage it from a plate that has several notches in it and move the lever forward or backward to engage or disengage the lock. Forward movement of the lever

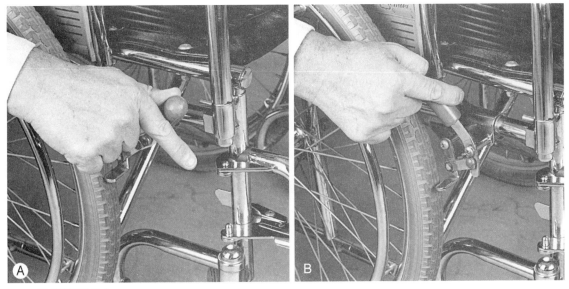

■ FIGURE 7–8
Toggle lock for the wheels. *A,* Moving the lever forward engages the lock; *B,* moving it backward disengages the lock.

locks the chair, and rearward movement disengages the lock, and there may be one or two positions to lock the wheel. The most forward position locks the chair fully; when the second position is used, the chair wheels are only partially locked. This device should not be used as a brake to stop or retard the motion of the chair.

A vertical extension can be attached to either type of lock to assist those who have poor trunk control or limited function in an upper extremity. By using the extension, the patient can operate the lock without leaning or reaching excessively.

Auxiliary Lock for a Reclining Back Chair An auxiliary lock is necessary to release the back and to increase the wheelbase when the back is reclined. An at-

tendant is needed to engage and disengage the lock (Fig. 7–9).

Caster Locks Caster locks are used to lock the caster wheels before a transfer. These locks have a pin or small flat metal bar that engages a hole or notch located in a metal ring attached to the caster wheel. This is an optional item for most wheelchairs.

BODY RESTRAINTS

Lap (Waist) Belt The lap belt (i.e., *restraint*), attached to the frame of the chair, is designed to prevent the user from falling out of the chair. As the name implies, this strap crosses the user's lower abdomen or

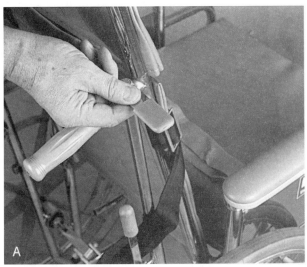
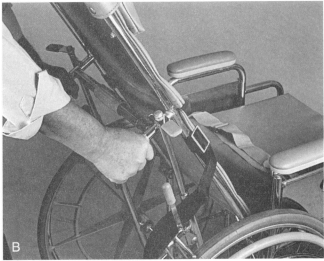

■ FIGURE 7–9
Auxiliary lock for the back of a reclining wheelchair.

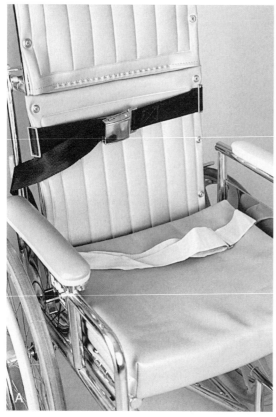

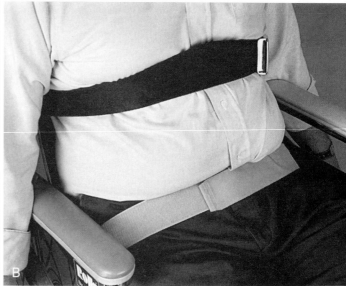

■ **FIGURE 7–10**
Lap and chest belts of a wheelchair.

pelvis, similar to an airplane or automobile lap belt. The buckle may be located in back of the chair to prevent patient access to it.

Chest Belt The chest belt is attached to the frame of the chair at midchest level to increase trunk stability, prevent the user from falling out of the chair, and maintain him/her in an upright posture. It may be combined with a lap belt for greater security. The buckle may be located in the back of the chair to prevent patient access to it (Fig. 7–10).

(*Note:* These belts are provided to protect the patient who has inadequate balance or trunk stability while seated. They are not appropriate for use as a method to restrain a patient in the chair for a prolonged time. Federal and state regulations and guidelines regarding the use of belts or straps as restraints must be followed.)

WHEELS AND TIRES

Caster Wheels Caster wheels are usually located at the front of the chair to permit changes of direction and turns. They are usually either 5 or 8 inches in diameter and may have solid rubber, *pneumatic* (air-filled), or *semipneumatic* (partially air-filled) tires (Fig. 7–11). Pneumatic or semipneumatic tires provide a smoother, more comfortable ride and function better on rough and soft surfaces such as sand, gravel, and grass, but they also may require greater energy expen-

diture by the user to propel the chair because they are wider than solid tires and create more friction.

Drive or Rear Wheels Drive wheels are used to propel the chair. They may have solid rubber, semipneumatic, or pneumatic tires (Fig. 7–12). Some pneumatic tires are manufactured to specifically reduce or prevent the occurrence of a flat tire. The handrim may be molded to the wheel rim or separated from the rim. In addition, the handrim may have ver-

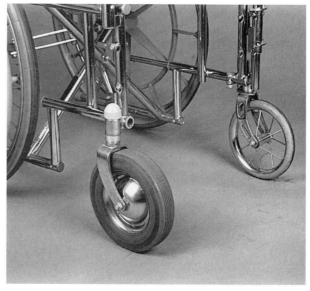

■ **FIGURE 7–11**
Caster wheels of a wheelchair.

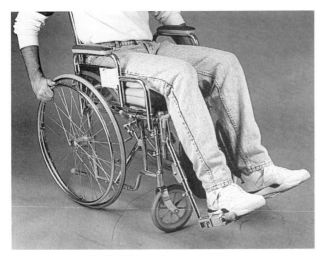

■ **FIGURE 7–12**
Drive wheels of a wheelchair.

tical, horizontal, or angled projections, or it may be coated with plastic to enable the user to propel the chair with greater ease when he/she has decreased hand function.

One-Arm-Drive Chair The one-arm-drive chair may be used for *independent propulsion* when the user has only one functional upper extremity and no functional lower extremities. Two handrims are attached to the same wheel (Fig. 7–13*A*). The outer, larger rim propels the far rear wheel, and the inner, smaller rim propels the near rear wheel. When the user grasps and moves both handrims simultaneously, the chair is propelled in a straight line forward or backward (see Fig. 7–13*B*). Use of one handrim independently causes the chair to turn. A linkage bar connects the two drive wheels (see Fig. 7–13*C*). This chair is heavier than a standard chair and more difficult to fold.

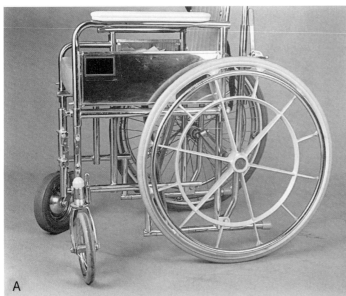

A

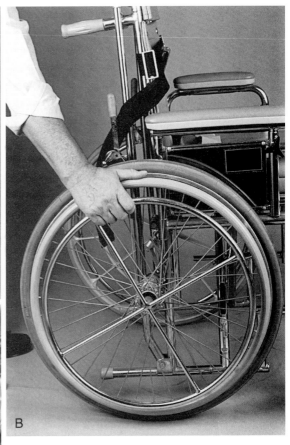

B

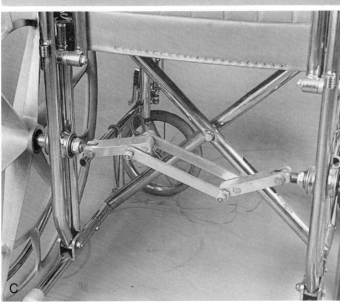

C

■ **FIGURE 7–13**
One-arm-drive wheelchair.

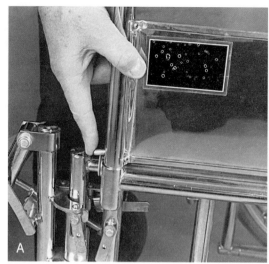

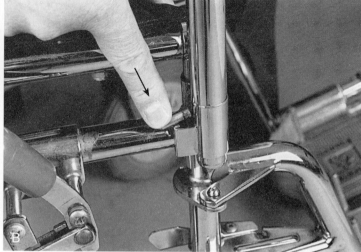

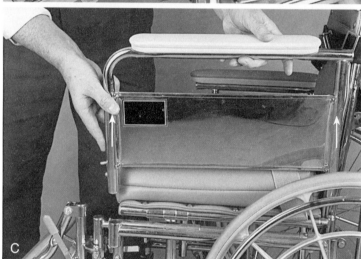

■ **FIGURE 7–14**
Removable arm, with pin lock and release.

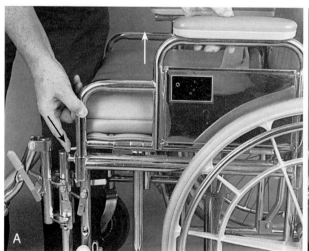

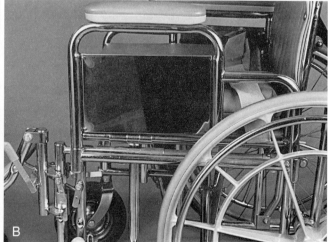

■ **FIGURE 7–15**
Desk (or cut-out) arm, with pin lock and release.

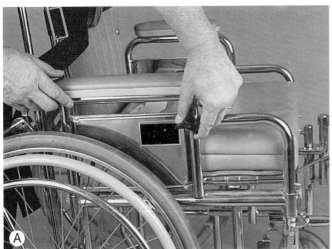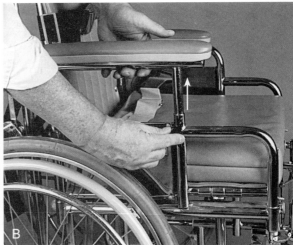

■ **FIGURE 7–16**
Adjustable armrest.

ARMRESTS

Fixed Armrests Fixed armrests are permanently attached to the chair frame. They are recommended for users who will be performing standing transfers and have no need to remove the armrest.

Removable or Reversible Armrests Removable or reversible armrests are recommended for users who will perform a lateral swinging or sliding transfer in a sitting posture. The armrest can be reversed to temporarily narrow the distance between the armrest panels and is usually secured to the frame by a pin-in-hole lock (Fig. 7–14).

Desk or Cut-out Armrests Desk armrests are recommended for persons who desire to position the wheelchair close to a permanent surface such as a desk, table, or countertop. These armrests can usually be reversed to improve anterior support when the user performs a standing transfer (Fig. 7–15).

Adjustable Armrests Adjustable armrests are used by persons who need to adjust the armrest height for different activities or when cushions with different thicknesses or bulky outer garments are used. Typical adjustments include a friction adjustment, accomplished by loosening and tightening a knob or by a pin-in-hole adjustment. Hand function is necessary to adjust the armrest height (Fig. 7–16).

FRONT RIGGING, LEG REST, AND FOOTREST COMPONENTS

Fixed Footrests Fixed footrests are attached permanently to the chair frame and are immovable. The footrest or foot plate can be elevated or raised from a horizontal to a vertical position when the user rises, sits, or desires to place his/her feet on the floor.

Swing-away/Removable Leg Rest Disengagement of a locking mechanism allows the front rigging to be pivoted outward, and lifting the leg rest removes the front rigging from the chair frame (Fig. 7–17). There are several different locking mechanisms available, including a pin lock and a pressure release lever. This feature is used to allow the user to position the chair closer to objects during transfers and to provide greater unimpaired space at the front of the chair for his/her feet.

Elevating Leg Rest The entire front rigging can be elevated and maintained at different heights. This is useful for the patient who is unable to fully flex his/her knees or when knee flexion must be avoided for various reasons. A calf panel is attached to the leg rest to support the lower leg (Fig. 7–18A,B). The leg rest remains elevated by a serrated cam or small gear, which engages a serrated piece of metal on the leg rest (see Fig. 7–18C,D). Lowering of the leg rest is usually accomplished by pushing on a lever that releases the adjustment lock (see Fig. 7–18E). The speed of the leg rest as it lowers must be controlled by another person, who supports the leg rest with one hand as it descends. Be careful to protect the patient's lower extremity when it is lowered because the weight of the leg will cause it to descend rapidly if the patient cannot control its descent. This precaution is especially important when a lower extremity has a cast applied.

The front rigging can usually be pivoted outward or removed from the chair to aid with transfer activities, and the length of the leg rest can be adjusted to accommodate the patient's lower extremity when it is elevated. When one or both lower extremities are elevated, the chair will have a greater tendency to tip

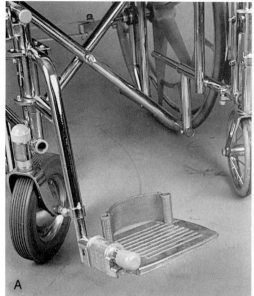

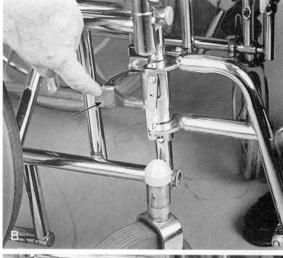

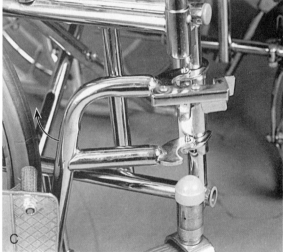

■ **FIGURE 7–17**
Swing-away leg rest, with release and lock control.

backward because the COG of the chair is altered; therefore, the user must be careful when propelling the chair up an incline. Too strong or too rapid movement of the rear wheels is apt to cause the caster wheels to be lifted from the surface.

Footrest The footrest, also called a foot plate, is available in various shapes and sizes depending on the patient's needs. It may have a toe or heel loop to help maintain the foot on the footrest (Fig. 7–19A). The heel loop prevents the foot from sliding backward, and the toe loop prevents the foot from moving forward. The heel loop should be moved forward before the footrest is raised to prevent damage to the heel loop fabric and allow the footrest to be fully raised before a standing transfer or folding the chair (see Fig. 7–19B,C). The footrests should always be elevated before a standing transfer or before movement of a patient into or out of the chair.

A strap may be used between the two leg rests instead of heel loops to prevent posterior movement of the patient's legs. These straps may have various shapes or configurations (e.g., a single strap, a double strap, or an "H" strap).

RECLINING WHEELCHAIRS

Semireclining Semireclining wheelchairs allow the back of the chair to be adjusted to various positions from fully upright to 30 degrees of extension. Usually there are two adjustment knobs on either side of the back frame that are used to release and adjust the position of the back. The chair back will usually be higher than on a standard chair, and a removable head support is necessary to support the user's head when he/she is reclined. Elevating leg rests are necessary components of this chair for user comfort and to maintain stability of the chair. If the leg rests do not elevate, the chair will tend to tip backward when it is reclined because of a shift in the relative position of the user's COG and the base of support of the chair. A bar

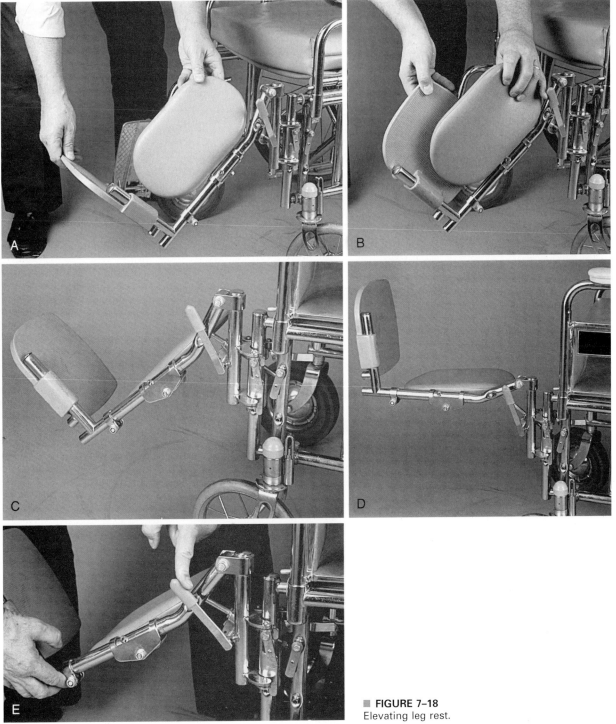

■ **FIGURE 7–18**
Elevating leg rest.

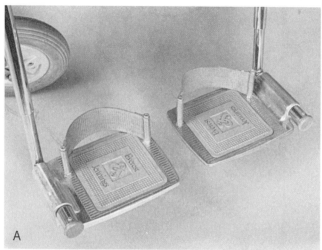

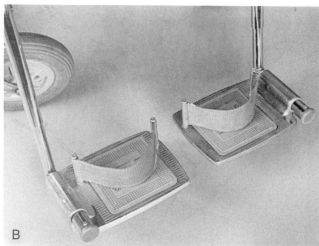

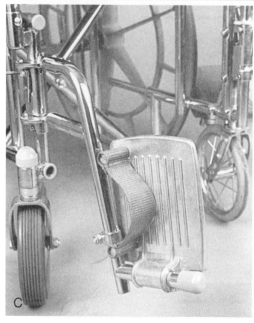

■ **FIGURE 7–19**
Footrests (footplates).

across the back adds support to the back frame (Fig. 7–20).

Fully Reclining Fully reclining wheelchairs allow the back to be adjusted to various positions from vertical to fully horizontal (Fig. 7–21A). Adjustment knobs or levers located on either side of the back frame are used to adjust the position of the back. A headrest and elevating leg rests are necessary components as described previously (see Fig. 7–21B). In addition, the rear wheels will be located more posteriorly than on a standard chair, or they may move back as the chair is reclined to increase the wheelbase (i.e., increase the base of support of the chair) and stability of the chair (Fig. 7–22). (*Note:* The reclining wheelchair is used for the person who must recline periodically while seated in the chair. Persons with lower extremity circulatory problems, who cannot tolerate an upright position because of decreased circulation, or who need

to relieve skin pressure but cannot perform pressure relief independently may find a reclining chair beneficial.)

EXTERNALLY POWERED WHEELCHAIR

This type of wheelchair is powered by one or more deep cycle batteries that provide stored electrical energy to one or more belts that drive or propel the chair. The motorized chair is available for persons with insufficient strength or motor control in the extremities to propel a standard chair. Various controls are available to operate the chair, including those operated by the patient's hand, chin, head, tongue, or mouth; more sophisticated microprocessor control systems are in use. The chair may have a proportional drive system, in which the speed is

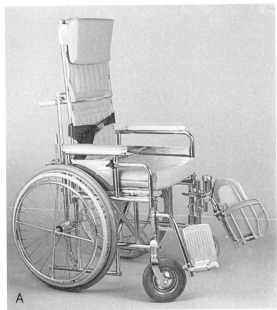

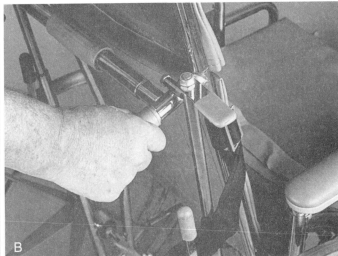

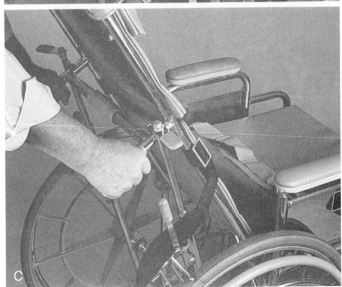

■ **FIGURE 7–20**
Semireclining wheelchair.

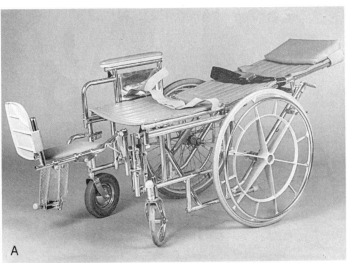

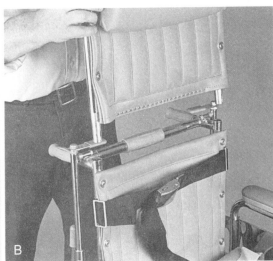

■ **FIGURE 7–21**
Fully reclining wheelchair.

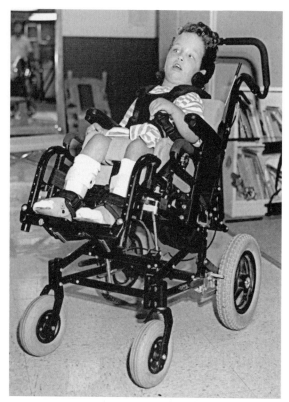

■ **FIGURE 7–22**
Child in an adjustable, reclining wheelchair.

SPORT/RECREATIONAL WHEELCHAIR

These wheelchairs have specific features such as low backrests; solid, lightweight frames; canted (angled) rear wheels; lower and narrow seats; and an overall low profile to make the chair more functional for the user. Many of these chairs are custom fabricated for the user depending on the sport or recreational activity in which he/she participates (Fig. 7–24A,B).

FOLDING WHEELCHAIRS

Many wheelchairs can be folded for storage or to transport them. To fold the chair, the footrests must be raised after the heel loops have been moved forward. The chair is folded by pulling up on the seat rails or on hand loops attached to the seat rails (Fig. 7–25A). An alternative method is to grasp the midline of the front and back of the seat upholstery and lift upward (see Fig. 7–25B,C). However, this method may cause damage to the upholstery if it is used excessively. After the chair has been folded, the seat upholstery can be positioned downward between the seat rails.

The back support bar of the reclining chair must be released or removed before folding this type of chair (see Fig. 7–25D). You will have to examine the bar to determine how to release it. The bar must be replaced and secured in place before a patient is placed in the chair.

To unfold the chair, lift the rear wheels from the floor by lifting on the push handles and gently begin to pull the push handles away from each other (see Fig. 7–25E). When the chair is partially unfolded, re-

directly related to the pressure applied to the control device (i.e., as more pressure is applied, there is greater speed), or it may have a microswitch system, in which the speed is preset so the chair will move only at that speed regardless of the amount of pressure that is applied to the control (Fig. 7–23A to C).

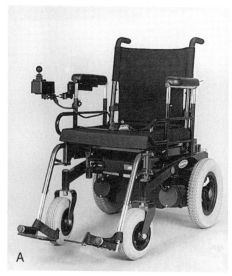

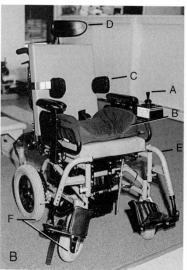

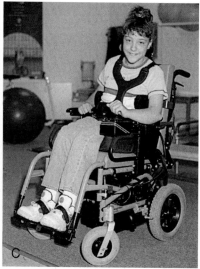

■ **FIGURE 7–23**
A, Externally powered wheelchair. B, A youth-size, externally powered wheelchair with (A) "joystick" control, (B) molded seat cushion, (C) side panels, (D) head support, (E) swing-away leg rests, and (F) semipneumatic tires. C, Youth seated in chair shown in B, showing yoke-type trunk restraint.

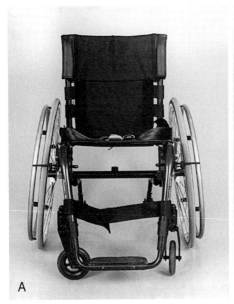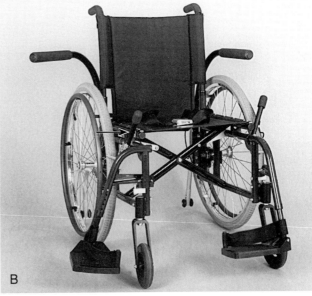

■ **FIGURE 7–24**
A, Sport-style wheelchair with the angled (canted) drive wheels, solid frame, low back rest, and lack of armrests. *B,* Current use, lightweight-style wheelchair with swing-away front rigging *(left),* swivel armrest *(left),* and wheel lock applied *(left).*

place the rear wheels on the floor and complete the unfolding by pushing down evenly on each seat rail (see Fig. 7–25*F,G*). If the chair is to be unfolded on a carpet, it may be necessary to unfold it with the rear wheels elevated throughout the entire process because the rear wheels will be difficult to separate when they are on the carpet.

A folded chair can be wheeled (transported) most easily by elevating the caster wheels and wheeling the chair on the rear wheels, using the push handles for control.

When the folded chair is to be lifted, the fixed or solid portion of the frame should be used. *Caution:* Do not lift the chair using any of the removable components, such as the armrests or front rigging, because they may be disengaged from the chair.

FUNCTIONAL ACTIVITIES

The person who will use a wheelchair for mobility should be instructed in the proper use and care of the chair. The projected use of the chair should be based on the person's goals, needs, and anticipated lifestyle. The many functional activities the person will have to learn should be practiced using proper safety and protective or guarding techniques. It may be necessary to visit the environment in which the person will function to identify the usual, unusual, and special activities the person should be taught.

Figure 7–26 illustrates the major components of a

standard wheelchair and the nomenclature of these components.

Operation of Wheelchair Components Each wheelchair user should be taught to operate the wheel locks; remove and replace the armrests; swing away, remove, and replace the front rigging; and elevate and lower the foot plates before performing other activities. The instructions may be verbal, demonstrated, written, or illustrated; a videotape can also be used. The user of the chair should not be expected to inherently understand how to perform these activities, and instructions should be given to each user along with an opportunity for the user to practice and demonstrate his/her ability to perform these activities. The person with functional use of the upper and lower extremities, normal trunk control, and normal balance should not experience difficulty learning and performing these tasks. However, the person with functional loss of use of the extremities, decreased trunk control, and decreased balance may require several practice sessions to be able to perform these tasks safely and proficiently.

INDEPENDENT PROPULSION

Bilateral Upper Extremities The user grasps the handrims at the top of the wheels (the 12 o'clock position) and pushes forward or pulls backward with equal force on each wheel (Fig. 7–27*A*). To turn, the user can hold one handrim and pull or push on the

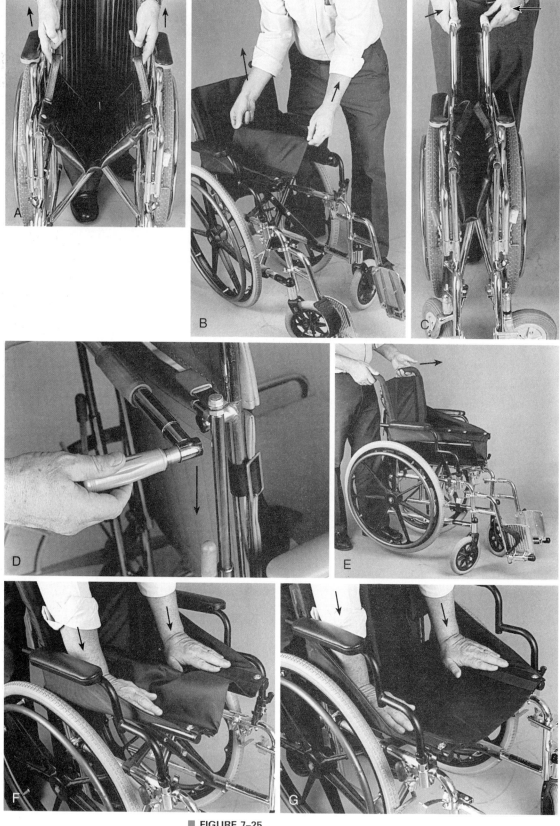

■ **FIGURE 7–25**
Folding and unfolding the wheelchair.

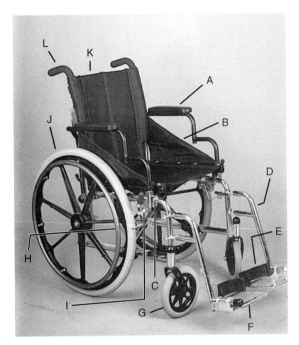

■ FIGURE 7–26
Wheelchair components. A, Armrest. B, clothing guard. C, Front rigging release. D, Front rigging. E, Heel loop. F, Footplate (footrest). G, Caster wheel. H, Handrim. I, Wheel lock. J, Drive wheel. K, Back upholstery. L, Push handle.

opposite handrim; to turn more quickly, he/she simultaneously pushes forward on one handrim and pulls back on the opposite handrim.

One Upper Extremity and One Lower Extremity The user grasps the handrim at the top of the wheel and pushes forward or pulls back, using the functional foot to pull or push simultaneously (see Fig. 7–27B). The foot also serves as a "rudder" to assist with turning while the user holds the handrim (see Fig. 7–27C). The use of one upper extremity and one lower extremity, usually on the same side, is an excellent method for a patient with hemiplegia as a result of a cerebrovascular accident or traumatic brain injury.

Bilateral Lower Extremities The user uses the heels and soles of his/her feet or shoes to propel the chair forward and backward and uses the feet as a "rudder" to turn to the left or right. This method is rarely used but would be of value for any user with reduced function of both upper extremities and poor trunk control and who is unable to ambulate.

The user should be instructed verbally and by demonstration how to propel the chair forward and backward, turn to the left and to the right, and turn the chair in a half or complete circle. Practice of these techniques will be required for the user to become independent and safe. These activities should be practiced initially on a smooth, flat surface, rather than on a carpet, and in a space that is free of objects. Eventu-

ally, the person should practice on carpeting or a rough surface and should attempt to maneuver around objects or in a congested area.

ASSISTED FUNCTIONAL ACTIVITIES

Assisted Level-Surface Propulsion When propelling a patient in a wheelchair, use the push handles to move and control the chair. To turn the chair, hold one push handle and push or pull on the other push handle. For example, to turn to the left, hold the left push handle and push on the right push handle, or hold the right push handle and pull on the left push handle. Do not push the chair and then release the push handles; you should always maintain control of the chair when it is moving and you are propelling it, particularly when moving down an incline or ramp. Start and stop chair movement smoothly, and avoid a sudden or abrupt start or stop. In most settings and environments, you should use the right side of the corridor or sidewalk when propelling the chair. Use caution when you reach the corner of a wall, especially when there is no mirror to view oncoming traffic or hazards that might be in the next corridor. Also use caution when you move the chair through any doorway because the patient's feet and chair footrests project in front of the chair, making them susceptible to being struck and injured.

In those situations in which it is necessary or desirable to tip the patient and propel the chair on its rear wheels, be certain to inform the patient of your intentions before you tip the chair. Finally, be certain the chair is secure and stable, with the footrests elevated, before the patient enters or exits the chair using a standing transfer. The chair wheels should be locked, or you should hold the push handles if the patient can enter or exit the chair independently and safely.

Elevation of the Caster Wheels To elevate the caster wheels, stand behind the chair and push down and forward with one foot on one tipping lever while pushing down and back with both hands on the push handles (Figs. 7–28 and 7–29). Once the chair is tipped, you will be able to control it with the push handles. The chair can be propelled while the caster wheels are elevated (Fig. 7–30). *Caution:* The person in the chair should be warned before being tipped, and the entire procedure should be described to him/her before it is performed. Reverse the procedure to lower the caster wheels to the floor, and retard the effect of gravity as the caster wheels descend. You must be certain you have the physical strength to perform this procedure and control the chair when it is tipped. Your use of proper body mechanics will be very important when you perform this procedure.

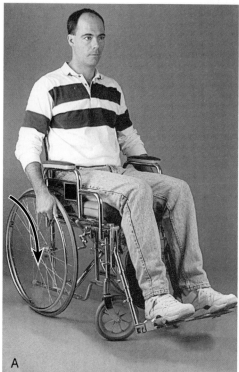

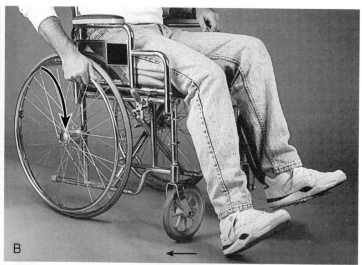

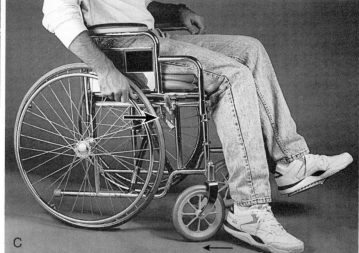

■ **FIGURE 7–27**
A, Independent propulsion by a patient using both upper extremities. B and C, Independent propulsion by a patient using one upper and one lower extremity.

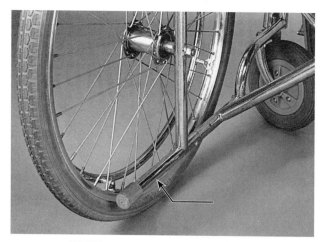

■ **FIGURE 7–28**
Tipping lever for elevation of caster wheels.

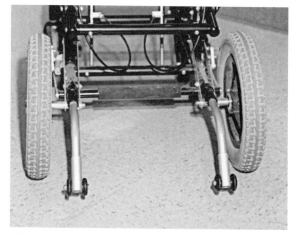

■ **FIGURE 7–29**
Antitipping extensions in position to prevent the chair from tipping backward. The extensions can be rotated upward or removed.

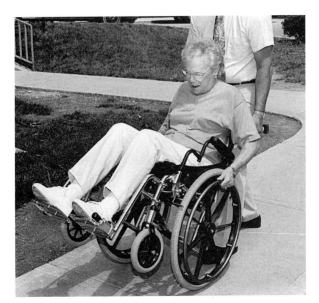

■ **FIGURE 7–30**
Propelling a wheelchair while it is reclined on the drive wheels.

Ascending a Single Elevation (Curb) Forward Position the chair facing the curb, and elevate the caster wheels as described previously (Fig. 7–31). Move the chair forward on its rear wheels until they contact the curb lip and the caster wheels are above the surface of the curb. Carefully lower the caster wheels, as described previously, onto the surface and then roll the chair forward so the rear wheels ascend the curb and all four wheels are on the upper level of the curb. (*Note:* The person in the chair can assist by leaning the trunk forward and pushing forward on the handrims as the chair is elevated and rolled up onto the curb. The person must have control of his/her trunk musculature, adequate balance, and functional use of the upper extremities to assist with this activity.) This method is the easiest to use, provides the greatest control of the chair, and requires the least effort by the caregiver.

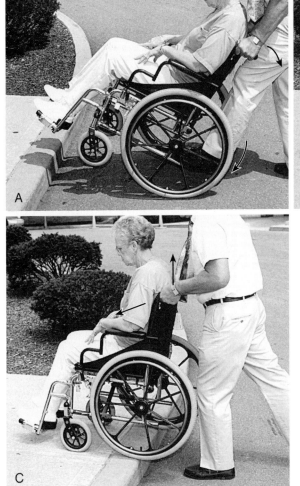

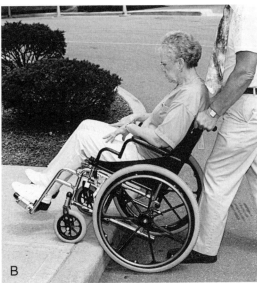

■ **FIGURE 7–31**
Ascending a curb forward.

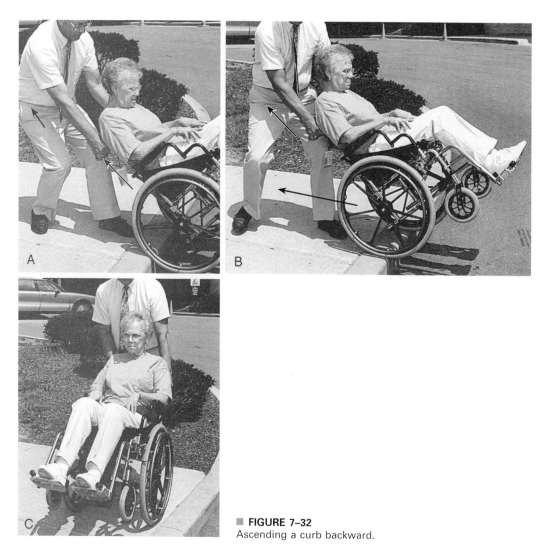

■ **FIGURE 7–32**
Ascending a curb backward.

Ascending a Single Elevation Backward Position the chair so that the rear wheels contact the curb, and tip the chair back so that the caster wheels are elevated (Fig. 7–32). Pull on the push handles so that the chair ascends the curb on its rear wheels, and then turn the chair 90 degrees to the left or right or pull it backward until the caster wheels are positioned over the upper level of the curb. Gently lower the caster wheels using the tipping lever and push handles. (*Note:* The person in the chair can assist by pulling back on the handrims as the chair is pulled up and over the curb. Maintain the chair in a tipped position until all four wheels are positioned over the surface above the curb.) This method is more difficult to perform because the effort needed to pull the chair up the curb and to control the chair is greater.

Descending a Single Elevation Backward Position the chair so the rear wheels are close to the edge of the curb (Fig. 7–33). Stand behind the chair and control the chair as it slowly rolls backward, with the rear wheels first, over the curb, while the caster wheels remain on the upper surface of the curb. The movement of the chair over and down the curb can be retarded if you use your thigh or the side of your hip against the back of the chair as it descends. When the rear wheels contact the street, turn the chair 90 degrees with the caster wheels elevated or roll it away from the curb until the caster wheels and front rigging clear the curb; then lower the caster wheels to the surface. *Caution:* Maintain the chair in a reclined position until the caster wheels and front rigging clear the curb. (*Note:* The person in the chair can assist by providing friction with his/her hands against the handrims and by leaning the trunk forward as the chair rolls over and down the curb.) This method is the easiest to perform because it provides greatest control of the chair and requires least effort by the caregiver.

Descending a Single Elevation Forward Position the chair with the caster wheels close to the edge of the curb. Tip the chair onto its rear wheels and control the chair as it rolls forward over the curb by pulling back on the push handles (Fig. 7–34). The chair must be maintained in a tipped position until the rear wheels are on the surface at the bottom of the curb. When the

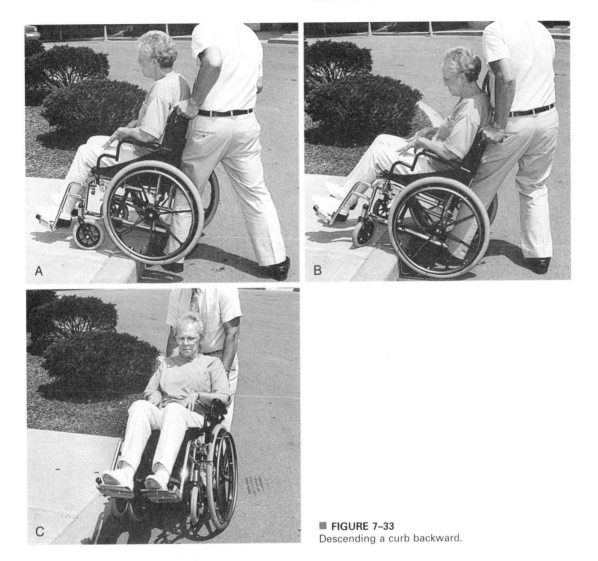

■ **FIGURE 7–33**
Descending a curb backward.

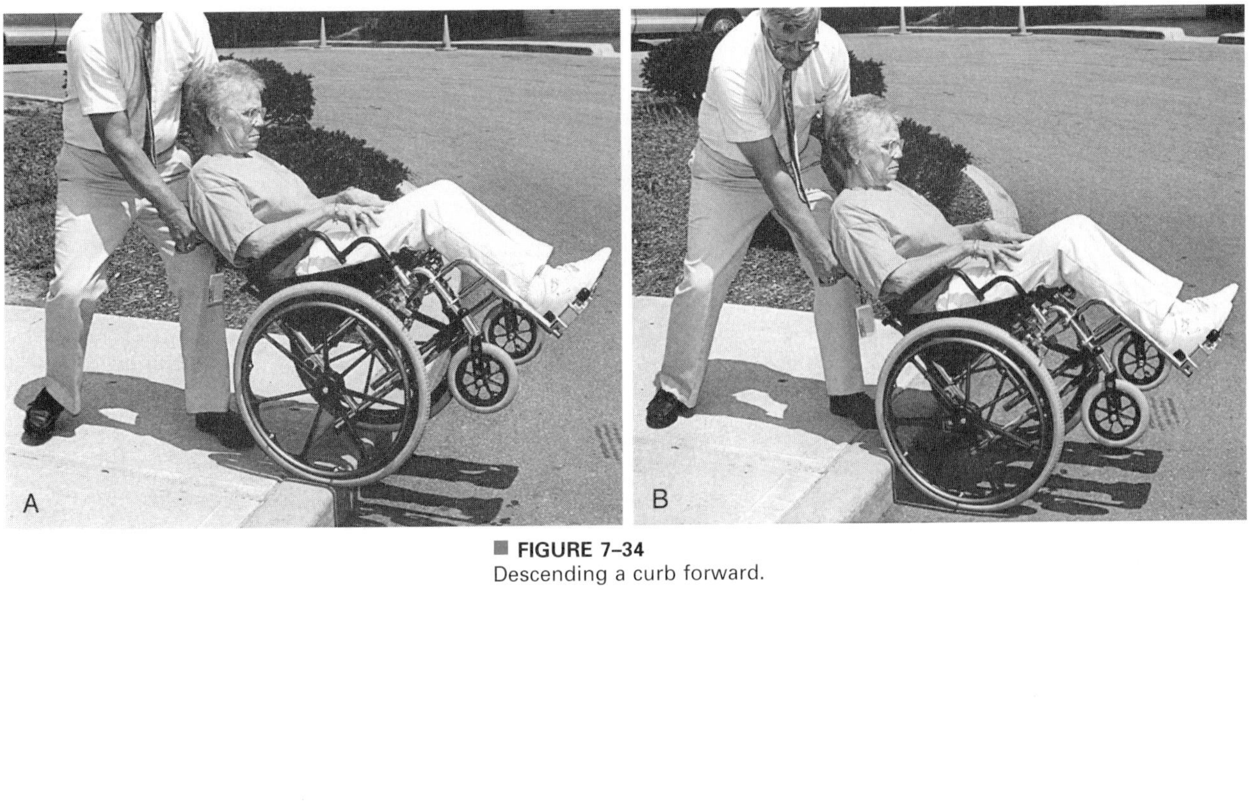

■ **FIGURE 7–34**
Descending a curb forward.

PROCEDURE 7 – 2
Assisted Ascending and Descending a Curb With a Wheelchair

For these activities, you should explain the activity to the patient, instruct him/her on how and when to assist, and alert him/her as you initiate the activity.

1. Descending forward
   a. Position the chair with the caster wheels at the edge of the curb; the patient should be seated back in the chair. Stand on the sidewalk surface.
   b. Tip the chair onto its rear wheels using the push handles and tipping lever.
   c. Wheel the chair forward and allow it to roll over the edge of the curb as you pull back on the push handles; the patient can assist to control the movement of the chair by providing friction to the handrims with his/her hands.
   d. After the rear wheels are on the street, lower the caster wheels using the push handles and tipping lever.

2. Descending backward
   a. Position the chair with the rear wheels at the edge of the curb; the caster wheels remain in contact with the sidewalk surface. Stand on the street surface.
   b. Allow the rear wheels to roll over the edge of the curb until they contact the street; control the movement of the chair with one hip against the back of the chair. The patient can assist to control the movement of the chair by providing friction to the handrims with his/her hands.
   c. Elevate the caster wheels until they have cleared the curb as you back up or turn the chair to one side.
   d. Lower the caster wheels onto the street surface using the push handles and tipping lever.

3. Ascending forward
   a. Position the chair facing the curb with the foot plates about 6 inches from the curb face. Stand on the street surface.
   b. Tip the chair back using the push handles and tipping lever. Wheel the chair forward until the rear wheels contact the curb, and lower the caster wheels to the sidewalk surface.
   c. Wheel the chair forward over the curb. The patient can assist by leaning forward slightly and pushing on the handrims until the rear wheels are on the sidewalk surface.

4. Ascending backward
   a. Position the chair so its back is toward the curb and the rear wheels contact the curb. Stand on the sidewalk surface.
   b. Tip the chair back using the push handles; maintain this position.
   c. Pull the chair over the curb on its rear wheels. The patient can assist by pulling on the handrims as the chair ascends.
   d. Back or turn the chair to one side until the caster wheels are above the sidewalk surface. Lower the caster wheels using the push handles and tipping lever.

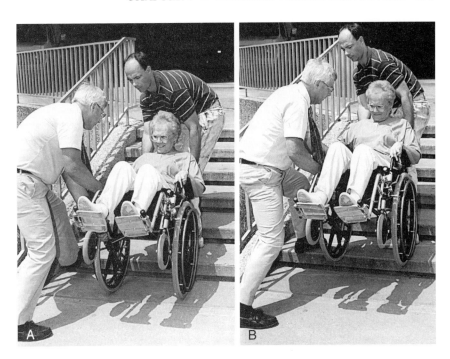

■ **FIGURE 7–35**
Ascending steps backward or descending
forward with two assistants.

rear wheels are on the street, the caster wheels are lowered gently. (*Note:* The person in the chair can assist by providing friction with his/her hands against the handrims as the chair rolls over and down the curb.) This is a difficult procedure and you must be certain you have the strength and ability to control the chair. Your use of proper body mechanics will be very important when you perform this procedure.

Practice each of these methods to determine which one is the most efficient and safest for you to perform. Perform each method with persons of different sizes and weights in the chair. By trying each method, you will be able to offer alternatives to a family member or other person who may eventually assist the user. Usually the movements that are the easiest to control and the safest to use are the ascending forward and descending backward movements (Procedure 7–2).

Ascending Multiple Elevations (Steps) Backward
(*Caution:* This activity is performed most safely using at least two persons other than the patient, and three persons will be required for a large or severely incapacitated patient.) Position the rear wheels so that they contact the bottom step, and elevate the caster wheels (Fig. 7–35*A*). The chair must be maintained in this tipped position as it is moved up the stairs. Pull the chair up and onto each step as described for ascending a curb backward. The persons who assist should stand on one or both sides of the chair and grasp the frame of the chair (see Fig. 7–35*B*). *Caution:* The assistants should not grasp any of the removable items of the chair such as the armrests or front rigging because these items could disengage from the chair. On com-

mand of the leader, all three people assist to roll the chair up the steps, one step at a time. The leader should indicate when the next step is to be ascended so that all persons work together. (*Note:* The person in the chair can assist by pulling back on the handrims on command [e.g., "Ready, pull"] [Fig. 7–36*A,B*].) At the top of the steps, turn the chair 90 degrees or roll it backward until it can be lowered onto its caster wheels. The person who controls the chair by grasping the push handles must use proper body mechanics by partially stooping, widening his/her base of support, and pulling, rather than lifting, on the push handles.

Descending Multiple Elevations (Steps) Forward
(*Caution:* This activity will be performed most safely if at least two persons assist and three persons will be required for a large or severely incapacitated patient.) Position the caster wheels at the edge of the top step, and tip the chair onto its rear wheels. Then slowly and carefully roll the chair until its rear wheels are at the edge of the step. The persons who assist should stand on one or both sides of the chair and grasp the frame of the chair. They should not grasp any of the removable items of the chair. On command of the leader, all three persons retard the motion of the rear wheels down to the next step. The chair must be maintained in this reclined position as it moves down the stairs. Stop the chair on each step to avoid developing momentum. (*Note:* The person in the chair can assist by providing friction against the handrims as the chair descends each step.) Lower the chair onto its caster wheels at the bottom of the steps. The person who controls the chair by grasping the push handles must use proper body mechanics as described previously.

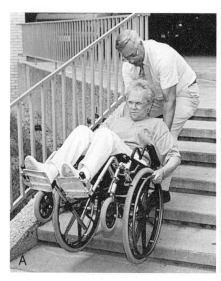
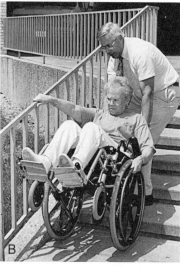

■ **FIGURE 7–36**
Ascending steps with one assistant.

Ramps, Inclines, and Hills

Ascending the Slope   You can push the chair forward on all four wheels or elevate the caster wheels and propel it either forward or backward on the rear wheels up the slope (Fig. 7–37). Pulling the chair up the slope backward with all four wheels in contact with the surface is not recommended because the patient may fall forward. For steep elevations, it may be necessary to zigzag up or down the incline by angling the chair to the left and then to the right up or down the incline. The person in the chair can assist in propelling the chair as described previously.

Descending the Slope   Elevate the caster wheels and retard the motion of the chair by holding the push handles as the chair descends forward, or leave all four wheels in contact with the ground and allow the chair to descend backward while retarding the motion of the chair with the side of your body against the back of the chair and your feet in a widened base of support. Allowing the chair to descend a steep slope forward with all four wheels in contact with the surface is not recommended because the patient may fall forward. The person in the chair can assist in retarding the motion of the chair by providing friction with his/her hands against the handrims.

Rough or Soft Surfaces   The most effective method to control and propel the chair over an uneven or soft surface is to elevate the caster wheels so only the rear wheels are in contact with the surface. The chair must be maintained in this tipped position as it is propelled over the surface.

Elevators   You can enter the elevator forward or backward. Many persons prefer to enter backward to be able to use the selector panel, to avoid facing the back wall of the car, and to avoid having to turn the chair around to exit the car. However, entering the elevator backward and exiting the elevator forward places the lower extremities at risk if the door panels

close prematurely or if there is limited access to the corridor into which the person exits. Furthermore, the caster wheels may lodge in the space between the elevator floor and the corridor surface, and the traffic in the corridor cannot be observed until the patient has completely exited the elevator. When the patient exits the car backward, his/her lower extremities are still at risk of being struck by the door panels, and it may be difficult to turn in the corridor because of limited space or traffic. However, the patient will be able to view the traffic in the corridor easily, and it will be easier to move the rear wheels over the space between the surface of the floor and the elevator car surface. You must be certain the chair is completely out of the elevator car before you attempt to turn it. This is particularly important when one or both of the patient's lower extremities are elevated. You may need to position your body against the edge of the door or to request someone in the car to use the "door open" control button to keep the door open as the patient enters or exits the car.

Many elevator locations have exterior wall mirrors to view the corridor before you exit the car. You should be familiar with the safety devices in the elevator car, such as the panel control to maintain the door open, and the emergency door opening items, such as a photoelectric beam or pressure sensors in the edge of the door. You should observe whether the floor of the elevator car and the corridor surface are level. If the two surfaces are not level, you may need to elevate the caster wheels to safely enter or exit the car.

Escalators   The person in a wheelchair should avoid using an escalator except in an extreme emergency. If the escalator is the only means to ascend or descend from one level to another, extreme caution will be required to maintain the person's safety.

The person, assisted by a caregiver, can ascend forward so the caster wheels are on the step above the

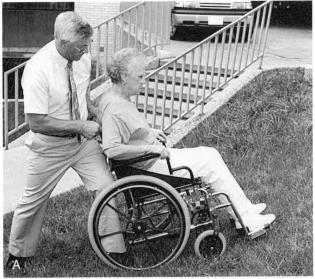

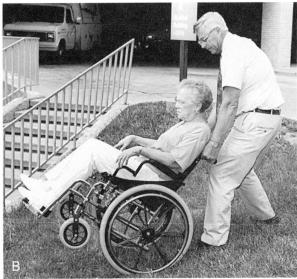

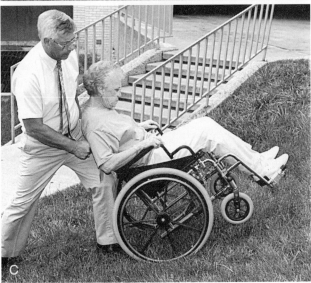

■ **FIGURE 7–37**
Ascending and descending a slope. *A,* Forward or backward on all four wheels. *B,* Backward or forward on two wheels. *C,* Forward or backward on two wheels.

rear wheels. He/she should be instructed to lean forward and grasp the moving handrails if the width of the escalator permits. The caregiver remains behind the chair to prevent it from tipping backward. When the level surface at the top of the escalator is reached, the caster wheels will contact it so that the chair can be propelled forward.

The person, assisted by a caregiver, can descend forward with the caster wheels elevated so that only the rear wheels contact the moving step. The person should be instructed to lean back in the chair and grasp the moving handrails if the width of the escalator permits. The caregiver remains behind the chair to prevent it from tipping backward. When the level surface is reached, the rear wheels are rolled onto it, and the caster wheels are lowered so the chair can be propelled forward. (*Note:* It will be necessary to allow sufficient distance from the front rigging of the chair to avoid contact with other persons using the escalator.)

Caution: This should not be considered to be an

ordinary activity for a person in a wheelchair, and extreme care must be used to prevent possible injury. It is recommended that two persons be used to control the chair: one in front and one behind the chair.

Doors and Doorways You can move a patient through a doorway forward or backward. Remember that problems or situations similar to those described for entering and exiting an elevator may occur with moving through a doorway.

Entering Forward If the door opens toward you, position the patient at a slight angle so he/she is nearest to and facing the edge of the door that will open (i.e., facing the farthest door frame). Open the door wide enough so the chair will pass between the door frame and the edge of the door. If the door has a *self-closing device,* you will have to use one foot or one hand to hold the door open as the chair moves through the doorway. Before you move the patient into the room or corridor, observe the area for traffic or other hazards.

If the door opens away from you, position the patient at a slight angle so he/she is near to the door and faces the nearest door frame (i.e., faces the door frame opposite to the frame with the hinges attached). Open the door wide enough for the chair to pass through, and hold the door open if it has a self-closing device. Follow the other precautions described previously to protect the patient.

Entering Backward If the door opens toward you, position the patient so his/her back is toward the opening edge of the door with the chair at a slight angle away from the edge of the door. Open the door wide enough for the chair to pass through, and pull the chair through the doorway. After the chair has passed completely through the doorway, turn the chair so the patient faces forward.

If the door opens away from you, position the patient so his/her back is toward the opening edge of the door with the chair at a slight angle toward the door frame. Open the door wide enough for the chair to pass through, and pull the chair through the doorway. Follow the other precautions described previously to protect the patient. (*Note:* If there is a raised threshold, it may be easier to move the chair through the doorway backward because the larger rear wheels will roll over the threshold better than the caster wheels. If you move the chair leading with the caster wheels, it may be necessary to elevate the caster wheels to clear the threshold.)

INDEPENDENT FUNCTIONAL ACTIVITIES

Elevation of the Caster Wheels ("Wheelie" or "Pop-up") Elevation of the caster wheels is necessary so the wheels can clear objects on the floor, sidewalk, or ground and to ascend/descend curbs and curb cutouts. The patient must have sufficient upper extremity strength and coordination and the ability to maintain his/her sitting balance when performing the activity. Practice will be required, and the patient should be protected so he/she does not fall backward during practice sessions. A demonstration of the technique by another patient or by you is usually helpful and should be performed for all patients.

Instruct the person to pull back quickly and equally on both handrims, and then abruptly stop the rearward motion of the rear wheels by firmly grasping the handrims (Fig. 7–38). The person should not attempt to propel the chair backward but should develop a rearward movement momentum of the chair. The caster wheels will lift from the floor because of the abrupt stopping of the rearward motion of the chair. This action will occur because of the principles associated with Newton's first law of motion. This law

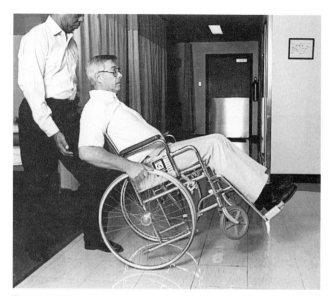

■ **FIGURE 7–38**
Elevation of the caster wheels by the person in the wheelchair (a "wheelie").

indicates a body will remain at rest or in motion in a straight line until acted on by a force. Once the chair and the person in it start in motion backward, they will continue to move backward even when a force (i.e., the hands grasping the handrims) stops the motion. The person will continue to move backward, with the axles of the rear wheels acting as a fulcrum, and the chair frame, with the person seated in it, will rotate backward, causing the caster wheels to elevate. The patient's first attempts may only briefly lift the caster wheels a few inches. Over time and with continued practice, while being guarded or otherwise protected, many patients will be able to balance on the rear wheels and may be able to propel the chair in this position.

When the caster wheels are elevated, small forward movements of the handrims will cause a rearward movement of the chair frame and seat and small backward movements of the handrims will cause a forward movement of the chair frame and seat. The patient should be taught and should practice these motions to maintain a balanced position.

During practice sessions, you should stand behind the patient, tip the chair to find his/her balance point, and protect him/her from falling backward. You must be alert when the patient performs the "wheelie" independently so you are always prepared to prevent the chair from tipping back too far. A rope properly measured to prevent the chair from tipping backward too far, attached to the push handles and running through a ceiling pulley or eye bolt, can also be used to protect the person as this activity is practiced. A patient with only one functional upper extremity probably will not be able to perform this activity because it will not be possible to generate sufficient force to gen-

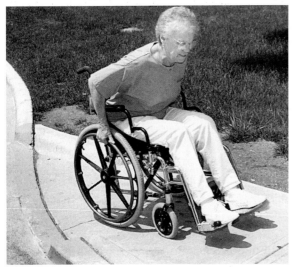

■ **FIGURE 7–39**
Ascent of a ramp by the person in the wheelchair using both upper extremities.

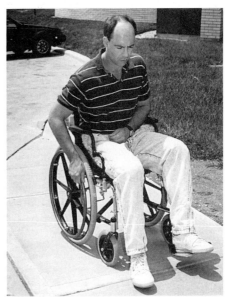

■ **FIGURE 7–40**
Ascent of a ramp by a patient using one upper and one lower extremity.

erate rearward momentum of the chair frame and still safely control the chair.

Ramps or Inclines

Ascending Forward When the patient propels the chair with both upper extremities, instruct him/ her to move the hips forward in the chair, lean the trunk forward, and push equally on the handrims using a smooth forward motion (Fig. 7–39). He/she will have to reposition the hands on the handrims to progress up the ramp. It is important for the patient to lean forward to move his/her COG forward and to decrease the possibility of tipping backward.

When the patient propels the chair using one upper extremity and one lower extremity, instruct him/ her to move the hips forward in the chair seat and to lean the trunk forward (Fig. 7–40). Instruct him/her to use the upper and lower extremities the same as they are used on a level surface, although it may be necessary to use the lower extremity for more power than is required on a level surface. The chair is apt to move to the left or right depending on the position of the caster wheels and the extremities used to propel the chair. If the patient propels the chair with his/her right extremities, the chair may deviate to the left; it may deviate to the right if the patient's left extremities propel the chair. This activity can be performed more easily by many patients if they ascend backward or if a handrail is available to grasp and pull on.

Descending Forward When the patient propels the chair with both upper extremities, instruct him/ her to position the hips to the rear of the seat and to maintain the trunk erect (Fig. 7–41). The person must be instructed to retard the forward motion of the chair by applying equal friction with the palms of the hands

on the handrims and to avoid catching the fingers in the spokes of the wheel. This can be accomplished by using only the palms against the side of the handrims and keeping the fingers extended. If uneven pressure is applied by the person's hands on the handrims, the chair will turn toward the wheel to which the greatest pressure is applied. Some persons may be able to descend using a "wheelie" position. This is an advanced technique, and you must guard the patient during all practice sessions.

When the patient propels the chair using one upper extremity and one lower extremity, instruct him/ her to position the hips to the rear of the seat and maintain the trunk erect. Instruct him/her to retard

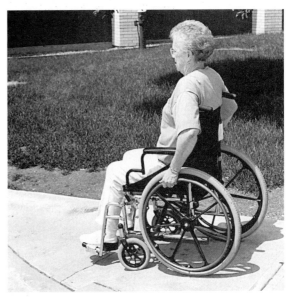

■ **FIGURE 7–41**
Descent of a ramp by a patient using both upper extremities.

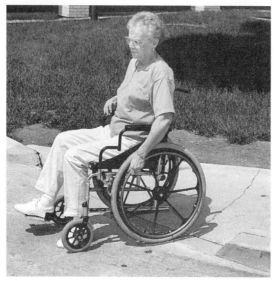

■ **FIGURE 7–42**
Backward ascent of a curb cut-out using one upper and one lower extremity.

the forward motion of the chair by applying friction of the palm of the hand against the handrim. Some additional friction may be applied by sliding the sole of the shoe on the surface. He/she will need to use the functional foot to guide the chair because friction on only one handrim will cause the chair to drift or roll toward the side to which the friction is applied. For example, when friction is applied to the right handrim, the chair will tend to deviate to the right; when the friction is applied to the left handrim, it will deviate to the left. This may be a difficult activity for a patient to perform and master safely because of this problem.

Ascending Backward Ascending backward is recommended for the person who uses one upper and one lower extremity for propulsion. Instruct the person to pull back on the handrim and push with the functional foot and lower extremity (Fig. 7–42). He/she should maintain the trunk erect with his/her back positioned in the chair seat. One complication with this procedure is the patient is unable to see directly the progress of the chair. He/she can be instructed to look behind the chair periodically or to locate a fixed object in front of him/her and use it as a guide to maintain the chair's direction.

Ascending or Descending Steep Inclines It may be necessary to instruct the person to zigzag or angle up or down the incline—that is, to propel up or down the incline at an angle to the right for several feet and then propel at an angle to the left for several feet. This pattern is continued until he/she reaches the top or bottom of the incline.

Curbs

Ascending Forward The person who is able to perform a "wheelie" can be instructed to position the chair close to and facing the curb. Then he/she performs a partial "wheelie" to elevate the caster wheels onto the upper surface of the curb. He/she should lean forward and propel the chair onto the curb by pushing strongly and equally on the handrims. Some persons may be able to remain in a "wheelie" position and propel the chair up onto the curb on the rear wheels. However, this is an advanced technique and will require many hours of practice for most patients. *Caution:* If the caster wheels are not elevated high enough or if they are not placed on the upper level of the curb, the footrests are apt to strike the front of the curb. When this happens, the person's body will move forward, and he/she may fall out of the chair. When the caster wheels are placed on the upper level, the person must maintain his/her weight forward to avoid tipping backward.

Descending Forward Instruct the person to approach the edge of the curb and, when the caster wheels reach the edge, perform a "wheelie." Instruct him/her to roll the rear wheels over the edge of the curb until they rest on the surface below the curb, and then lower the caster wheels onto the lower surface. *Caution:* This technique creates a risk that the person may tip backward, or the chair may drop forward if the "wheelie" position is not maintained and it should be attempted only by those persons who are able to control the balance and position of the chair. You must guard the person very carefully when he/she practices descending or ascending the curb forward.

Descending Backward Instruct the person to turn the chair so that the curb edge is behind the chair and to wheel the chair to the edge of the curb; he/she leans the trunk forward and allows the rear wheels to slowly and gradually roll over the edge of the curb by retarding the movement of the chair with hand friction on the handrims. When the rear wheels are on the lower surface, instruct him/her to perform a "wheelie" and roll back away from the curb to clear the footrests from the curb. Then he/she lowers the caster wheels to the surface. If the patient is unable to perform a "wheelie," he/she wheels the chair backward until the caster wheels are on the same level as the rear wheels. When this technique is used the foot plates will probably strike and rest on the curb as the chair is moved away from the curb. This can damage or cause malalignment of the foot plates. *Caution:* There is a danger that the person may tip backward as the "wheelie" is performed or when the footrests are on the upper level of the curb. The person must lean the body forward to reduce this danger.

(*Note:* Independent ascent and descent of a curb require excellent strength, balance, and coordination and a great amount of practice before the person is able to perform the activity safely and independently. You must guard the patient during the practice sessions by remaining behind the chair and being ready

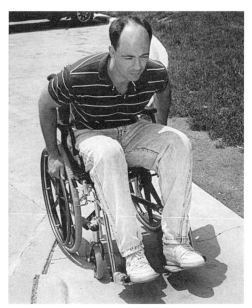

■ **FIGURE 7–43**
Forward ascent of a curb cut-out using both upper extremities.

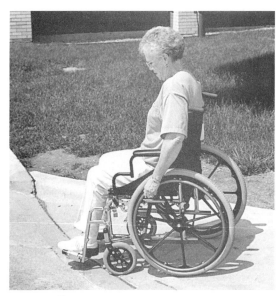

■ **FIGURE 7–44**
Forward descent of a curb cut-out.

to react to excessive forward or backward movement of the chair or the person to prevent a fall or injury.)

Curb Cutouts

Many curb cutouts have a relatively narrow area where the cutout meets the street. If the person does not align the caster wheels of the chair properly with this area, it may be difficult to ascend the cutout forward because the footrests may contact the surface, the chair may tip back when the caster wheels contact the surface, or the chair may stop abruptly when the foot plate or caster wheels contact this area. The person should be instructed to observe the cutout before attempting to use it so he/she will be prepared for the difficulties that could occur owing to the construction of the cutout.

Ascend Forward Instruct the person to use the same positions and techniques described for ascending an incline or ramp (Fig. 7–43). Some persons may be able to perform a "wheelie" and ascend the cutout on the rear wheels. This is an advanced method, and you will have to guard the person during practice sessions. If the cutout is steep or uneven with the street surface, it may be necessary for the person to perform a partial "wheelie" to elevate the foot plates over the edge of the cutout so the caster wheels will rest on the cutout surface. The person who uses one upper and one lower extremity to propel the chair may find it necessary to ascend backward. *Caution:* If the person ascends forward and the foot plates strike the cutout surface before the caster wheels rest on it, he/she may fall forward or lose his/her balance forward.

Descend Forward Instruct the patient to use the same positions and techniques described for an incline or ramp (Fig. 7–44). Some persons may be able to per-

form a "wheelie" and descend on the rear wheels of the chair. This is an advanced technique, and you will have to guard the person during practice sessions. If the cutout is steep or uneven with the street surface, the foot plates may strike the street surface before the caster wheels rest on it; this may cause the person to fall forward or lose his/her balance forward.

Descend Backward Instruct the person to use the same positions and techniques described for descending a curb or incline backward by keeping all four wheels in contact with the cutout (Fig. 7–45). (*Note:* Patients who use one upper extremity and one lower extremity to propel the chair should use the same techniques as described for an incline or ramp.)

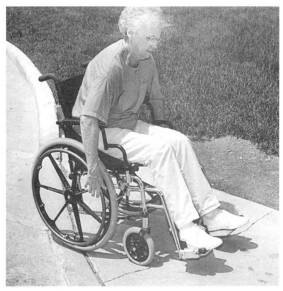

■ **FIGURE 7–45**
Backward descent of a curb cut-out.

Doors

The user of a wheelchair should be taught how to open a door with a self-closing device and proceed through the doorway, as well as how to open and proceed through the doorway and close a door without a self-closing device. He/she should also practice propelling the chair through the doorway until the activity can be accomplished safely and efficiently.

The door with a self-closing device poses problems for the wheelchair user because it offers resistance when it is opened and will be closing as the chair proceeds through the doorway. Therefore, the user will need to learn specific techniques to assist him/her to open the door, to keep it open as he/she moves through the doorway, and to avoid personal injury from the force of the self-closing device. If the resistance of the self-closing device or the size or weight of the door is excessive, or if the space available to open the door and manipulate the chair is limited, it may be necessary for the user to seek assistance with this task.

If the user intends to pass through an automatic, self-opening door (i.e., an electronically operated door) that swings on its hinges and opens toward the user, he/she must be cautioned to remain far enough away from the door so the front rigging of the chair or his/her feet will not be struck by the door as it opens. He/she should also practice propelling the chair over a raised threshold, which is often associated with exterior doors. It may be necessary to have the patient enter or exit backward to lead with the rear wheels of the chair and make it easier to cross the threshold. When he/she enters forward, it may be necessary for him/her to perform a partial "wheelie" to elevate the caster wheels over the threshold.

Self-Closing Door Opening Outward (Away From the Person)   Instruct the person to position the wheelchair to face the door at an angle toward the frame of the doorway containing the latch, if space permits (Fig. 7–46A). If space does not permit the person to angle the chair, instruct him/her to approach the door forward and as near as possible to the edge that will open. (*Note:* The door will not need to be opened as far if the person can propel through the doorway at an angle.) He/she reaches for the door knob, latch, or *crash bar* to open the door with a quick, firm push (see Fig. 7–46B). The door may be opened wider than necessary with one push, but it may need to be opened with a series of short pushes until it is opened wide enough for the chair to pass through the doorway. (*Note:* Some self-closing devices provide greater resistance when a forceful push is used to open the door.)

Because of the resistance offered by the self-closing device, the patient may need to stabilize the wheelchair so it does not roll backward before pushing on the door. This can be done by holding one handrim, locking one wheel, or holding onto the door frame (see Fig. 7–46C). The patient may be able to quickly propel the chair through the doorway before the door closes, but it is more likely that he/she will need to keep the door open to move through it (see Fig. 7–46D). This can be done by using the rubber bumper at the end of the front rigging, by holding the crash bar, or by using a series of pushes on the door or crash bar to keep the door open as he/she passes through the doorway (see Fig. 7–46E). The patient must protect his/her foot and hand nearest to the door when proceeding through the doorway.

Self-Closing Door Opening Inward (Toward the Person)   Instruct the patient to position the wheelchair to face the door at an angle toward the frame of the door with the hinges, if space permits (Fig. 7–47A). If space does not permit the patient to angle the chair, instruct him/her to approach the door forward and near to the edge that will open. He/she reaches for the door knob or latch to open the door with a quick, firm pull; it may need to be opened with a series of short pulls until it is opened wide enough for the chair to pass through the doorway (see Fig. 7–47B). The same techniques and precautions described previously to keep the door open, stabilize the chair, and propel the chair through the doorway can be applied to this activity. The person can use one hand on the door frame to pull the chair quickly through the doorway, and the rear wheels can be used to prevent the door from closing until the chair is completely through the doorway (see Fig. 7–47C to E). (*Note:* This will be an extremely difficult task for the patient who does not have functional use of both upper extremities and good trunk control.)

Regular Door, No Self-Closing Device   Instruct the patient to position the wheelchair as described for the door that opens outward or inward. Because there is no self-closing device, the patient will not need to use strong force to open the door and should open the door only wide enough for the chair to pass through the doorway. It will be necessary to turn the chair or the patient will need to turn his/her body to close the door once the chair has passed through the doorway. If the patient can move through the doorway at an angle, the door will not need to be opened as wide as it would if he/she moves straight through the doorway.

Elevators

The user of a wheelchair should be taught and should practice entering and exiting an elevator car. He/she may enter and exit forward or backward depending on the space available in the car and in the area outside the car, such as the corridor or entryway. You should caution him/her to be observant and aware of some specific problems associated with an elevator. For instance, the floor of the elevator and the surface of the corridor or entryway may be uneven; that is, the car may stop slightly above or below the outside surface. This may make it difficult for the person to enter

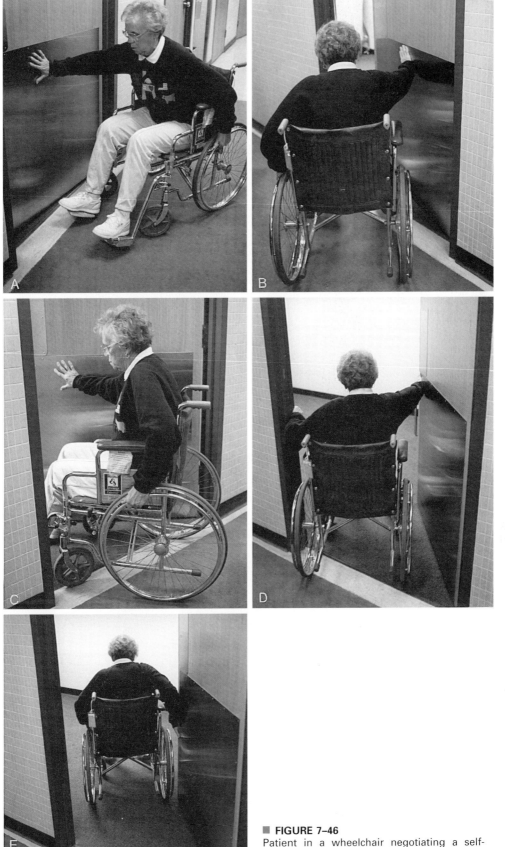

■ **FIGURE 7–46**
Patient in a wheelchair negotiating a self-closing door that opens away from her.

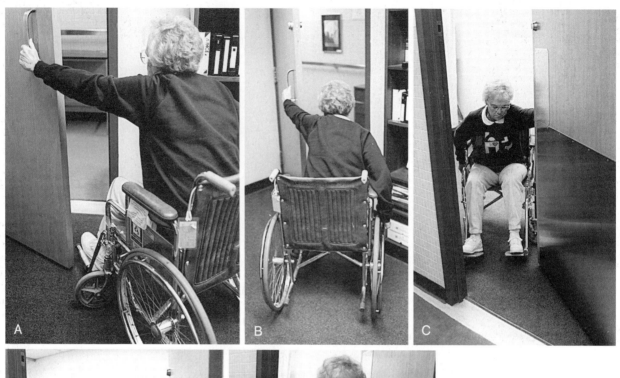

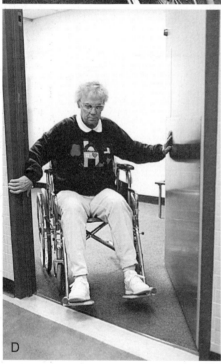

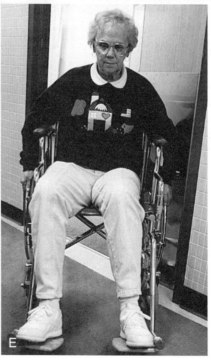

■ **FIGURE 7–47**
Patient in a wheelchair negotiating a self-closing door that opens toward her.

or exit the car, because the caster wheels may not roll over the elevated surface, or the chair could stop abruptly or tip forward. If this problem occurs, the person should enter and leave by leading with the rear wheels.

A second problem is a space between the front edge of the car floor and the outside surface. The caster wheels may drop into this space if they are turned to the side, and it may be difficult for the patient to extract them. If this problem occurs, the person should enter and leave the car with the caster wheels directed straight forward. Most of the informa-

tion provided previously in the section on assisted use of an elevator also applies to the independent use of it, and the person will need to decide whether to enter and exit forward or backward. He/she should be instructed to approach the external panel with the control pads or buttons with the wheelchair positioned at an angle or parallel to the wall containing the panel. This will enable him/her to reach the control pads or buttons more conveniently. If he/she approaches the wall directly forward, the front rigging will prevent the chair from being close to the control panel, and the person will have to lean forward to reach the

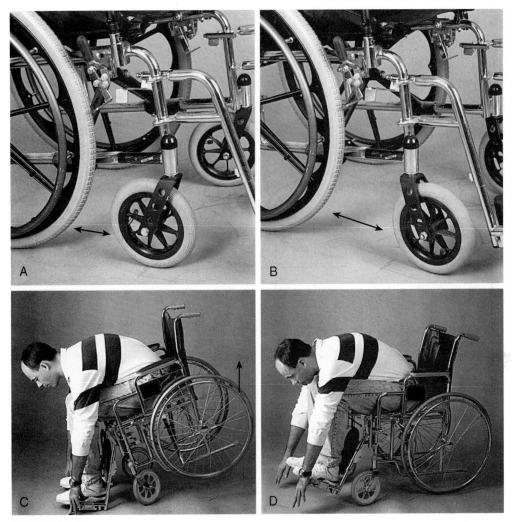

■ **FIGURE 7–48**
Patient in a wheelchair reaching for an object on the floor. *A,* Improper position of wheels. *B,* Proper position of wheels. *C,* Person reaching forward with wheels in improper position. *D,* Person reaching forward with wheels in proper position.

panel. Furthermore, it may not be possible to reach the pads or buttons that are located at the top of the panel, and assistance from another person may be required.

Once the person is inside the car, he/she may have to request another passenger to activate the desired floor designation pad or button. When exiting the car, it may be necessary to request another passenger to activate the "door open" control so the patient can be given more time to exit safely.

The person should be taught to recognize automatic door-opening devices such as a photoelectric beam or pressure sensors in the edge of the elevator doors. Remind the person that his/her feet and lower extremities project in front of the chair and are relatively unprotected from various objects in the environment, including the doors of an elevator. Therefore, the patient must be aware of the potential hazards or objects that could cause an injury to his/her feet and lower extremities. Also remind the patient that the handrims and rear wheels can provide protection, provided his/her hands and arms are placed within the area between the two wheels (e.g., in the lap or on the armrests). The rear of the chair is protected by the push handles and by the posterior position of the rear wheels. The front of the chair is somewhat protected by the rubber bumpers on the distal portion of the front rigging; however, the feet may project beyond the bumper.

Reaching an Object on the Floor in Front of the Chair Instruct the person to position the caster wheels in a forward position to increase the base of support of the chair (Fig. 7–48*A,B*). He/she should lock the rear wheels and shift the hips forward in the chair. Some persons may prefer to place their feet on the floor, but the feet can remain on the foot plates while the activity is performed. From this position, the person can reach forward for the object (see Fig. 7–48*C,D*). *Caution:* Instruct the person how to position

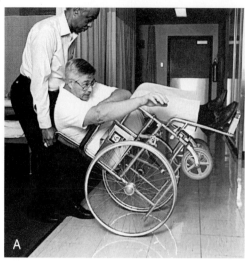 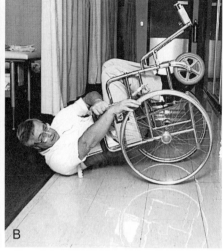

■ **FIGURE 7–49**
Instructing a patient in a wheel-chair how to fall backward.

the caster wheels and how to maintain trunk control while reaching forward. The caster wheels can be positioned by maneuvering the chair until they face forward, thereby increasing the distance between the back of the caster wheel and the front of the rear wheel. The person may need to control his/her trunk position by holding onto a push handle, the back frame, the seat frame, the armrest, or the upper position of the front rigging. The specific site chosen will depend on the patient's condition and abilities.

If the object weighs more than 5 to 10 pounds, the chair is apt to tip forward onto the footplates when it is lifted from the floor, or the person may have difficulty lifting the object and returning to an erect posture. This activity should be considered relatively unsafe and should be used primarily in an emergency. It is imperative to have the caster wheels positioned *forward* before the patient attempts this task. A safer procedure is to teach the patient to reach for and lift the object with the chair positioned at the side and parallel to the object.

Falling Backward When the chair tips backward, instruct the person to prevent the knees and thighs from hitting his/her face by placing one forearm across them with the hand holding the opposite armrest (Fig. 7–49*A*). He/she should flex his/her neck and reach forward with the free arm to promote trunk flexion (see Fig. 7–49*B*). He/she should not attempt to reach backward for protection, because this will increase the speed of the fall and the possibility of injury to the upper extremities and head. The push handles of the chair will strike the ground before the back of the chair, but it is important for the person to keep his/her head and trunk forward. Grasping an armrest with one hand will help to keep him/her in the chair. The feet are apt to fall off the footrests and the lower legs may dangle below the seat, as the chair tips back.

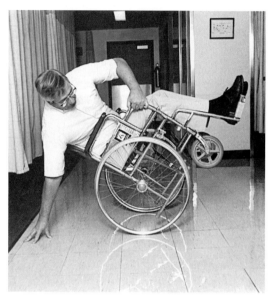

■ **FIGURE 7–50**
Patient returning to an upright sitting position.

Returning to an Upright Sitting Position Instruct the person to remain in the chair and lock the rear wheels. He/she places one hand on the floor behind the chair and reaches with the other arm across the body to the opposite seat rail or armrest (Fig. 7–50). The person uses the hand on the floor to "walk" forward, keeping the head and trunk flexed to move the chair to an upright position. When the chair has been elevated to its highest point a rapid, strong push with the hand on the floor while reaching forward with the other arm and flexing the head and neck will assist in tipping the front of the chair down. (*Note:* This is an advanced activity that will require a great amount of practice. A lap belt may be necessary during the practice sessions, and an assistant will be needed to help the patient attain an upright position; many patients may not be able to perform this activity independently.)

P R O C E D U R E 7 – 3
Protective Fall From a Wheelchair

These procedures should be described and demonstrated by the caregiver before the patient attempts them; when the patient practices the activity, he/she must be guarded closely, and protective mats should be placed on the floor.

1. Backward fall
   a. The patient quickly grasps an opposite armrest with one hand, allowing his/her forearm to rest on the thighs.
   b. He/she tucks the chin toward the chest and reaches *forward* with the free upper extremity.
   c. He/she remains in a semiflexed position and allows the push handles to contact the floor.
   d. To return to an upright position, he/she remains in the chair, locks the rear wheels, places one hand on the floor behind the chair, grasps an opposite armrest with the free upper extremity, and "walks" the hand on the floor forward while keeping the head and trunk flexed.
   e. Using the fingers, he/she pushes strongly and reaches forward with the opposite upper extremity to move the chair to an upright position.
   f. An alternate method is to remove his/her body from the chair, position the chair on all four wheels, and reenter the chair using one of the techniques presented in Chapter 6, providing no serious injury has occurred.

2. Forward fall
   a. The patient reaches forward with both upper extremities.
   b. When the hands contact the floor, he/she bends (flexes) the elbows to absorb some of the force of the fall.
   c. He/she attempts to turn or pivot the pelvis to land on one hip *or,* if the knees contact the floor first, he/she attempts to "side sit" on one hip.
   d. To return to the chair, the chair is positioned on all four wheels, and he/she reenters the chair using one of the techniques presented in Chapter 6, provided that no serious injury has occurred.

Alternatively, instruct the person to remove his/her body from the chair, place the chair upright, and enter the chair forward or backward as described in Chapter 6.

Falling Forward Instruct the person to hold an armrest with one hand and reach toward the floor with the other hand. This technique may cause the chair to fall on top of the person if he/she holds the armrest too long; therefore, some patients prefer to reach forward with both hands simultaneously for protection. Instruct the patient to absorb the force of the fall by flexing the elbows after the hands are on the floor. The knees may strike the floor with excessive force, and injury may result, unless the person is taught to turn his/her body so

he/she lands on the lateral side of a hip (Procedure 7–3).

Moving From the Wheelchair to the Floor and Returning to the Wheelchair Techniques for the patient to use to move from the wheelchair to the floor and return to the wheelchair are presented in Chapter 6. These techniques allow the patient to plan and somewhat control the movement from the wheelchair to the floor and return to the wheelchair. They should not be confused with the information related to falling forward or backward while seated in a wheelchair. However, a review of that material may provide some ideas you could offer the patient to assist him/her to develop methods of self-protection should he/she fall from the chair.

GENERAL CARE AND MAINTENANCE

A wheelchair will function best when it is maintained properly. The user should be encouraged to read and follow the instructions contained in the maintenance manual supplied by the manufacturer or distributor. Periodic cleaning of exposed metal with a nonabrasive metal polish or automobile wax and cleaning of the upholstery using an appropriate fabric cleaner or damp cloth is recommended. The chair should not be immersed in water or sprayed with a hose, and it should be wiped dry after exposure to rain, snow, or other types of moisture. The cross-brace center pin should be lubricated with a molybdenum-based grease every 6 months. Do not use light oil because it will collect dirt particles and will not provide long-lasting lubrication. The arm insert posts and the front and rear post slides (i.e., the open tubing into which the armrest posts insert) should be lubricated periodically with a silicone spray such as WD-40 or with a small amount of paraffin. The wheel bearings can be lubricated only if they are removed from the wheels. A high-quality bearing grease should be used as the lubricant. Do not oil the bearings, because oil will decrease the effectiveness of the grease that is in the bearings, and the overall lubrication will be decreased. It may be best to have these items inspected and lubricated by a reputable dealer or repair service.

Frequent visual inspection of the frame, upholstery, wheels, joints, tires, and other parts of the wheelchair will enable early detection of signs of wear or disrepair. Pneumatic tires should be checked for proper inflation at least monthly. Wheel spokes should be tested for tightness, and loose ones should be tightened to maintain proper rim shape and support. *Caution:* Improper tightening of the spokes may distort the shape of the rim, and it may be best to have this adjustment performed by a reputable dealer or repair service. The user and his/her family members should be encouraged to read the owner's manual periodically for information about proper maintenance. The facility where the chair was purchased and the manufacturer are additional sources of information about proper chair maintenance. In many large cities, wheelchair repair or service facilities are available and can be found in a telephone directory; additional information may be available from a health care facility. The patient and his/her family should be encouraged to perform proper maintenance and repair the chair promptly to enhance its function and longevity.

SUMMARY

When a wheelchair is a person's primary means of *locomotion*, it must fit and function properly to enhance his/her independence. The caregiver should be able to evaluate and confirm the fit of the wheelchair and to determine its mechanical condition and level of function. The potential adverse effects of an improperly fitting wheelchair should be recognized by the caregiver and explained to the user. These problems should be corrected or modified as soon as possible to avoid injury, discomfort, or reduced independent function.

The caregiver should become competent in the management and handling of the chair so he/she can demonstrate to and instruct others in the proper techniques or procedures. The person using the chair should be instructed to use the chair independently, including how to perform as many functional activities as possible within his/her abilities. Instruction in the proper maintenance and care of the chair should be provided.

■ SELF-STUDY/DISCUSSION ACTIVITIES

1. Discuss the potential adverse effects on the user of an improperly fitted wheelchair in relation to seat width, seat depth, leg length, armrest height, seat height, and back height.

2. Describe how you would teach a patient to propel a standard wheelchair on a level surface using (1) both upper extremities and (2) one upper extremity and one lower extremity. Consider how the person will turn and move backward.

3. List the primary components of a standard wheelchair.

4. Describe how you would confirm the fit of the wheelchair with the patient seated in the chair.

5. Describe how you would teach a patient to elevate the caster wheels (i.e., perform a "wheelie" or "pop-up").

6. For persons with hemiplegia of the left upper and lower extremities, paralysis below the level of the T10, bilateral midthigh amputations (no prostheses), or paralysis below the level of the C3, outline what wheelchair and components are required, and explain your rationale for your selection.

Chapter 8

Ambulation Aids, Patterns, and Activities

After studying this chapter, the reader will be able to:

1 Identify various types of ambulation aids.

2 Describe the advantages and disadvantages of various types of ambulation aids.

3 Describe and perform the two-point, four-point, three-point, three-one–point, and modified two-point and four-point gait patterns.

4 Describe the advantages and disadvantages of the previously cited gait patterns.

5 Teach a patient to perform any of the gait patterns cited, using appropriate equipment for his/her condition.

6 Describe and perform various functional activities.

7 Teach a patient to perform the functional activities appropriate for his/her condition, using proper ambulation aids.

■■■ K E Y   T E R M S

Affected: Attacked by disease; afflicted.

Ambulation: Act of walking or being able to walk.

Ambulation aid: A piece of equipment (e.g., crutch, cane, or walker) used to provide support or stability for a person as he/she walks.

Axilla: Armpit.

Axillary crutches: Wooden or metal crutches, adjustable or nonadjustable, that fit under a person's upper arms and into his/her axilla with a handpiece to grasp.

Bilateral: Pertaining to two sides.

Crab cane: A cane with three or four feet that forms a wider base of support than the single crutch tip; also referred to as a *three-* or *four-footed, quad,* or *hemi cane.*

Dorsiflexion: Backward flexion or bending, as of the hand or foot; for example, when the top of the foot (dorsum) approaches the lower leg/ankle, dorsiflexion has occurred.

Forearm crutches: Wooden or metal crutches with a full or half cuff that fits over a person's forearms and with a handpiece to grasp; also known as *Lofstrand* or *Canadian crutches.*

Four-point gait: The repetitive, alternate, reciprocal forward movement of an ambulation aid (e.g., a crutch or cane) and a person's opposite lower extremity.

Functional activities: Activities identified by an individual as essential to support his/her physical and psychological well-being and to create a personal sense of well-being.

Gait: The manner or style of walking.

Immobilizer: An object or apparatus that immobilizes or prevents motion, such as a cast or brace.

Monitor: To check constantly on a given condition or phenomenon, such as blood pressure or heart or respiration rates.

Parallel bars: Wooden or metal bars, adjustable or nonadjustable, that are horizontal and parallel to each other and attached to vertical uprights to provide a stable, nonmobile support for a person who requires an ambulation aid.

Pelvis: The lower portion of the trunk of the body.

Platform attachment: Wooden or metal crutches with an adjustable or nonadjustable platform for a person's forearm to rest on and aid in weight bearing.

Posterior: Toward the rear of an object.

Reciprocal: Corresponding but reversed on both sides.

Riser: A vertical piece of wood joining two steps: the back of the step.

Scapular: Pertaining to the scapula.

Styloid process: Long and pointed bony projection.

Three-one–point gait: One lower extremity is full weight bearing, and the opposite lower extremity is partial weight bearing; bilateral canes, crutches, or a walker are used to partially support the person's weight as he/she bears weight on the partial weight-bearing lower extremity; the full weight-bearing lower extremity advances independently, and the ambulation aids and partial weight-bearing lower extremity advance simultaneously.

Three-point gait: One lower extremity is full weight bearing and the opposite lower extremity is non–weight bearing; bilateral crutches or a walker are used to support the person's weight as he/she advances the weight-bearing lower extremity.

Tripod position: The use of three points as supports, such as a cane or crutch tips and a person's feet, with the tips in front of and to the side of the person's feet to form a base of support when the person stands.

Trochanter: A broad, flat surface on the femur at the upper end of its lateral surface (greater trochanter).

Two-point gait: The repetitive, simultaneous, reciprocal forward movement of an ambulation aid (e.g., a crutch or cane) and a person's opposite lower extremity.

Ulnar: Pertaining to the ulna, one of the two bones of the forearm.

Unilateral: Pertaining to one side.

Walker: An ambulation aid, usually with four contacts that are placed on the floor and a frame to support the patient's weight and provide stability during ambulation.

INTRODUCTION

An individual may require *ambulation aids* to compensate for impaired balance, decreased strength, alteration in coordinated movements, pain during weight bearing on one or both of the lower extremities, absence of a lower extremity (with or without prosthetic replacement), or altered stability; to improve functional mobility; to enhance body functions; and to assist with fracture healing. Selection of the proper ambulation devices and gait pattern is important to provide optimal security, safety, and function with the least expenditure of energy.

ORGANIZATION OF AMBULATION ACTIVITIES

GENERAL PREPARATION

It is important that planning and organization occur before initiating *ambulation* activities. The caregiver must be aware of the patient's problems and abilities; his/her goals and expectations of ambulation; the selection, measurement, and fit of the equipment needed for each patient; and the selection, practice, and progression of specific *gait* patterns and activities required by each patient (Box 8–1). Providing safety and protection to each patient through the use of proper guarding techniques, precautions, and instructions is necessary (Box 8–2). Finally, you may need to prepare the patient physically or mentally to perform the activities on which you and he/she decide.

PREPARATION FOR AMBULATION

After an assessment of the patient, it may be necessary to improve the patient's balance, coordination, flexibility (range of motion), strength, or endurance before initiating ambulation. A discussion of specific exercises or techniques to accomplish any of these activities is beyond the scope of this text. However, it is important to know the primary muscles required for ambulation with bilateral crutches when the patient will use a three-point or non–weight bearing (NWB) gait pattern. In the upper extremity, the *scapular* stabilizers, shoulder depressors, shoulder extensors, elbow extensors, and finger flexors are the most important muscles to strengthen. The scapular, shoulder, and elbow muscles support the body's weight and assist in moving the body, and the finger flexors are used to grasp the handpiece or handgrip of the device. In the weight-bearing lower extremity, the hip extensors and abductors, knee flexors and extensors, and the ankle *dorsiflexors* are the most important muscles to strengthen. The muscles of the hip and knee provide support and stability during weight bearing (e.g., the stance phase), whereas the ankle dorsiflexors position the foot so it clears the ground during forward motion of the extremity (i.e., the swing phase). Other muscles of the upper and lower extremity are also needed, but those cited are the most significant (Box 8–3).

For most patients, ambulation should be initiated with *parallel bars* to provide maximal security, stability, and safety. The gait pattern the patient is to use should be explained and demonstrated to the patient before it is attempted. Ambulation is a motor skill, and it is important that you provide instruction and the patient practice the activity to reduce his/her anxiety and fear and to increase the safety of the activity. The

BOX 8–1

Preparation for Ambulation Activities

1. Review the patient's medical record for information to assist in planning the ambulation activities. What information will be particularly important to you?
2. Assess or evaluate the patient to determine his/her limitations and capabilities to assist in planning the preambulation activities and gait pattern.
3. Determine the appropriate equipment and pattern based on the medical record, your assessment, and the goals of treatment.
4. Prepare the patient for ambulation (e.g., explain the pattern, obtain consent, and improve physical abilities).
5. Remove items in the area that may interfere with ambulation to maintain a safe environment.
6. Verify the initial measurement of the equipment to ensure a proper fit and determine that the equipment is safe. For example, tighten loose nuts and bolts, be certain spring adjustment buttons are secure, and examine rubber tips for dirt or cracks in the rubber.
7. Always apply a safety belt to the patient.
8. Be certain the patient is mentally and physically capable of performing the selected gait pattern.
9. Explain and demonstrate the gait pattern for the patient; ask the patient to describe the pattern, how it is to be performed, and what he/she is expected to do. Do not ask the patient whether he/she understands your instructions. Instead, require the patient to explain the procedure or activity in his/her words to verify that he/she truly understands and comprehends your instructions.
10. Use the safety belt and the patient's shoulder as points of control when guarding the patient.
11. Maintain proper body mechanics for yourself and the patient.

equipment selected must fit the patient properly and be in safe condition. When parallel bars are used, you should remain inside the bars to guard and assist the patient most effectively and to reduce the risk of injury to yourself.

If only partial weight bearing (PWB), rather than full weight bearing (FWB), is permitted, a temporary device with a microswitch connected to an audible

---

Precautions for Ambulation Activities

1. Be sure the patient wears appropriate footwear; do not allow the patient to ambulate while wearing slippers or loosely fitting shoes or while not wearing shoes. These conditions can lead to patient insecurity and injury.
2. *Monitor* the patient's physiologic responses to ambulation frequently and evaluate his/her vital signs, general appearance, and mental alertness during the activity. Compare your findings to normal values to determine the patient's reaction to the activity.
3. Avoid guiding or controlling the patient by grasping his/her clothing or his/her upper extremity. These items are insufficient to protect the patient.
4. Anticipate the unexpected, and be alert for unusual patient actions or equipment problems; anticipate that the patient may slip or lose his/her stability or balance at any time.
5. Guard the patient by standing behind and slightly to one side of him/her, and maintain a grip on the safety belt until the patient is able to ambulate independently and safely.
6. Do not leave the patient unattended while he/she is standing, because he/she may not be as stable as he/she appears or indicates to you, and he/she could fall.
7. Protect patient appliances (e.g., cast, drainage tubes, intravenous tubes, and dressings) during ambulation.
8. Be certain the area used for ambulation is free of hazards, such as equipment or furniture, and the floor or surface is dry. Safe conditions must be maintained to reduce the risk of injury to the patient.

---

alarm can be attached to the patient's shoe. The microswitch can be adjusted to cause the alarm to sound when the predetermined amount of weight bearing is exceeded. Another method to determine the amount of weight bearing is to have the patient place the PWB extremity on a scale. Instruct the patient to bear weight to the predetermined amount of weight bearing indicated on the scale. The patient must be able to proprioceptively remember and repeat a similar amount of weight bearing during ambulation. The patient's ability to partially bear weight should be reevaluated on the scale periodically to determine the amount of weight bearing the patient is using.

If a "touch-down" or "toe-touch" gait is requested, the patient should be encouraged to use a heel-strike gait or place the foot flat with minimal weight bearing, rather than using a toe-touch gait. The toe-touch pattern is an abnormal pattern because it positions the foot in plantar flexion at the beginning of the weight-bearing (stance) phase of the pattern. The normal gait pattern requires the heel to contact the floor first, so a heel-strike approach should be taught.

The patient must be protected during ambulation and *functional activities* through the use of proper guarding techniques by the caregiver or assistant. During the early gait training session, a safety belt should be applied to the patient's waist, and the caregiver should avoid grasping any part of the patient's clothing when guarding (Fig. 8–1). When the patient can safely perform independent ambulation activities, the safety belt may be removed. The judgment of the caregiver as to when the patient is able to ambulate independently and safely is critical. You must observe the patient carefully, noting any problems with balance, coordination, strength, or endurance, to determine his/her ability to perform safely and independently.

During ambulation the caregiver should be positioned behind and slightly to one side of the patient; one hand grasps the safety belt, and one hand rests on or is positioned in the area of the lateral upper shoulder. There are many proponents who believe the caregiver should initially stand behind and to the side of

---

Major Muscle Groups Used for Non–Weight-Bearing Ambulation

1. Upper trunk
   a. Scapular depression
   b. Scapular stabilizers
2. Lower trunk
   a. Trunk extensors
   b. Trunk flexors
3. Upper extremity
   a. Shoulder depressors
   b. Shoulder extensors and flexors
   c. Elbow extensors
   d. Finger flexors
4. Weight-bearing lower extremity
   a. Hip abductors
   b. Hip extensors
   c. Knee extensors
   d. Ankle dorsiflexors

Note: Strength, flexibility, endurance, and motor control of these groups should be evaluated before ambulation training and deficiencies should be corrected so the ambulation activity can be performed safely.

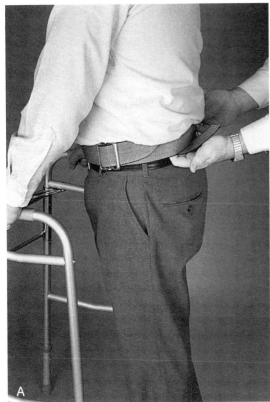

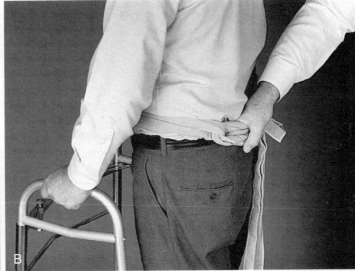

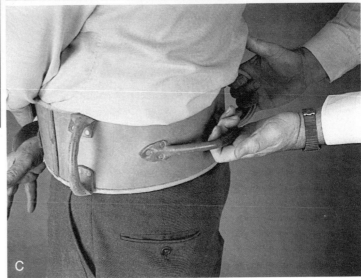

■ **FIGURE 8–1**
Caregiver grasping a correctly applied safety belt.

the patient's *affected* or weakest side or lower extremity. Using the hand nearest to the patient, grasp the safety belt with your fingers under the belt, palm up, and forearm supinated. The hand farthest from the patient is used to control his/her upper shoulder (Fig. 8–2). Some persons prefer to use their dominant hand on the safety belt, regardless of the patient's disability, and may stand nearer to the patient's stronger extremities.

During ambulation the lower extremity that is farthest from the patient should be positioned between the patient's lower extremity and the crutch or cane, whereas the lower extremity that is nearest to the patient remains behind the patient. For example, if you stand behind and to the patient's left side, your right hand would hold the safety belt, your left hand would control the patient's left shoulder, your left foot would be between the left crutch and the patient's left foot, and your right foot would trail behind the patient. You must learn to move forward in step with the patient. If the patient falls backward, pivot toward the patient and widen your stance to provide a stable support toward which the patient can be guided. If the patient falls to either side, guide the patient toward an upright, centered position. If the patient falls forward, step forward with your outside lower extremity and lower the patient to the floor using the safety belt. Other specific guarding techniques are presented later in this chapter (Procedure 8–1).

EQUIPMENT

Ambulation aids are designed to improve a person's stability by expanding his/her base of support, to reduce weight bearing on one or both lower extremities, and to permit mobility. Stated another way, they help the patient compensate for decreased balance, strength, or coordination or a decreased ability to bear weight on one or both lower extremities, and they reduce pain during ambulation.

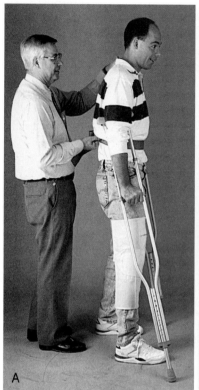
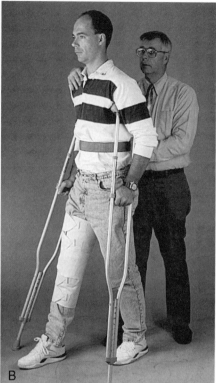
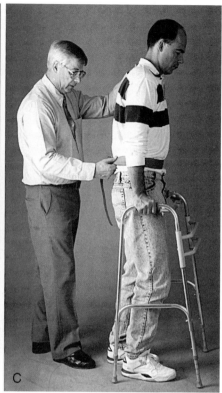

■ **FIGURE 8–2**
The caregiver's hand nearest to the patient grasps the safety belt; the other hand controls the shoulder.

PROCEDURE 8 – 1
Guarding a Patient During Ambulation

1. Apply a safety belt on the patient before ambulation.
2. Stand behind and slightly to one side of the patient (i.e., toward weak or affected extremity); remain close.
3. Grasp the safety belt with one hand; use your other hand to guard at the patient's shoulder. DO NOT GRASP THE PATIENT'S ARM OR CLOTHING.
4. Position your feet anterior-posterior; place your outside foot between the patient's foot and assistive aid and forward of your other foot; your inside foot trails your outside foot as the patient moves forward.
5. Move forward as the patient moves forward; maintain your outside foot forward of your inside foot as you move forward.
6. If patient loses balance forward, pull him/her toward you using the safety belt and your hand on his/her shoulder; assist patient to regain his/her balance and stability.
7. If patient loses balance backward, position your body behind the patient with feet anterior-posterior; allow him/her to lean against the side of your body; assist patient to regain his/her balance and stability.

The basic categories of ambulation aids, given in order from greatest to least in their amount of support or stability are parallel bars, walkers, crutches, single crutches, bilateral canes, and single canes. A patient may need to initiate ambulation with an aid that provides maximal stability or support but restricts mobility. As the patient's ability or condition improves, he/she may be able to progress to an aid that provides less stability or support and allows greater mobility. The decision regarding which type of aid to use, when to change to a different aid, and the type of gait pattern to use will be made by the clinician. Criteria to consider include the environment in which the patient will ambulate, the expected or desired ambulation activities, and the prognosis for improvement or regression of his/her condition and abilities.

Parallel Bars Parallel bars are used when maximal patient stability and support are required. Many gait patterns are initiated in parallel bars, and the evaluation of the fit of the ambulation aid is frequently performed in bars. The bars severely limit mobility, and the patient must progress to another ambulation aid to be mobile. The bars should be adjusted so a proper fit for each patient is accomplished.

Walkers *Walkers* are used when maximal patient stability and support, along with mobility, are required. Various styles are available, and most have four support legs/feet; some may have two or more wheels, and most can be adjusted for proper fit. Walkers are lightweight, and some can be folded for storage. Disadvantages of the use of a walker include the following:

1. It may be difficult to store or transport.

2. It is difficult or impossible to use on stairs.

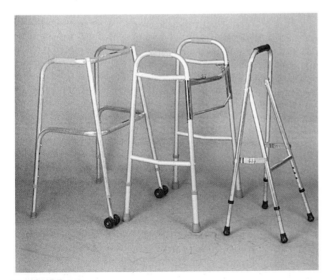

■ **FIGURE 8–3**
Three types of walkers *(left to right):* the wheeled, folding, and "Hemi" walkers. All are adjustable.

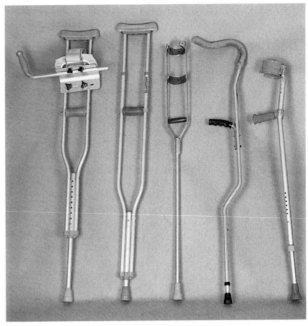

■ **FIGURE 8–4**
Five types of crutches *(left to right):* the forearm attachment, adjustable aluminum, triceps, offset adjustable, and forearm adjustable (Lofstrand or Canadian crutches).

3. It reduces the speed of ambulation.

4. It may be difficult to perform a normal gait pattern.

5. It can be difficult to use in narrow or crowded areas.

Types include standard (adjustable, nonadjustable), *reciprocal,* stair-climbing, wheeled, folding, and one-handed ("hemiplegic") (Fig. 8–3).

Axillary Crutches *Axillary crutches* are used for persons who need less stability or support than that provided by parallel bars or a walker. They allow greater selection of gait patterns and ambulation speed and provide good stability and support. Most crutches are composed of wood or aluminum and can be easily adjusted for proper fit. They are relatively easily stored and transported and can be used in narrow or crowded areas or for stairs. Disadvantages include the following:

1. They are less stable than a walker.

2. They can cause injury to axillary vessels and nerves if used improperly.

3. They require good standing balance.

4. Elderly patients may feel insecure with them.

5. Functional strength of the upper extremities and trunk muscles is required for most gait patterns.

Types include standard (adjustable, nonadjustable), offset, and triceps (elbow extension) (Fig. 8–4).

Forearm Crutches *Forearm crutches*, also referred to as *Lofstrand* or *Canadian crutches*, are used when the stability and support of an axillary crutch are not required but more stability and support than can be provided by a cane are needed. They eliminate the danger of injury to axillary vessels and nerves and are more functional on stairs and in narrow, confined areas. It is relatively easy to store and transport these crutches, and the forearm cuff retains the crutch on the forearm when the patient reaches for an object. Disadvantages include the following:

1. They provide less stability and support than axillary crutches, a walker, or parallel bars.
2. They require good standing balance and good upper body and upper extremity strength for many gait patterns.
3. The forearm cuff makes it difficult to remove the crutch.
4. Elderly patients may feel insecure with them.

Types include standard (adjustable, nonadjustable) (see Fig. 8–4).

Platform Attachment A *platform attachment* is used for individuals who are unable to bear weight through their wrists and hands; who have severe deformities of the wrists or fingers, making it difficult to grasp the handpiece of a regular crutch; who have a below-elbow amputation; or who are unable to extend one or both elbows passively. Disadvantages include the following:

1. The patient loses the use of his/her triceps to elevate and maintain his/her body during the swing phase.
2. Another person may need to apply them.
3. They are less effective on stairs.

Types include a platform that can be attached to an axillary or forearm crutch or to a walker; it is sometimes referred to as a "trough" or "shelf" (see Fig. 8–4).

Cane A cane is used to compensate for impaired balance or to improve stability. A cane is more functional on stairs and in narrow, confined areas, and it can be stored and transported more easily than crutches or a walker. Disadvantages include the following:

1. A cane provides very limited stability because of its small base of support.
2. Two canes do not provide sufficient stability to perform a *three-point gait* pattern, but they can be used to perform other gait patterns.

Types include "J," "T," pistol grip, offset shaft, three- or four-legged/footed (sometimes referred to as

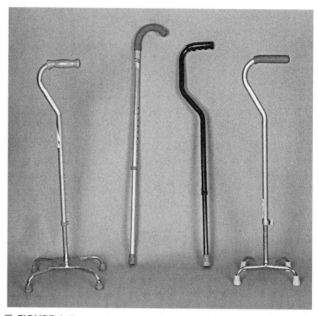

■ **FIGURE 8–5**
Four types of canes *(left* to *right):* four-footed adjustable ("crab" or "Hemi"), J-top adjustable, offset adjustable, and another four-footed adjustable ("crab" or "Hemi").

a *quad, Hemi,* or *crab cane*), and Walkane (walk cane) (Fig. 8–5).

MEASUREMENT AND FIT

There are several methods that can be used to initially measure the various ambulation aids. If the initial measurement is performed with the patient in a position other than standing, the fit of the aid must be evaluated and confirmed when the patient stands. An aid that does not fit the patient properly will adversely affect the patient's ability to perform a gait pattern and may result in an unsafe or unstable pattern. The position to use to confirm the fit of the aid is described in another section of this chapter.

Parallel Bars Each bar should be adjusted to provide 20 to 25 degrees of elbow flexion when the patient stands erect and grasps the bars approximately 6 inches anterior to his/her hips. The bars should be approximately 2 inches wider than the patient's greater *trochanters* when he/she is centered between the bars. The elbow flexion can be estimated by adjusting the bar so its top is even with the patient's greater trochanter or with the patient's wrist crease or *ulnar styloid process* when the patient stands erect and the upper extremity is straight along the side.

Canes The length of the cane can be determined with the patient standing or supine. The handgrip of the cane should be placed at the level of the patient's greater trochanter or the wrist crease of the ulnar

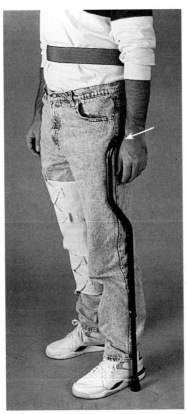

■ FIGURE 8-6
Measurement for proper fit of a cane.

styloid with the arm straight along the side. Place the cane parallel to the femur and tibia with the foot (tip) of the cane on the floor or at the bottom of the heel of the shoe (Fig. 8–6). A tape measure can be used to determine the distance from the patient's greater trochanter to the heel with the hip and knee straight, which determines the length of the cane.

Forearm Crutch   The length of the crutch can be measured as described for the cane to determine the height of the handpiece with the patient supine or standing (Fig. 8–7A). The top of the forearm cuff should be located approximately 1 to 1½ inches distal to the olecranon process when the patient grasps the handpiece with the cuff applied to the forearm and the wrist in neutral flexion-extension (Fig. 8–7B).

Axillary Crutch   Several methods can be used to measure this aid.
Length of Crutch
1. If the height of the patient is known, multiply the height by 77% (e.g., 70 inches × 77% = 53.90, or 54 inches) *or* subtract 16 inches from the height (e.g., 70 inches − 16 inches = 54 inches) and use the resulting value for the overall crutch length (i.e., axillary rest to tip).
2. With the patient supine, use a tape to measure the distance from the anterior axillary fold (crease of the armpit) to a point approximately 6 to 8 inches

lateral to the patient's heel for the overall crutch length.
3. With the patient sitting and his/her upper extremities abducted at shoulder level, with one elbow extended and one elbow flexed to 90 degrees, measure from the olecranon process of the flexed elbow to the tip of the long finger of the hand of the opposite upper extremity; this determines the overall crutch length.

These methods should provide similar results, but there may be a difference in the measurements. You will have to select the method that provides the best result consistently. This measurement is an estimate of the length of the crutch and will have to be confirmed with the patient standing.

Handpiece Height   With the patient supine, measure from the greater trochanter, from the wrist crease, or from the ulnar styloid process with the arm by the side and the elbow extended to the heel of the shoe; hold the tape next to the side of the lower extremity. Use this value to position the handpiece by measuring up from the rubber tip of the crutch to the handpiece. An alternative method is to measure from the anterior axillary fold to the patient's trochanter or ulnar styloid with the arm along the side. Use this value to position the handpiece by measuring downward from the center of the axillary rest to the handpiece.

Parallel Bar Method   Stand the patient in parallel bars with the head erect, shoulders level and relaxed, upper extremities grasping the parallel bars, trunk erect, hips straight, *pelvis* level, knees slightly flexed, and feet flat on the floor. Use this position to measure from a point at the anterior axillary fold to a point on the floor approximately 2 inches lateral and 4 to 6 inches anterior to the patient's toes for the overall crutch length.

It will be necessary to ask the patient or another person to hold one end of the tape at the *axilla* as you extend the tape to the floor. To determine the handpiece height, the crutch should be positioned in the patient's axilla with the tip forward and lateral to the patient's toes. The patient should have approximately 20 to 25 degrees of elbow flexion when he/she grasps the handpiece while keeping the shoulders level and relaxed. The slight amount of elbow flexion will allow the patient to lift or support the body by extending the elbows during the non–weight-bearing phase of the three-point gait pattern and to maintain a comfortable elbow position when other gait patterns are used. To obtain the most accurate measurement and fit, the axillary pad, handpiece pad, and crutch tip should be applied before all measurements are made and the fit is confirmed, and the patient should wear shoes.

ALTERNATIVE METHOD   Position the patient in the parallel bars as described previously. Using a crutch with push-button ("quick fit") length and handpiece adjustments, position the crutch in the axilla and

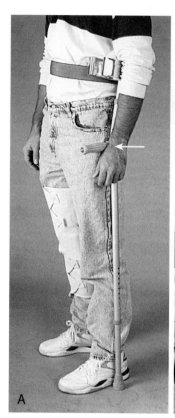

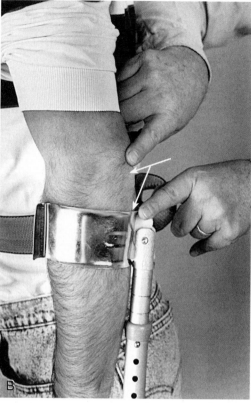

■ **FIGURE 8–7**
Measurement for proper fit of a forearm crutch.

along the patient's side. Adjust the handpiece at the level of the wrist crease, or greater trochanter, or ulnar styloid process; then position the tip approximately 2 inches lateral and 4 to 6 inches anterior to the forefoot (toes), and adjust the length so that there are approximately two finger breadths between the axillary rest and the bottom of the axilla. Have the patient grasp the handpiece, and evaluate the amount of elbow flexion and the length of the crutch with the crutch in the proper forward, *tripod position*. Readjust the crutch as necessary to obtain the proper length and handpiece position.

Any one of these methods should provide an initial measurement, which should be evaluated and confirmed with the patient standing. Do not rely on these measurements to be exact or final. The fit must be evaluated with the person standing with the ambulation aid properly positioned.

Common errors associated with the measurement or evaluation of fit of axillary crutches are listed in Box 8–4.

Walker The height of the walker can be determined with the patient standing or supine. The handgrip of the walker should be placed level with the patient's wrist crease, ulnar styloid process, or greater trochanter, with the walker positioned in front of and along the patient's sides and with the patient's arms straight along the sides (Fig. 8–8). The feet of the walker should be resting on the floor or even with the heels; the hips and knees should be straight, and shoes

BOX 8–4

Common Errors in Fitting of Axillary Crutches

1. The patient elevates or hunches his/her shoulders, and the crutches are improperly measured. The crutches will be too long when the patient stands properly.
2. The patient depresses or drops his/her shoulders or flexes the trunk at the hips, and the crutches are improperly measured. The crutches will be too short when the patient stands properly.
3. The patient flexes or extends his/her wrist, and the handpiece is improperly positioned too high.
4. The measurements are made without the patient wearing shoes or without the crutch tips or axillary pads in place. The crutches will be improperly measured and will be too long as a result.
5. The crutch evaluation is made without the patient in the tripod position. The crutches may be too short or too long depending on how the patient stood initially.

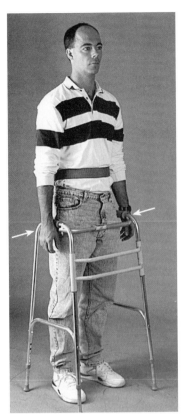

■ **FIGURE 8–8**
Measurement for proper fit of a walker.

should be worn. A tape measure can be used to determine the distance from the patient's greater trochanter to the heel, with the shoe on and with the hip and knee straight. This value is used to adjust the height of the walker by measuring from the floor to the top of the handpiece with the walker resting on its feet on the floor or on a higher surface such as a treatment table.

CONFIRMATION OF FIT

Improper fit is apt to cause decreased stability, increased energy expenditure, decreased function, and decreased safety for the patient.

The evaluation of the fit of crutches can be performed only with the patient standing with his/her head erect, shoulders relaxed and level, trunk erect, hips in extension, pelvis level, knees slightly flexed, and feet flat on the floor. The crutch tips are positioned approximately 2 to 4 inches lateral and 4 to 6 inches anterior to the toes or forefoot; the elbows should be flexed approximately 20 to 25 degrees when grasping the handpiece with the wrists in a neutral position. This position forms a triangle of the crutch tips and the patient's foot or feet and is called the tripod position. This position provides the best base of support and starting position for most crutch gait patterns, especially the three-point and three-one patterns (Fig. 8–9).

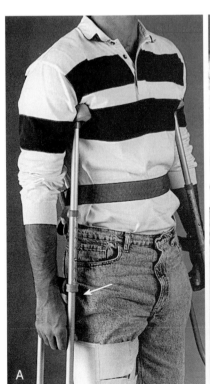
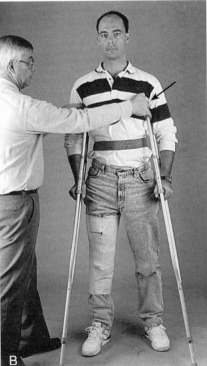
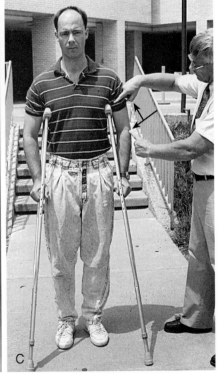

■ **FIGURE 8–9**
Measurement and confirmation of the fit of axillary crutches.

PROCEDURE 8 – 2
Confirmation of the Fit of an Ambulation Aid

Each aid should be evaluated for fit with the patient standing with his/her head erect, shoulders relaxed and level, trunk erect, pelvis level, knees flexed slightly, and feet (foot) flat.

1. Axillary crutches
   a. Position the axillary rest in the axilla; position the tips approximately 2 inches lateral and 4 to 6 inches anterior to the toe of the shoe(s).
   b. Have the patient grasp the handpieces with the wrists straight (avoid wrist flexion or extension).
   c. Evaluate for space between the top of the axillary rest and the floor of the axilla; it should be approximately 2 inches.
   d. Observe the angle of elbow flexion; it should be approximately 20 to 25 degrees.

2. Forearm crutches
   a. Have the patient grasp the handpieces with his/her forearms inserted in the forearm cuffs.
   b. Position the crutch tips approximately 2 inches lateral and 4 to 6 inches anterior to the toe of the shoe(s).
   c. Observe the angle of elbow flexion; it should be approximately 20 to 25 degrees.
   d. Observe the position of the upper edge of the cuff; it should be approximately 1 to 1.5 inches below the olecranon process.

3. Walker
   a. Position the walker in front of the patient so the rear feet are approximately opposite to the toe of the shoe(s).
   b. Have the patient grasp the handpieces; observe the angle of elbow flexion; it should be approximately 20 to 25 degrees.

4. Cane
   a. Position the cane so the tip is approximately 2 inches lateral and 4 to 6 inches anterior to the toe of the shoe(s).
   b. Observe the angle of elbow flexion; it should be approximately 20 to 25 degrees.
   c. The width of the bars, if it can be adjusted, should provide approximately 2 to 4 inches of space between the patient's hips and the rail on each side.

The fit of a walker, cane, and forearm crutches should also be confirmed with the patient standing. There should be approximately 20 to 25 degrees of elbow flexion when the patient grasps the handpiece and positions the device in preparation for ambulation. The tips of the forearm crutches and cane(s) are placed forward approximately 4 to 6 inches and approximately 2 to 4 inches lateral to each forefoot. The rear tips of the walker should be placed opposite to the midportion of the patient's feet (foot). The patient's posture should be similar to that described for the crutch fit evaluation. The initial fit of the aid may need to be revised after the patient has ambulated several times. As the patient becomes stronger, more skilled, and more proficient, the initial fit of the aid may no longer be comfortable or efficient. It will be necessary to observe the patient as he/she ambulates to determine whether the aid continues to fit properly. The aid should be adjusted if it is not providing proper function to avoid the development of bad gait habits or an unsafe gait pattern (Procedure 8–2).

TILT TABLE

A tilt table may benefit persons who need to physiologically accommodate to an upright position due to a variety of conditions, such as prolonged recumbence; disturbance in balance, proprioception, kinesthesia, lower extremity circulation; or generalized weakness. A tilt table is particularly useful because it can be elevated gradually and maintained at any position between horizontal and completely vertical. Changes in elevation levels are accomplished manually or mechanically; a scale or protractor attached to the frame can be used to measure the elevation angle the person attains and tolerates. The ability to gradually elevate a person from a horizontal to an upright position and to allow him/her to adapt or adjust to any given elevation provides a safe method for the body to accomplish physiological accommodation for upright activities (Fig. 8–10).

The person's vital signs should be measured before treatment to establish baseline values, especially for blood pressure and pulse rate. His/her vital signs should be measured each time he/she progresses to higher elevation, and a log of the values should be maintained as part of the records. Excessive increases or decreases in the blood pressure and pulse rate are usually indicators the person is experiencing difficulty adapting to an upright position. Other indicators of the person's intolerance include changes in consciousness, excessive perspiration, facial pallor, edema formation in the lower legs, decrease in or loss of pedal pulses, complaints of nausea or numbness or tingling in the lower extremities, and dizziness. A person whose condition limits his/her capacity or ability to return venous blood from the lower extremities or abdomen to the heart may benefit from the application of elastic bandages or elastic hose to the lower extremities or from an abdominal binder.

Although it is the circulatory system that is primarily conditioned, bowel and bladder function may also be affected in a positive manner due to the effect of gravity. In addition, it has been theorized that standing on a tilt table may assist in promoting or maintaining bone density in the lower extremities, especially for the person with a complete spinal cord injury. However, research studies have not provided conclusive evidence this effect occurs. Finally, many persons who have used a tilt table have indicated their mental outlook was improved because they were able to assume a semi-upright or fully upright position even if only for a brief period. Other activities can be performed by the person while he/she is standing, depending on the amount of function he/she has in the upper extremities, his/her mental status or capacity, and the maximum elevation he/she can tolerate. An adjustable over-the-bed table or a lap board attached

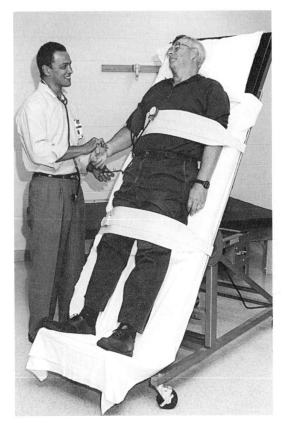

■ **FIGURE 8–10**
Use of a tilt table; caregiver measures pulse rate and blood pressure.

to the frame of the tilt table can be used to support items such as reading or writing materials, food and utensils, communication devices, personal hygiene materials, games, cards, and similar items. Thus, the person can be somewhat active while standing rather than merely standing. Strengthening and range-of-motion exercises can be performed, and some lower extremity muscle groups can be positioned so a prolonged passive stretch force can be applied to them.

Usually, it will not be necessary to elevate the person to 90 degrees to assist him/her in adapting to or accommodating an upright position. An elevation of approximately 70 to 80 degrees for 15 to 20 minutes should be sufficient; however, you must consider each person individually. When the person is elevated above 80 degrees he/she will sense that he/she is falling forward. This occurs because his/her center of gravity (COG) will be shifted forward due to the pressure from the surface of the table against his/her back. The compensatory function of the anterior-posterior curves of the body is negated by the table surface; thus, he/she senses a forward position change has occurred. The frequency and duration of treatment sessions with a tilt table vary depending on the person's condition or diagnosis, his/her response to the treatment, and his/her ability or capacity to adapt to, accommodate, or tolerate an upright position. A session may be as brief as 5 or 10 minutes or as long as 1 hour, and they may occur once or twice per day or on alternate days (Procedure 8–3).

PARALLEL BAR ACTIVITIES

Most patients should initiate their gait training in parallel bars, because they provide maximal stability, security, and safety. After the patient has practiced the pattern in the parallel bars, he/she will be able to perform the selected gait pattern with ambulation aids with greater ease and safety. It is important that the height and width of the bars be adjusted properly for each patient for safety and efficiency.

MOVING FROM SITTING TO STANDING

The necessary components of the activity of moving from sitting to standing are forward movement of the body to the center or front portion of the seat, proper foot placement, forward inclination of the trunk, flexion of the hips, extension of the neck and spine, forward movement of the pelvis to initiate an erect posture, and extension of the hips and knees to attain the final standing posture. These activities assist the individual in shifting the COG over and within the base of support and to align the trunk and to move the COG from a lower to a higher position. To return to sitting, the patient will have to incline the trunk forward, combined with hip and knee flexion and extension of the neck and spine; move the knees forward; and flex the hips and knees to lower the body into the chair seat. These same principles should be applied to standing transfers.

STANDING IN PARALLEL BARS

Prepare and instruct the patient to do the following:

1. Position and lock the wheelchair in front of the bars with a safety belt applied.
2. Remove his/her feet from the footrests, lift the footrests, and swing away the front rigging or remove it, if possible.
3. Position desk type arms with the higher portion forward, if these are one of the features of the chair.
4. Move the body forward to the middle or the front edge of the seat by either alternately lifting each hip or side of the pelvis and moving it forward or by leaning against the back of chair and sliding the

hips forward, then moving the trunk forward. If the patient can move each hip forward alternately, he/she will be more independent in preparing to stand and adjusting the position of the body.
5. Position the foot of the stronger lower extremity slightly *posterior* to the foot of the affected or involved lower extremity so that the stronger extremity will be in the best position to assist to raise or elevate the patient from the chair seat. (*Note:* For some patients, it may be desirable to place their feet parallel to each other or to position the foot of the weaker lower extremity posterior to the other foot. You will have to try each position with some patients to determine which one is most effective.)
6. Place both hands forward on the armrests of the chair with the trunk inclined forward (i.e., "the nose over the toes" position).
7. Simultaneously push down with the upper and lower extremities while leaning the trunk forward and then continue to stand by extending the hips and knees and alternately placing each hand onto a parallel bar. Do not allow the patient to use the bars to pull himself/herself to a standing position, because when the bars are not available, the patient will not have a stable object on which to pull. The ability to stand independently is enhanced when the patient is taught to stand by pushing on the chair armrests while simultaneously using the lower extremities to elevate the body.

BALANCE AND PREAMBULATION ACTIVITIES

1. The patient stands and slowly shifts his/her weight from side to side and forward and back while maintaining the shoulders and pelvis in line and the trunk erect. He/she should hold each position change for 3 to 5 seconds.
2. At first the patient should be taught to briefly and alternately lift the hands from the bars to promote a sense of the decreased support he/she will experience when the ambulation aid is moved; later, both hands can be lifted simultaneously. The patient may be taught to perform a "push-up" using the bars to improve his/her arm strength and to experience the sense of effort required to support the body when the lower extremities are not in contact with the floor or ground. The patient may be taught to alternately or simultaneously lift his/her opposite upper and lower extremities to simulate a particular gait pattern or to increase balance when support and stability are decreased. Other exercises to improve the patient's strength, endurance, and coordination can be performed with him/her

PROCEDURE 8 – 3
Tilt Table

1. Explain the procedure to the patient and obtain consent; measure the person's vital signs.

2. Position him/her supine on the table; place a rolled towel beneath each knee; position his/her feet flat on the footboard approximately shoulder width apart. The upper extremities may be positioned parallel to the sides of the body, and they may be placed beneath or remain free from the chest strap or they may rest on an over-the-table support or be supported by slings attached to the table frame. A pillow under the head will add to his/her comfort until he/she is elevated to approximately 75 degrees, at which time it may be more comfortable if the pillow is removed.

3. Apply one restraint strap over the lower thighs (just proximal to the patellae) and one strap across the mid or upper thorax; a towel may be placed beneath each strap for protection and comfort; the strap buckles should be positioned so they do not contact the patient. *Note:* When the lower strap is applied over the distal thigh, rather than directly over the patellae, pressure to the patellae can be avoided. If desired, a third strap can be applied over the abdomen or pelvis. *Caution:* An abdominal strap should not be used in place of a chest strap, especially for a person who lacks functional trunk and hip extensors. An abdominal strap, without a chest strap, will not prevent the upper body from falling forward at elevations at which gravity has a forward force effect (i.e., approximately 65 to 75 degrees). If a chest strap is not in place, the person must have sufficient strength and control of the trunk and hip extensors to maintain his/her body erect.

4. Elevate the table to a position tolerated by the person; maintain that position for several minutes; measure and log his/her vital signs; inquire about his/her status (i.e., "How do you feel?" "Are you comfortable?").

5. If his/her condition is stable, raise the table to a new elevation; measure and log his/her vital signs; evaluate his/her tolerance to the new position; maintain the position for several minutes.

6. Repeat this process based on his/her ability to tolerate and accommodate to becoming more erect; continue to measure and log his/her vital signs; decrease elevation of the table when it is apparent he/she is unable to tolerate a given elevation. *Caution:* Signs and symptoms of intolerance to being upright include loss of consciousness, excessive increase in pulse rate (tachycardia) or excessive decrease in blood pressure (hypotension), facial pallor, excessive perspiration, or complaints of nausea, dizziness, or sensory changes in the lower extremities. Be observant for signs and symptoms of autonomic hyperreflexia and postural (orthostatic) hypotension. (Refer to Chapter 11 for information about these conditions.) *Note:* Several sessions may be required for the person to become tolerant to an upright position.

7. To conclude a treatment session, return him/her to horizontal; observe him/her and inquire about his/her status; measure and log his/her vital signs; observe and palpate the lower extremities for edema or circulatory responses (i.e., pedal pulses, color, temperature).

8. Document your activities and findings as necessary.

in the bars. The selection of specific exercises should be based on the patient's disability and residual abilities and the particular gait pattern to be used, and the exercises should be designed to improve his/her ambulation skills.

3. The patient should practice the selected gait pattern in the bars; he/she should be taught and should practice moving forward, backward, and sideward and turning to the right and to the left.

4. The patient should practice the selected gait pattern using the proper ambulation aid. The aid may be used with the patient inside the bars, or the patient may use one bar and one ambulation aid.

You should guard the patient by using a safety belt and proper protective techniques. It is recommended that you remain inside the bars with the patient for optimal control and safety.

BASIC GAIT PATTERNS

Selection of the appropriate gait pattern will depend on the patient's balance, strength, coordination, functional needs, weight-bearing status, and energy level. The advantages and disadvantages of several patterns are presented (see Box 8–4).

Four-Point Pattern The *four-point gait* pattern requires the use of *bilateral* ambulation aids. The pattern uses an alternate and reciprocal forward movement of the ambulation aid and the patient's opposite lower extremity (i.e., right crutch, then left foot; left crutch, then right foot) (Fig. 8–11). This is a very slow but stable pattern and is the safest one to use in crowded areas. It requires low energy expenditure and can be used when the patient requires maximal stability or balance. It approximates a normal gait pattern, but the patient must ambulate slowly.

Two-Point Pattern The *two-point gait* pattern requires the use of bilateral ambulation aids. The pattern uses a simultaneous and reciprocal forward placement of the ambulation aid and the patient's opposite lower extremity (i.e., right crutch and left foot; left crutch and right foot) (Fig. 8–12). This is a relatively stable pattern and can be performed more rapidly than the four-point gait. It requires relatively low energy expenditure and is very similar to a normal gait pattern. However, it also requires coordination by the patient to move one upper extremity and its opposite lower extremity forward simultaneously. The patient can ambulate more rapidly but with less stability than with the four-point pattern (Fig. 8–13).

Modified Four-Point or Two-Point Pattern These patterns require only one ambulation aid and are used for the patient who has only one functional upper extremity or who uses only one ambulation aid. The aid is held in the upper extremity opposite to the lower extremity that requires protection. This will widen the

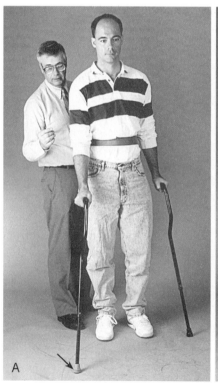
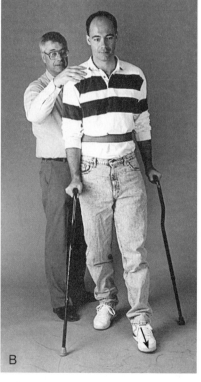

A   B

■ **FIGURE 8–11**
Four-point gait pattern.

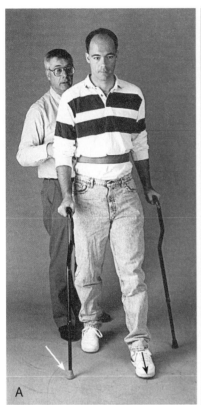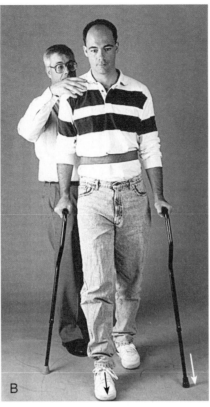

■ **FIGURE 8–12**
Two-point gait pattern.

base of support and assist in shifting the patient's COG away from the protected lower extremity. This pattern is sometimes referred to as a "hemi" gait or "hemi" pattern. The patient performs the pattern in the sequences described for the four- and two-point pattern, but only one ambulation aid is used; thus the pattern is "modified" (Fig. 8–14).

Three-Point Pattern The three-point gait pattern requires bilateral ambulation aids or a walker but cannot be performed with bilateral canes. The pattern should be referred to as a "step-to" or "step-through" pattern rather than a "swing-to" or "swing-through" pattern. It is used when the patient is able to bear weight on one lower extremity but is non–weight bearing (NWB) on the opposite lower extremity.

The walker or crutches and the NWB extremity are advanced, and then the patient steps up to the walker or through the crutches (Fig. 8–15). It is a less stable pattern than the patterns described previously or the three-one pattern, but rapid ambulation is possible. It requires good strength in the upper extremities, trunk, and one lower extremity, and energy expenditure is quite high because of the need to use the upper extremities to lift, support, and propel the body. The patient should be taught to step through the crutches and to control the movement of the trunk and lower extremities with his/her normally functioning musculature. This will reduce energy expenditure and increase the patient's balance and stability.

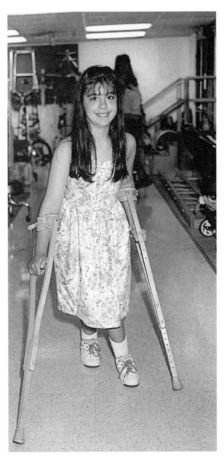

■ **FIGURE 8–13**
Adolescent ambulating with forearm crutches; a two- or four-point pattern is demonstrated.

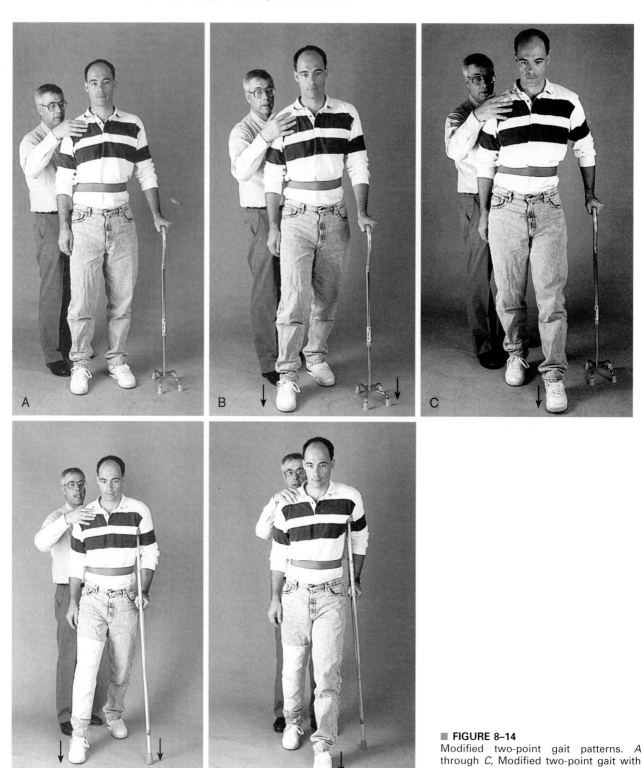

■ **FIGURE 8–14**
Modified two-point gait patterns. *A* through *C,* Modified two-point gait with cane. *D* and *E,* Modified two-point gait with an axillary crutch.

Note: It is recommended that the terms "swing-to" and "swing-through" not be used in conjunction with the three-point pattern. These terms are better suited for the patient who is unable to actively use the muscles of the lower trunk and lower extremities during ambulation and who must "swing" the trunk and lower extremities "to" or "through" the crutches to ambulate. These gait patterns are associated most frequently with the patient with a spinal cord injury or a developmental disability that requires the patient to use the upper extremities to support and provide the force necessary to lift and move the

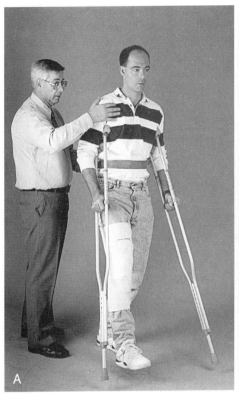
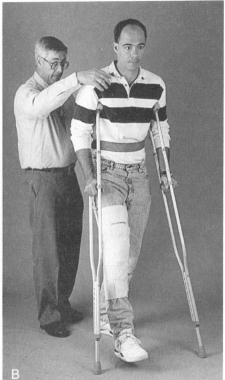
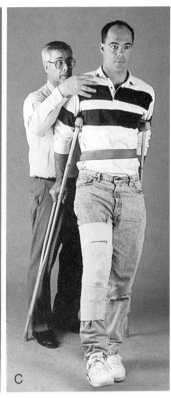

■ **FIGURE 8–15**
Three-point gait pattern.

body forward without assistance from the lower extremities.

Three-One–Point, or Modified Three-Point Pattern
The *three-one–point gait* pattern requires the use of bilateral ambulation aids or a walker. The pat-

tern is used when the patient is permitted FWB on one lower extremity but only PWB on the other lower extremity. The walker, crutches, or canes are advanced simultaneously with the PWB lower extremity (Fig. 8–16*A*). Then the FWB lower extremity is advanced while the patient distributes his/her body

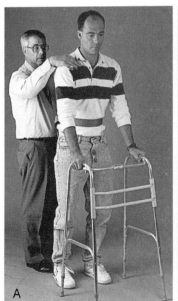
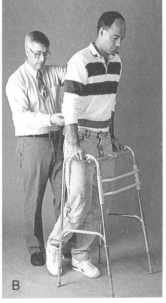
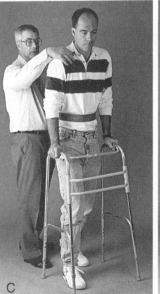
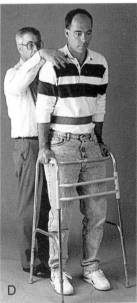

■ **FIGURE 8–16**
Three-one, or modified three-point, gait pattern.

weight onto the aid, partially bearing weight on the protected lower extremity (see Fig. 8–16*B–D*). It is a more stable pattern than the three-point pattern and requires less strength and less energy expenditure than the three-point pattern, but it is a slower pattern. It allows the affected lower extremity to be exercised while maintaining some weight bearing on it. These can be positive features and benefits depending on the patient's diagnosis or condition (Procedure 8–4).

P R O C E D U R E   8 – 4
Ambulation Patterns With Assistive Aids

A. Four-point—Assistive aid (AA) and opposite lower extremity (foot) advance *alternately;* bilateral canes, crutches, or reciprocal walker may be used. RF/LF = right/left foot.

	(L)	(R)
4.	AA	<u>RF</u>
	LF	AA
3.	<u>AA</u>	
	LF	AA
		RF
2.	<u>LF</u>	AA
	AA	
		RF
1.		<u>AA</u>
	AA	
	LF	RF
Start	AA	AA
	LF	RF

B. Two-point—AA and opposite lower extremity (foot) advance *simultaneously;* bilateral canes, crutches, or reciprocal walker may be used.

	(L)	(R)
4.	<u>AA</u>	<u>RF</u>
	LF	AA
3.	<u>LF</u>	<u>AA</u>
	AA	RF
2.	<u>AA</u>	<u>RF</u>
	LF	AA
1.	<u>LF</u>	<u>AA</u>
	AA	RF
Start	AA	AA
	LF	RF

C. Three-point—AA advances *simultaneously* with the non–weight-bearing (NWB) lower extremity; then the full weight-bearing (FWB) lower extremity (foot) steps through the aids; bilateral crutches or walker may be used.

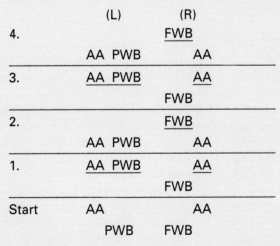

	(L)	(R)
4.	AA	AA
	FWB	
3.	FWB	
	AA	AA
2.	AA	AA
	FWB	
1.	FWB	
	AA	AA
Start	AA	AA
	FWB	

D. Three-one–point—AA and partial weight-bearing (PWB) lower extremity (foot) advance *simultaneously;* then the FWB lower extremity steps through the aids; bilateral cane, crutches, or walker may be used.

	(L)	(R)
4.		FWB
	AA PWB	AA
3.	AA PWB	AA
		FWB
2.		FWB
	AA PWB	AA
1.	AA PWB	AA
		FWB
Start	AA	AA
	PWB	FWB

E. Modified four-point—Only one AA is used; the AA and the opposite lower extremity (foot) advance *alternately;* the AA is held in the hand opposite the affected lower extremity.

	(L)	(R)
4.	LF	AA
	RF	
3.		AA
	RF	
	LF	
2.	RF	
	LF	AA
1.	LF	AA
	RF	
Start		AA
	LF	RF

continued

PROCEDURE 8–4, *continued*

F. Modified two-point—Only one AA is used; the AA and the opposite lower extremity (foot) advance *simultaneously;* the AA is held in the hand opposite the affected lower extremity.

	(L)	(R)
4.	LF	AA
		RF
3.		RF
	LF	AA
2.	LF	AA
		RF
1.		RF
	LF	AA
Start		AA
	LF	RF

PREAMBULATION FUNCTIONAL ACTIVITIES

Each patient will have to be instructed on how to perform the gait pattern he/she will use, as well as how to perform various functional activities. Actual requirements may vary from patient to patient depending on each person's goals, needs, problems, and abilities. Instruction and practice in various functional activities such as using stairs, curbs, inclines, ramps, and doors; sitting into and standing from different types of chairs or other seating items (e.g., armless chairs, low chairs and sofas, soft chairs and sofas, toilets, automobile seats, theater seats, and benches); ambulating on rough, soft, or uneven surfaces (e.g., grass, carpeting, gravel, concrete); sitting on the ground or floor and returning to standing; protecting himself/herself at the time of a fall and returning to standing; using public transportation; crossing a street during the walk cycle of the traffic control system; and using an elevator and escalator should be considered for inclusion in the gait training program. The specific activities selected will depend on the patient's needs, goals, anticipated activities, problems, ambulation aid used, and his/her abilities (Fig. 8–17).

The caregiver must explain and demonstrate the activities to the patient and protect or guard the patient to reduce the risk of injury. Videotapes, instructional booklets or manuals, and observation of other skilled and competent patients are other methods of instruction that can be used.

The goal for most patients will be safe and independent performance of the functional activities he/she needs to accomplish. However, some patients may not become independent. In such instances a family member, friend, or coworker should be instructed in the proper way to assist and protect the person. In addition, the patient should be made aware of his/her limitations and of the risk of injury that would accompany an attempt at independent performance of an activity for which assistance is required. The caregiver should document the activities the patient is able to perform safely and independently. Any restrictions or limitations in the person's ambulation activities should be noted as well, and the family should be informed of them. This information is especially important for family members of young or elderly patients or patients who have decreased mental competence, which would interfere with the ability to make a competent decision or judgment.

The amount of time available to instruct the patient and to allow him/her to practice may be extremely limited as a result of restrictions on the patient's length of stay in the hospital. Many patients may be hospitalized for only a few days before they are discharged and return to their home. Thus, they may not have access to multiple treatment or practice sessions, and their opportunities to become proficient in functional activities will be minimal. Therefore, it may be necessary to provide written instructions and precautions related to functional activities for the patient and his/her family.

These precautions may include suggestions for the proper maintenance of equipment, such as inspecting the support tips of the device for wear or damage or dirt in the grooves, checking wing nuts for tension, inspecting the item for cracks or broken parts, and checking all spring adjustment buttons to be cer-

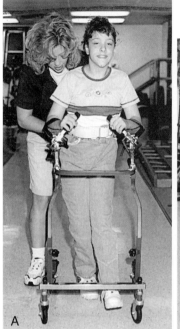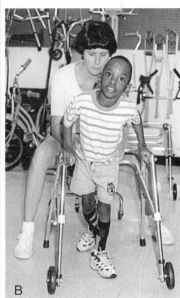

■ **FIGURE 8–17**
Children ambulating with adjustable wheeled walkers.

A   B

tain they are securely positioned in the holes provided. The patient should be cautioned that moisture on the support tips or ambulation on a wet floor could cause the tips to slip or slide. Loose objects, such as small area rugs, and waxed or polished floor surfaces are also threats to safety and should be avoided, if possible. Extra care should be taken during ambulation on grass or on rough or uneven surfaces and in an area crowded with furniture or other hazards or where there are many other persons (e.g., a busy hallway, store, or busy sidewalk).

Sidewalks that are wet or obstructed by rain or snow create special problems, and only the most proficient and cautious person should attempt to ambulate with assistive devices in these conditions. The patient should be made aware of the potential problems associated with doorway thresholds, the change from one type of surface to a different surface (e.g., from a linoleum surface to carpeted surface), and the stair tread overhang (stair lip).

These precautions are most important for the person who uses the assistive aid for maximal body support and stability, such as the person who is NWB on one lower extremity. However, all persons who use an ambulation aid should be provided with instructions to assist them in avoiding or reducing the risks to their safety caused by the conditions or factors cited. It is the caregiver's responsibility to discuss these precautions with the patient during the ambulation training program. In addition, you should inform the patient or his/her family how you can be contacted for advice or assistance after the patient has been released from the facility or has returned home. This information should be written and given to the patient or his/her family.

STANDING AND SITTING ACTIVITIES

Each patient must be taught to stand and return to sitting using his/her aid so this can be done safely, efficiently, and independently. The entire program or technique used may differ among patients, but there are many components that should be taught to all patients.

Before a patient attempts to stand, he/she must move his/her body forward in the chair seat. This will position his/her COG nearer to his/her base of support (i.e., the feet and lower extremities) so the person will be able to stand more easily and will have better balance once he/she is standing. Most patients find it easier to stand if they place the foot of the unaffected or stronger lower extremity slightly posterior to the foot of the opposite lower extremity. This anterior-posterior position of the feet promotes a better "push-off" or lift from the stronger lower extremity as the person begins to stand. The position also provides a wide base of support when the person is standing and approximates the foot position most people use to stand from a chair. If both lower extremities have essentially equal strength and weight-bearing capacity, the foot of the dominant lower extremity is usually positioned most posteriorly (Fig. 8–18A).

The patient should be taught to use the upper extremities to push simultaneously with the lower extremities to elevate the body. The hands should be placed on the chair armrests and positioned anterior to the hips. This allows the patient to push upward and forward to move the hips and trunk forward and toward the base of support (see Fig. 8–18B), and also enables the patient to use the most stable object for support as he/she initiates the movement to stand. The

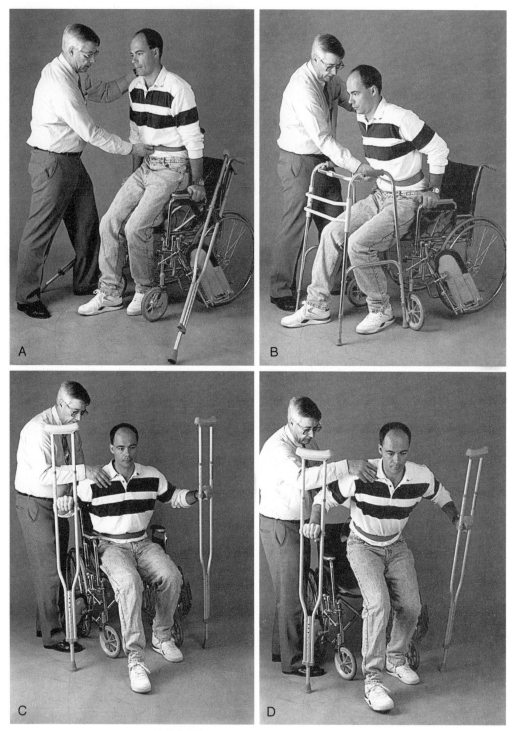

■ **FIGURE 8–18**
Methods used to stand from a wheelchair.

more advanced patient may be able to stand using the ambulation aid rather than the chair armrests. However, this method requires excellent strength, coordination, and balance to perform the activity safely (see Fig. 8–18C,D).

The patient should be taught to incline the trunk forward as he/she pushes with the upper and lower extremities. This will shift his/her COG forward and eventually over his/her base of support, leading to a relatively stable standing position.

When the person returns to the chair, the process is reversed. The foot of the stronger lower extremity is positioned nearest to the chair seat, with the patient facing away from the chair. He/she lowers himself/herself into the chair using the upper and lower extremities to control the movement. The trunk is inclined

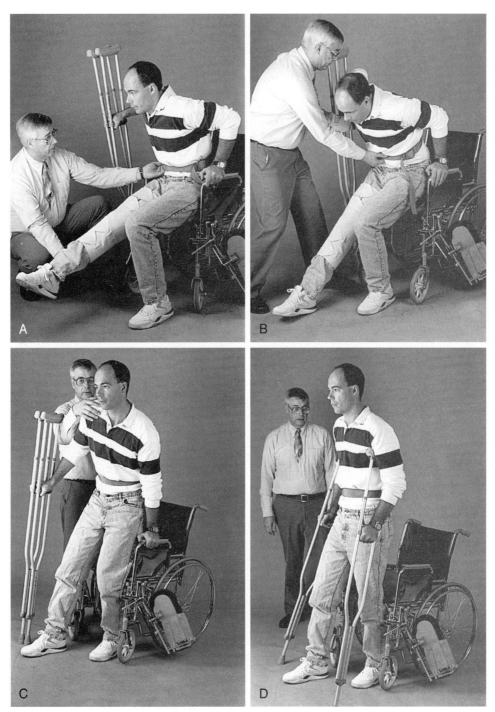

■ **FIGURE 8–19**
Patient rising from a sitting position with axillary crutches.

forward to maintain the COG over the base of support and to avoid striking the back of the chair with the upper back before the buttocks are on the chair seat. The person who attempts to sit without inclining the trunk forward will be unstable and will have difficulty controlling the movement of his/her body into the chair.

Axillary Crutches For standing, instruct the patient to move his/her hips forward to the middle or front portion of the chair seat.

The foot of the stronger or unaffected lower extremity is positioned slightly posterior to the foot of the other lower extremity. If the knee of the most affected lower extremity cannot be flexed, the patient should be taught to slide the heel forward prior to attempting to stand, or the caregiver may have to support the lower extremity as the patient stands (Fig. 8–19A).

The patient holds both crutches with the hand on the same side as the most affected lower extremity.

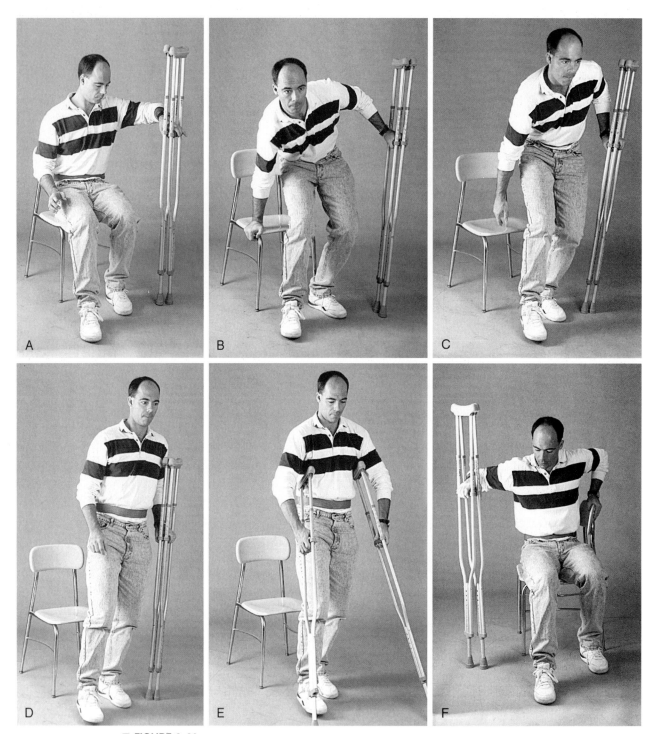

■ **FIGURE 8–20**
Patient using axillary crutches to rise from a sitting position in a chair without arms.

The crutches are placed opposite to the foot of the stronger lower extremity. This widens the patient's base of support, so when he/she stands, his/her vertical gravity line will be located between the crutches and the strong lower extremity (see Fig. 8–19B). The patient simultaneously pushes down with the upper extremities and the strongest/least affected lower extremity and leans forward as he/she stands (see Fig. 8–19C).

After the patient is standing, the free hand

reaches for one crutch, held in the opposite hand, and places it in the axilla on the side of the body of the hand that is not holding the crutches. He/she then positions the remaining crutch into the opposite axilla (see Fig. 8–19D).

An alternative method is to hold the crutches with the hand on the same side of the body as the unaffected lower extremity. This narrows the base of support but increases the force the patient is able to use to stand. The ipsilateral upper and lower extremities function simultaneously to lift the patient upward. The patient pushes from the armrest, seat, or back of chair with the opposite hand to assist with the stand (Fig. 8–20).

To return to sitting, the patient is instructed to approach the chair and then pivot on the strongest/least affected lower extremity so his/her back is toward the chair (Fig. 8–21). He/she steps back until the posterior thigh of the strongest/least affected lower extremity touches the front of the chair seat (see Fig. 8–19D).

The patient alternately removes the crutches from the axillae and holds them with the hand on the same side of the body as the most affected lower extremity to widen the base of support and increase stability (see Fig. 8–19B). An alternative method is to have him/her hold the crutches with the hand on the same side of the body as the strongest/least affected lower extremity as described previously.

The patient uses the free hand to grasp the armrest of the chair and lowers his/her hips into the chair using the upper extremities and the least affected lower extremity. If the knee of the most affected lower extremity cannot be flexed, the patient should allow it to slide forward as he/she sits. The crutches are placed on the floor, and he/she moves back in the chair. (*Note:* Instruct the patient to avoid placing the crutches against a wall, table, or chair, because they are likely to

slide and fall to the floor, which could damage the crutches or injure someone nearby.)

Forearm Crutches To stand, instruct the patient to perform the process discussed for standing with axillary crutches.

After the patient is standing, he/she reaches with the free hand, grasps the handpiece of one crutch, and positions the crutch lateral and anterior to the foot on the same side as the hand holding the crutch (Fig. 8–22). Then he/she positions the second crutch lateral and anterior to the other foot. When each crutch is positioned, the forearm cuff is applied alternately to each forearm.

An alternative method can be used for the patient with good strength, coordination, and balance but usually cannot be performed by elderly, weak, unstable, or debilitated patients. For this method, the patient moves the hips forward to the middle or front portion of the chair seat. The foot of the strongest/least affected lower extremity is positioned slightly posterior to the foot of the other lower extremity. He/she grasps the handpiece of each crutch in each hand, and the crutch tips are positioned lateral and anterior to each foot. He/she simultaneously pushes down with the upper extremities and the strongest/least affected lower extremity, leans the trunk forward, and stands (Fig. 8–23).

To return to sitting, the patient is instructed to perform the same process discussed for axillary crutches. An alternative method is to instruct the patient to perform all activities described for sitting with axillary crutches before removing the crutches. Then the patient alternately removes the cuff from each forearm but retains his/her grasp on each handpiece. The patient lowers himself/herself into the chair using the upper and lower extremities, places the crutches on the floor, and moves back into the chair seat.

Walker For standing, the patient is instructed to move the hips forward to the middle or front portion of the chair seat. The foot of the strongest/least affected lower extremity is positioned slightly posterior to the foot of the other lower extremity. The walker is positioned directly in front of the chair with the open side toward the patient. The patient grasps the chair armrests in front of the hips. This position provides the greatest stability and allows the patient to use the upper and lower extremities most effectively to stand.

To stand, the patient simultaneously pushes down with the upper extremities and the strongest lower extremity, leans forward, and stands (see Fig. 8–24A). If he/she has started with both hands on the chair armrests, one hand is moved onto the handgrip of the walker when he/she is partially standing, and then the

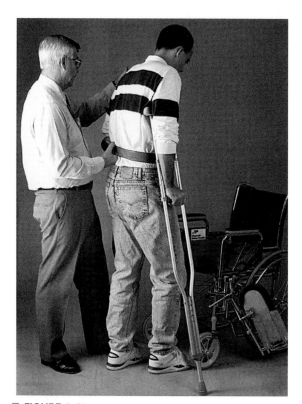

■ **FIGURE 8–21**
Patient approaching a wheelchair using axillary crutches.

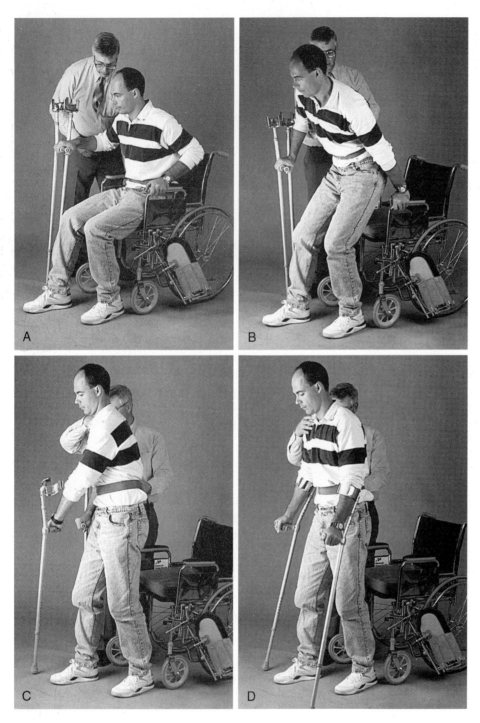

■ **FIGURE 8–22**
Patient standing from a wheelchair using forearm crutches.

opposite hand moves to the other handgrip (Fig. 8–24B).

An alternative method is to instruct the patient to preposition his/her body and feet and place one hand on one handgrip of the walker and the other hand on the chair armrest in front of the hips (Fig. 8–24C). However, this position can be unsafe if the patient attempts to pull himself/herself to a standing position using the walker only, because the walker is not secure on the floor. Furthermore, if he/she attempts to push down with the upper extremities on the handgrips,

he/she may experience difficulty, because the upper extremities will be too high to exert a strong downward force.

To return to sitting, the patient is instructed to approach the chair and pivot on the strongest/least affected lower extremity so his/her back is toward the chair and the walker remains in front of him/her (Fig. 8–25A,B).

The patient steps back until the back of the strongest/least affected lower extremity touches the front of the chair seat. He/she reaches one hand at a time for

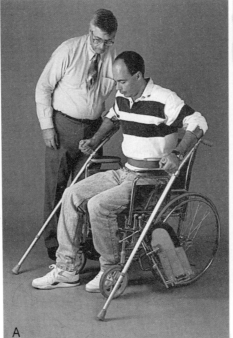
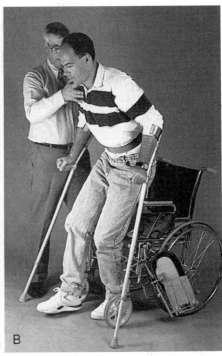

■ **FIGURE 8–23**
Patient standing from a wheelchair using forearm crutches (alternative method).

each armrest of the chair. Once the patient has both hands on the armrests of the chair, he/she can control the lowering of the body into the chair using the upper and lower extremities. This method provides the greatest stability for the patient because the chair is more secure and stable than the walker (see Fig. 8–25C–E).

An alternative method is to instruct the patient to reach one hand to the armrest while the other hand remains on the walker handgrip (Fig. 8–26). This method offers less stability than the previous method because the walker is not as secure as the chair. However, some patients may perform better using this method. The patient lowers the hips onto the chair using the upper extremities and the strongest/least affected lower extremity and then positions himself/herself in the chair by moving the hips back into the seat. If the chair does not have arms, the patient can be

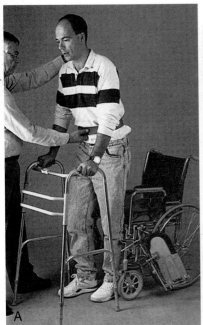
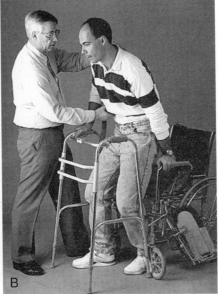
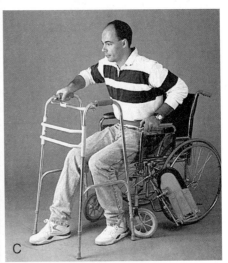

■ **FIGURE 8–24**
Patient standing from a wheelchair using a walker.

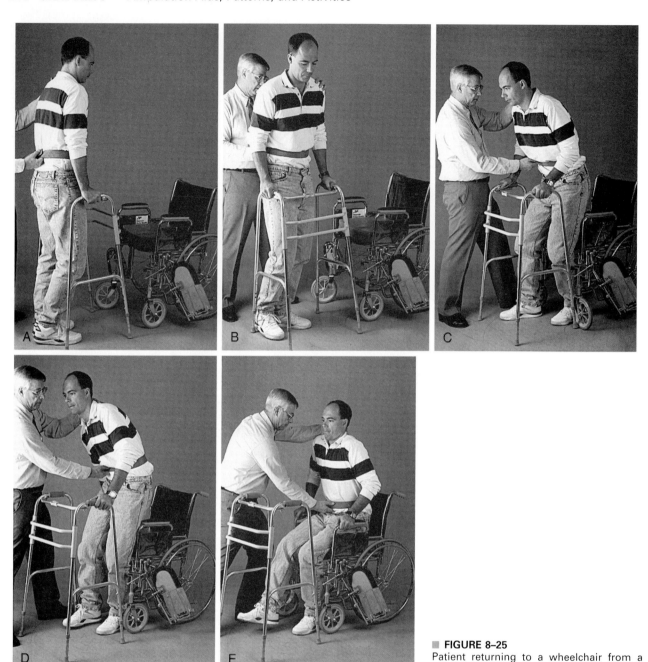

■ **FIGURE 8–25**
Patient returning to a wheelchair from a walker.

taught to use the handgrips of the walker to assist to raise or lower the body using the alternative methods previously described. It is important to teach the patient to push down on the walker handgrips and to avoid pulling or pushing the walker. This method should not be considered safe for patients who are weak or mentally confused or have poor balance or decreased strength in the upper and lower extremities.

Canes　For standing, instruct the patient to move his/her hips forward to the middle or the front portion of the chair seat. The foot of the strongest/least

affected lower extremity is positioned slightly posterior to the foot of the other lower extremity. The patient places his/her hands on the armrests in front of the hips to be able to push with them to lift the body from the chair.

The standard cane is hooked over the front portion of the armrest. If a *unilateral* cane is used, it is placed on the armrest on the side of the stronger/least affected upper and lower extremity. The self-standing (three- or four-footed, crab, or Walkane) cane is placed next to the front of the armrest of the stronger/least affected upper and lower extremity (Fig. 8–27*A,B*). By positioning the canes as described, the

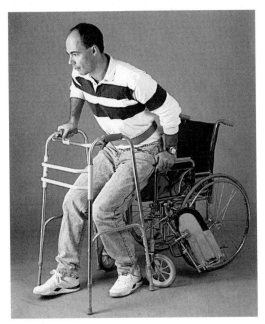

■ **FIGURE 8–26**
Patient returning to a wheelchair from a walker (alternative method).

patient will be able to use the aid with the upper extremity opposite to the weakest/most affected lower extremity. This widens the patient's base of support and allows some weight shift from the lower extremity onto the cane when both items are used during the weight-bearing (stance) phase of the gait pattern.

The patient simultaneously pushes down with the upper and lower extremities and leans the body forward to stand. He/she picks up the cane from the chair armrest or reaches for the self-standing cane (Fig. 8–27C–E).

(*Note:* If the chair does not have arms, the patient can be taught to hold the cane in the hand opposite to the weakest/most affected lower extremity and to use the other upper extremity to push against the chair seat or back to assist in standing.)

To return to sitting, instruct the patient to approach the chair and turn sideward, leading with the strongest/least affected upper and lower extremities. With the strongest/least affected extremities nearest to the chair, the cane is hooked over the armrest, or the self-standing cane is placed to the side or in front of the armrest the patient faces.

The patient first grasps the near and then grasps the far armrest and continues to pivot until his/her back is toward the chair. He/she lowers the hips into the chair seat using the strongest/least affected upper and lower extremities (Fig. 8–28). He/she then positions himself/herself in the chair by moving the hips back into the chair.

(*Note:* If the chair does not have arms, the patient can be taught to release the cane, allowing it

to fall sideward to the floor, and to reach to the chair seat or the back of the chair with the free upper extremity to assist to lower the body into the chair.)

The methods described for standing from and sitting into a chair should be safe and effective for the majority of patients who have average or normal strength, coordination, and balance. However, some patients may require the assistance of another person or the use of a firm, stable object (e.g., a chair with arms; a table; a handrail or grab bars; or a vanity, bed, or counter) to help them to stand or sit. The patient who uses a wheelchair may need to be taught to turn toward the chair and to face the chair after he/she is standing to grasp the crutches, which have been hooked over the push handles or armrests. Observing the patient or attempting different methods may be necessary to determine which method will be the safest and most independent for the patient. You must protect the patient when any of these methods are taught by using proper guarding techniques, including the application and use of a safety belt (Procedure 8–5).

SAFETY CONSIDERATIONS AND PRECAUTIONS

PATIENT PROTECTION AND GUARDING TECHNIQUES

The use of a safety belt is necessary during all initial level-ground and functional gait activities. The belt should be applied securely and grasped in the center at the patient's back. *Caution:* Do not use the patient's clothing, upper extremity, or personal belt for control. These items are not sufficiently strong or secure to provide a safe grasp site. If the safety belt has a buckle, the buckle should be positioned so it will not injure the patient if tension is applied to the belt (i.e., at the patient's side or in the back) (see Fig. 8–1).

Position During Level-Ground Ambulation Stand behind and slightly to one side of the patient. You may stand more toward the patient's weakest/most affected or strongest/least affected lower extremity depending on your own personal or facility philosophy or your own rationale and sense of control. A patient can be safety guarded and protected from either position, and you may find it helpful to practice both techniques (see Fig. 8–2A,B).

Grasp the safety belt from the bottom with one hand with your palm up and forearm supinated. Position your free hand above the patient's shoulder that

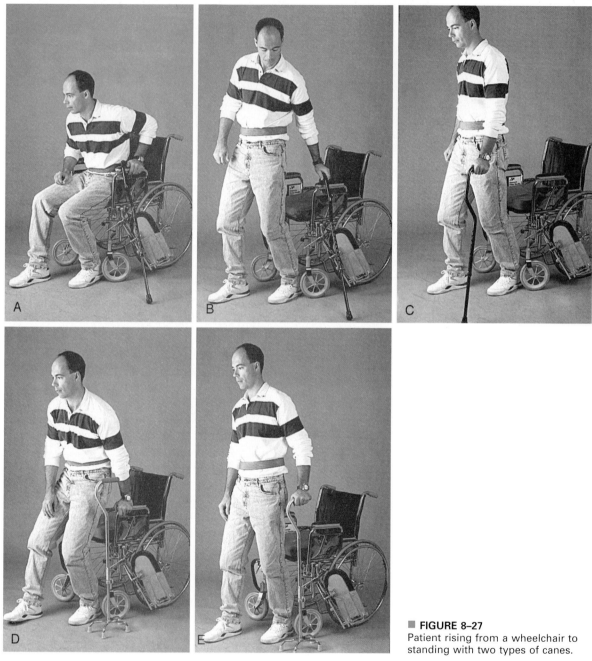

■ **FIGURE 8–27**
Patient rising from a wheelchair to standing with two types of canes.

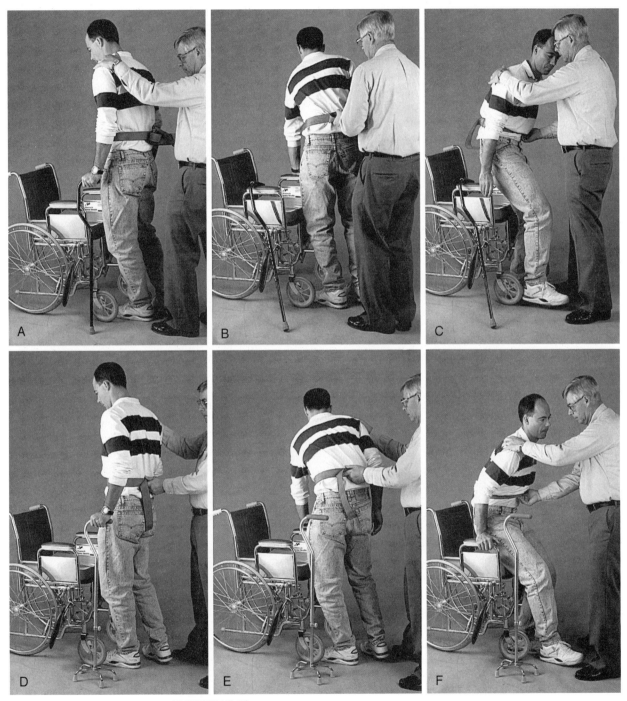

■ **FIGURE 8–28**
Patient returning to a wheelchair from standing with cane.

PROCEDURE 8–5
Independent Standing and Sitting With Assistive Aids

I. Cane: For descriptive purposes, assume the left upper and lower extremities are affected or weaker.
  1. Rise to stand
    a. The cane is positioned on the right side of the chair; a footed cane is placed slightly to the front and to the side of the right armrest, and a standard cane is hooked over the front portion of the armrest.
    b. He/she moves toward the front of the chair seat, positions his/her feet parallel or anterior-posterior and flat on the floor, and places the right hand on the armrest.
    c. To rise, he/she leans the trunk forward and pushes primarily with the right upper and lower extremities; the left extremities assist.
    d. He/she grasps the cane with the right hand and establishes his/her balance before ambulation.
  2. Return to sitting
    a. The patient approaches the chair and turns toward the chair, leading with his/her right upper extremities, until the right side is nearest the chair.
    b. He/she places a footed cane in front and to the side of the right armrest or hooks a standard cane over the armrest.
    c. He/she grasps the right armrest with his/her right hand and continues to turn until his/her back is toward the chair seat.
    d. He/she uses his/her right upper and lower extremities primarily to lower self into the chair slowly, then moves back in the chair.
II. Crutches: For descriptive purposes, assume the patient is non–weight bearing on the left lower extremity.
  1. Rise to stand
    a. The patient moves toward the front of the chair seat and places the right foot approximately 6 to 8 inches forward.
    b. He/she grasps the handpieces of both crutches in his/her left hand and positions the crutches vertically slightly in front and to the side of the chair; the right hand holds the armrest.
    c. To rise, he/she leans the trunk forward and pushes with both hands and right lower extremity.
    d. He/she establishes balance and uses the right hand to place one crutch in the right axilla; the remaining crutch is placed in the left axilla.
    e. The crutches are positioned to form a tripod before ambulation.
  2. Return to sitting
    a. The patient approaches the chair forward and turns, leading with the right extremities, until his/her back is toward the chair.
    b. He/she steps back until the edge of the chair seat contacts the right lower extremity.
    c. He/she removes the crutches, one at a time, from the axillae; grasps the handpieces with the left hand; and positions the crutches to the side and vertically.
    d. He/she grasps the right armrest with the right hand, lowers self into the chair slowly using his/her upper extremities and right lower extremity, and then moves back in the chair.

PROCEDURE 8–5, *continued*

III. Walker: For descriptive purposes, assume the patient has generalized weakness in the lower extremities.

1. Rise to stand
   a. The walker is positioned directly in front of the chair and close enough to be within the patient's reach when he/she stands.
   b. He/she moves toward the front of the chair seat, positions his/her feet parallel or anterior-posterior and flat on the floor; and places hands on front portion of armrests.
   c. To rise, he/she leans trunk forward and pushes with both hands and lower extremities.
   d. When standing, he/she reaches, one hand at a time, to grasp the handpieces on the walker and establishes balance before ambulation.

2. Return to sitting
   a. The patient approaches the chair forward and turns toward the chair, leading with the stronger extremities, until his/her back is toward the chair.
   b. He/she steps back until the front edge of the chair seat contacts one or both lower extremities.
   c. He/she reaches, one hand at a time, to grasp each armrest; lowers self into the chair slowly using his/her upper and lower extremities; and then moves back in the chair.

Note: *For each of these activities, the patient should be instructed to elevate the foot plates or swing the front rigging and lock the wheelchair before standing.*

---

is farthest from you so it will be ready to control the upper trunk if his/her balance is disturbed.

If you use this technique, you must be prepared to grasp the patient's shoulder quickly. Some clinicians apply an across-the-chest grasp to maintain optimal control. If this technique is attempted, you must be certain your arm is on the patient's chest and not over the anterior neck or throat.

An alternative method is to place your free hand, with very light pressure, on the patient's upper shoulder, but you must not restrict his/her movement or cause an alteration in balance.

Place your feet in an anterior-posterior position with your outermost lower extremity between the patient's lower extremity and the ambulation aid; position your opposite lower extremity posterior to the patient's nearest lower extremity. If you stand behind and toward the patient's right side, your right foot will be positioned forward, between the ambulation aid and his/her right foot, with your left foot trailing behind the patient (Fig. 8–29).

Move in the same direction with the patient but do not "cross-step" with your feet. Your outermost lower extremity moves with the ambulation aid, and your inside foot moves forward with the patient's lower extremities (see Procedure 8–1).

Be alert for unexpected or unusual movements by the patient (e.g., misplacement of the ambulation aid, slipping of the ambulation aid, a misstep, or slipping of the patient's foot), and be prepared to prevent a forward, backward, or sideward fall.

Guarding a patient by positioning yourself in front of the patient is not recommended, as this position does not allow you to move smoothly with the patient, it blocks the view of the patient, you cannot see objects behind you, and you must stay somewhat distant from the patient so that he/she has sufficient space to step. All of these factors make it more difficult to protect the patient (Procedure 8–6).

Position During Gait Training on Curbs, Stairs, and Ramps

Ascending Stairs Remain behind and slightly to the side of the patient in the area where there is the least protection for the patient. Use an anterior-posterior stance with your outside foot on the step on which the patient is standing and your inside foot on the step below the step on which he/she is standing. Grasp the safety belt with one hand and the handrail, if one is available, with your opposite hand (Fig. 8–30).

Advance your feet up one step after the patient has advanced one step, but maintain your feet in an anterior-posterior position as described previously. This process is repeated to ascend all the steps. Teach

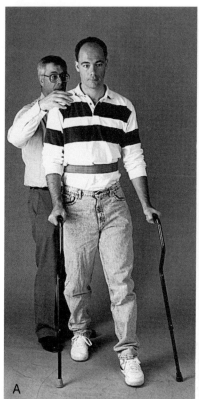 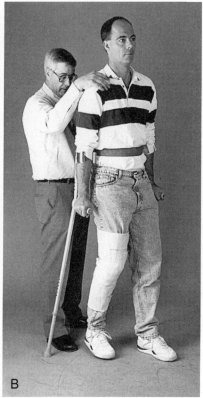 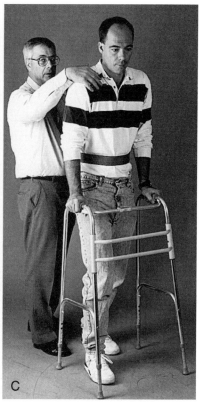

■ **FIGURE 8–29**
Correct position of the caregiver behind a patient with an ambulation aid.

PROCEDURE 8 – 6
Guarding Techniques: Standing and Level Surface Ambulation

I. General considerations
  A. The size, stature, weight, and strength of the patient and the caregiver may affect how the techniques presented are applied; modifications may be necessary.
  B. For some situations, it may be necessary to have two persons guarding.
  C. The patient should be instructed to release the ambulation aids and assist with protecting himself/herself when it is apparent he/she will not be able to remain in a balanced, upright position.
  D. If you are unable to maintain the patient in a balanced, upright position, you should assist him/her to a safe position (i.e., on the floor, on a step, on the ground, or into a chair).
II. Patient stands with ambulation aids
  A. Position yourself on the side opposite to the extremity with which the patient holds the aids and somewhat behind him/her.
  B. Grasp the safety belt with one hand; be prepared to use your other hand to control the trunk; maintain a wide base of support with your feet.
    1. He/she loses balance forward
      a. Pull back on the safety belt; use your other hand to pull the trunk upward and back; do not pull on the patient's clothing or arm.

      b. It may be helpful to push forward against the pelvis as you pull back on the trunk.

      c. Assist him/her to regain a balanced position, or if unable to maintain him/her upright, assist him/her to the floor or chair.

  2. He/she loses balance backward

      a. Push forward on the pelvis and trunk to assist him/her to regain a balanced position.

      b. If unable to maintain him/her upright, assist him/her to sit in the chair.

  3. He/she loses balance to one side, away from you

      a. Pull on the safety belt to move him/her toward you.

      b. Assist him/her to regain a balanced position or assist him/her to sit.

  4. He/she loses balance to one side, toward you

      a. Move your body so you face the patient's side; widen your stance; use your body to support him/her.

      b. Assist him/her to regain a balanced position or assist him/her to sit.

III. Level surface ambulation

  A. Position yourself somewhat behind and toward one side of the patient; position your outside foot between the ambulation aid and his/her foot; position your other foot so it trails as you walk.

  B. Grasp the safety belt with one hand; be prepared to use your other hand to control his/her trunk; do not use it to grasp his/her clothing or arm.

  C. *Note:* Many caregivers prefer to be positioned to the side of the patient that is weakest or at which the less functional extremity or extremities are located.

    1. He/she loses balance forward

      a. Pull back on the safety belt; turn your body sideward; widen your stance.

      b. Use your free hand to pull back on the upper trunk (i.e., shoulder or chest); position one hip against his/her pelvis.

      c. Assist him/her to regain a balanced position or assist him/her to the floor.

    2. He/she loses balance backward

      a. Turn your body so one side is toward him/her; widen your stance; allow him/her to be supported by your body.

      b. Use the safety belt and your other hand to control him/her.

      c. Assist him/her to regain a balanced position or assist him/her to the floor or ground.

    3. He/she loses balance to one side, away from you

      a. Pull on the safety belt to move him/her toward you.

      b. Allow him/her to lean against you for support.

      c. Assist him/her to regain a balanced position or assist him/her to the floor or ground.

    4. He/she loses balance to one side, toward you

      a. Turn your body so he/she can lean on you; use the safety belt and your other hand to control him/her.

      b. Assist him/her to regain a balanced position or assist him/her to the floor or ground.

Caution: When you pull on the safety belt, you must not pull too quickly or use excessive force. You should attempt to correct the movement of the patient by using a firm, smooth pull on the belt. If you pull with excessive force, you may cause further disturbance of the patient's balance. It is recommended you practice with an unimpaired individual, who can simulate various loss-of-balance movements, to assist you to develop a sense of the control needed when you use a safety belt.

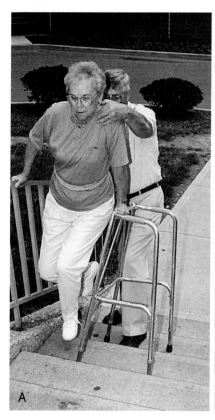
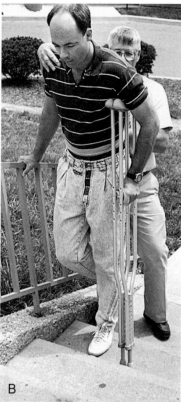

A   B

■ **FIGURE 8–30**
Guarding position for ascending stairs, three-point pattern.

the patient to stop and gain his/her balance on each step before progressing to the next step (Procedure 8–7).

(*Note:* If there is no handrail, grasp the safety belt with one hand and position your other hand anterior and above, but not touching, the patient's shoulder, as described for level-ground ambulation. In many instances, when no handrail is available, it is recommended that two persons guard the patient. One person is positioned in front of the patient, and another person is positioned behind or to the side. If you are alone with the patient, you should be prepared to use your free hand to gently push the patient's trunk forward if he/she loses his/her balance backward.)

Descending Stairs Stand in front and to the side of the patient in the area where there is the least protection for the patient. Use an anterior-posterior

---

P R O C E D U R E 8 – 7
Guarding Techniques for Stairs, Curbs, and Ramps

I. General considerations
   A. The size, stature, weight, and strength of the patient and the caregiver may affect how the techniques presented are applied; some modifications may be necessary, and in some situations, two persons may be required.
   B. The techniques presented for use on stairs are appropriate for use with curbs and ramps.
   C. Regardless of the technique used to guard a patient on stairs, you must prevent him/her from falling down multiple steps or forcing you to fall. Therefore, you must
      1. Maintain a wide stance with your feet; do not place both feet on the same step; use one hand to grasp the safety belt.

    2. Properly position yourself to maximally protect yourself and the patient.

    3. Anticipate the actions you will perform in case he/she loses balance when ascending or descending the stairs.

II. Ascending stairs: Guarding the patient from behind

  A. Position yourself behind and to one side of the patient

    1. If a handrail is used, position yourself to the side opposite it.

    2. If a handrail is not used, position yourself to the side at which the greatest danger or potential for injury exists should the patient lose his/her balance.

    3. *Note:* Many caregivers prefer to be positioned to the patient's weakest side or the side of his/her least functional extremity.

  B. Grasp the safety belt with one hand; be prepared to use your other hand to control the trunk or grasp the handrail, when it is available.

  C. Place your outside foot on the step he/she stands on; place your other foot on the step below.

    1. He/she loses balance forward

      a. Pull back on the safety belt; use your other hand to pull back on the trunk or to grasp the handrail.

      b. Assist him/her to regain balanced position.

      c. If he/she is unable to regain balance, assist to lower him/her to the steps or move him/her toward the handrail.

    2. He/she loses balance backward

      a. Turn your body sideward toward him/her; maintain a wide stance with your feet.

      b. Use one hand to press forward against his/her pelvis or trunk; use your other hand to grasp the handrail.

      c. Assist him/her to regain a balanced position or assist to lower him/her to the steps or move him/her toward the handrail.

    3. He/she loses balance to one side, toward you

      a. Use one hand or your shoulder to press against the trunk; use your other hand to grasp the handrail.

      b. Assist him/her to regain a balanced position or assist to lower him/her to the steps or move him/her toward the handrail.

    4. He/she loses balance to one side, away from you

      a. Use the safety belt to pull him/her toward you; use your other hand to control the trunk or to grasp the handrail.

      b. Assist him/her to regain a balanced position or assist to lower him/her to the steps or move him/her toward the handrail.

III. Descending: Guarding the patient from the front

  A. Follow general considerations IC, 1–3.

  B. Place your outside foot on the step onto which the patient will step; place your other foot on the step below.

  C. He/she loses balance forward

    1. Move in front of him/her but maintain a wide stance.

    2. Use your free hand to press back against the chest or to grasp the handrail; instruct him/her to look up and straighten his/her trunk or to release the aid(s) and grasp the handrail.

    3. Assist him/her to regain a balanced position or assist him/her to sit on a step.

  D. He/she loses balance backward

    1. Pull forward on the safety belt; use your other hand to grasp the handrail.

    2. Assist him/her to regain a balanced position or assist him/her to sit on a step.

continued

PROCEDURE 8-7, *continued*

    E. He/she loses balance to one side, toward you
1. Use one hand or your shoulder to press against the side of the chest to move him/her away from you; one hand grasps the safety belt.
2. Assist him/her to regain a balanced position, or assist him/her to sit on a step or instruct him/her to release the aid(s) and grasp the handrail.

    F. He/she loses balance to one side, away from you
1. Pull on the safety belt to move him/her toward you; use your other hand to grasp the handrail.
2. Assist him/her to regain a balanced position or assist him/her to sit on a step or instruct him/her to release the aid(s) and grasp the handrail.

IV. Descending: Guarding the patient from behind

    A. Follow general considerations IC, 1–3.

    B. Place one foot on the step on which the patient stands; place the other foot on the step below.

    C. He/she loses balance forward
1. Pull back on the safety belt; use your other hand to control the trunk or to grasp the handrail; maintain a wide stance with your feet.
2. Assist him/her to regain a balanced position or assist him/her to sit on a step or instruct him/her to release the aid(s) and grasp the handrail.

    D. He/she loses balance backward
1. Move so you are somewhat behind him/her; press forward at the pelvis; use your other hand to control the trunk or to grasp the handrail; maintain a wide stance with your feet.
2. Assist him/her to regain a balanced position or assist him/her to sit on a step or instruct him/her to release the aid(s) and grasp the handrail.

    E. He/she loses balance to one side, toward you
1. Use your body to support him/her and to prevent him/her from falling to the side.
2. Assist him/her to regain a balanced position or assist him/her to sit on a step or instruct him/her to release the aid(s) and grasp the handrail.

    F. He/she loses balance to one side, away from you
1. Pull on the safety belt to move him/her toward you; use your other hand to control the trunk or to grasp the handrail.
2. Assist him/her to regain a balanced position or assist him/her to sit on a step or instruct him/her to release the aid(s) and grasp the handrail.

Caution: When you pull on the safety belt, you must not pull too quickly or use excessive force. You should attempt to correct the movement of the patient by using a firm, smooth pull on the belt. If you pull with excessive force, you may cause further disturbance of the patient's balance. It is recommended you practice with an unimpaired individual, who can simulate various loss-of-balance movements, to assist you to develop a sense of the control needed when you use a safety belt.

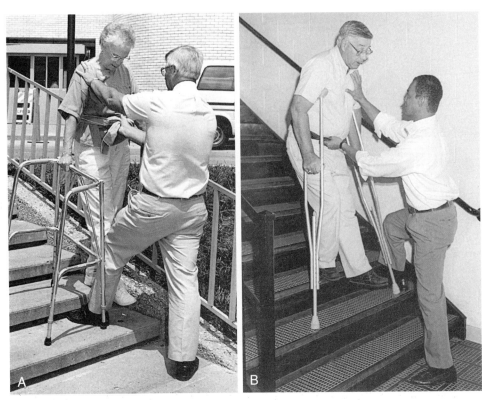

■ **FIGURE 8–31**
Guarding position for descending stairs, three-point pattern.

stance with your outside foot on the step to which the patient will step and your inside foot on the step that is one step lower. Some people prefer to widen their stride so the upper foot is on the step the patient is standing on and the lower foot is on the step below the step to which the patient will step (Fig. 8–31). This requires the person to span two steps, which will not be possible for women who wear skirts or for the person with a short stride. *Caution:* Do not stand with your feet parallel to each other and on same step directly below and in front or to the side of the patient. This position will be unstable if the patient falls forward because it does not provide a wide anterior-posterior base of support.

Grasp the safety belt with one hand and the handrail, if one is available, with the opposite hand. Step down one step with each foot after the patient has descended one step; repeat the process to descend all the steps. Teach the patient to stop and gain his/her balance on each step before he/she progresses to the next step. Do not allow the patient to develop momentum as he/she descends the stairs. A too-rapid descent is apt to lead to imbalance and increases the possibility of a fall. (*Note:* If there is no handrail, grasp the safety belt with one hand, and position your other hand above and anterior to, but not touching, the patient's shoulder. If your hand does touch the anterior shoulder, it must not restrain the patient's forward movement or cause him/her to alter his/her normal balance.)

Alternative Method Stand behind and to the side of the patient in the area where there is the least protection. Use an anterior-posterior stance with your outside foot on the step on which the patient is standing and your inside foot one step above the step on which the patient is standing (Fig. 8–32).

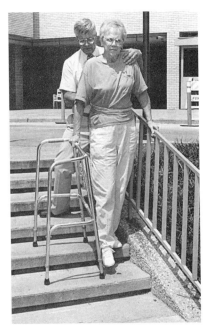

■ **FIGURE 8–32**
Guarding position for descending stairs (alternative method).

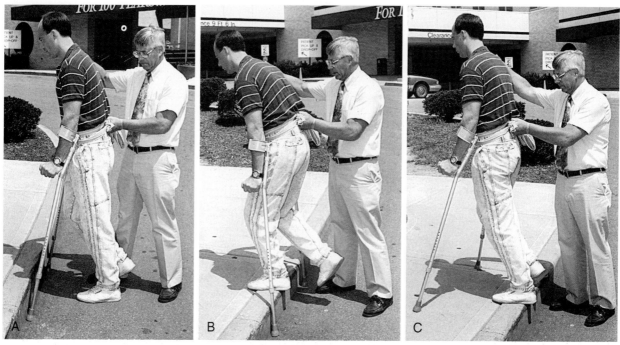

■ **FIGURE 8–33**
Guarding position for ascending a curb, three-point pattern.

Grasp the safety belt with one hand and the hand-rail, if one is available, with your opposite hand. Descend one step with each foot after the patient has descended one step. Teach the patient to stop and gain his/her balance on each step before he/she progresses to the next step.

(*Note:* Either of these techniques can provide safety for the patient. Most patients have a greater sense of security when someone is in front of them when they descend stairs. If you are behind the patient and he/she loses his/her balance forward, you can provide security by gently pulling back on the safety belt and the patient's shoulder; if necessary, sit him/her on the stair. You must avoid allowing the patient to pull you forward if he/she experiences a serious loss of balance.)

Ascending a Curb Stand behind and slightly to one side of the patient in an anterior-posterior stance. Grasp the safety belt with one hand, and position the other hand above and anterior to the patient's shoulder (Fig. 8–33). The patient steps up onto the curb, and then you step up onto the curb.

Descending a Curb Stand in front of and slightly to one side of the patient in an anterior-posterior stance. Place your outside foot on the curb and your inside foot on the surface onto which the patient will step.

Grasp the safety belt with one hand, and position your other hand anterior to the patient's shoulder or mid-chest. Move back as the patient steps down, and then reposition yourself behind the patient if he/she continues to ambulate.

An alternative is to stand behind the patient in an anterior-posterior stance and with your outside foot at the edge of the curb. Grasp the safety belt with one hand, and position your other hand anterior to the patient's shoulder (Fig. 8–34). The patient steps down, and then you step down. (*Note:* As explained previously, either technique can provide safety for the patient provided you are aware of and alert to the risks involved with each technique.)

Ascending and Descending a Ramp or Incline Stand behind the patient when he/she ascends the ramp, using the techniques previously discussed regarding the positioning of your feet and hands. You may position yourself behind or in front of the patient when he/she descends the ramp. However, regardless of the position you select, use the techniques previously presented regarding the position of your feet and hands.

ACTIONS IF THE PATIENT LOSES BALANCE OR FALLS

You must be alert and ready to act quickly should the patient lose his/her balance. Your protective reactions must be so well developed that you are able to react automatically to prevent or minimize injury.

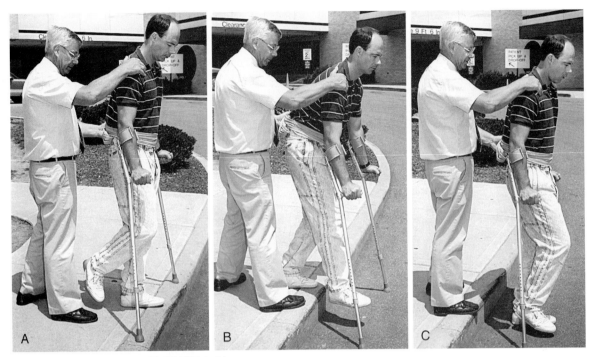

■ **FIGURE 8–34**
Guarding position for descending a curb, three-point pattern.

Proper guarding techniques must be practiced after you understand the rationale and basis for them. In many instances it will not be necessary or desirable to maintain the patient upright. Assisting the patient to the floor or onto a firm object is an accepted procedure, providing proper techniques are used and injury to the patient is minimized. Your primary responsibility is to provide a safe environment and treatment and to protect the patient from injury to the best of your ability.

Level-Ground Ambulation If the patient loses his/her balance forward in a trunk-flexed position, restrain the patient by firmly holding the safety belt; push forward against the pelvis, and pull back on the shoulder or anterior chest. Then assist the patient to regain his/her balance and to stand erect, providing it has been determined that the patient did not sustain any serious injury. In some instances it will be helpful to allow the patient to lean against you briefly. If the patient loses his/her balance backward, rotate your body so one side is turned toward the patient's back and your anterior-posterior stance is widened. Push forward on the patient's pelvis, and allow him/her to lean against your body. Then assist the patient to regain his/her balance and to stand erect.

If the patient falls forward, beyond the point where you can maintain him/her standing, instruct him/her to quickly release or remove the crutches and reach for the floor. Retard the forward motion by pulling back gently but firmly on the safety belt and the

patient's shoulder, but do not prevent the patient from reaching the floor (Fig. 8–35A). Step forward with your outside foot as the patient is moving toward the floor, and gently retard his/her descent (see Fig. 8–35B). Instruct the patient to cushion the fall by bending the elbows as the hands contact the floor and to lower himself/herself to the floor (see Fig. 8–35C). It may be helpful to instruct him/her to turn the head to one side as the fall occurs to avoid injuring the face (see Fig. 8–35D).

If the patient falls backward, beyond the point where you can maintain him/her standing, rotate your body so it is turned toward the patient's back and widen your anterior-posterior stance. Instruct the patient to release or remove the crutches, and allow him/her to briefly lean against your body or to sit on your thigh. It may be necessary to lower the patient onto the floor to a sitting position using the safety belt and proper body mechanics (Fig. 8–36).

Stairs

Ascending Stairs When you are positioned behind the patient and he/she loses balance forward, restrain him/her by gently and firmly pulling on the safety belt and his/her shoulder, or hold firmly to the handrail and the safety belt and pull gently and firmly on the safety belt. Move closer to the patient and maintain your anterior-posterior stance as you assist him/her to regain his/her balance and to stand erect. If you are unable to maintain the patient standing, instruct him/her to release the crutches and reach for

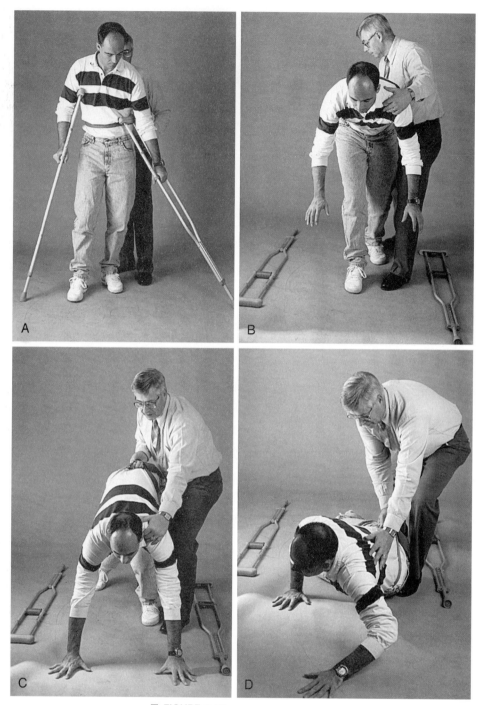

■ **FIGURE 8–35**
Guarding position for a forward fall.

the handrail. Lower the patient to the stair using the safety belt, or maneuver the patient toward the wall of the stairway.

If the patient loses balance backward, maintain your anterior-posterior stance, and press forward against the upper trunk or pelvis as you hold onto the handrail. Assist the patient to regain his/her balance and to stand erect. If you are unable to maintain the patient standing, instruct the patient to release the

crutches and grasp the handrail or lean forward. Allow the patient to lean against your body or sit on your thigh, or maneuver the patient toward the wall of the stairway. Regardless of which technique you use, you must prevent the patient from falling backward and causing you and him/her to fall down the stairs.

Descending Stairs When you are positioned in front of the patient and he/she loses his/her balance

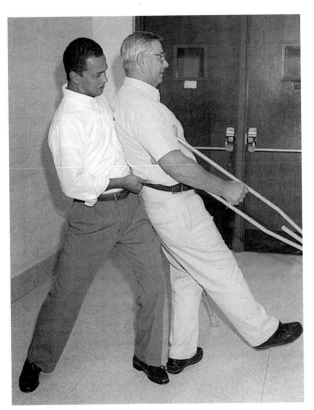

■ FIGURE 8–36
Guarding a person when balance is lost backward.

forward, restrain him/her by gently but firmly pushing on the shoulder or chest and gently but firmly pulling on the safety belt. You may prefer to hold firmly to the handrail and the safety belt and move your body toward the patient's chest. Assist the patient to regain his/her balance and to stand erect. If you are unable to maintain the patient standing, instruct the patient to release the crutches and grasp the handrail, or push on his/her pelvis and chest while grasping the handrail to maneuver him/her toward the wall of the stairway. Regardless of which technique you use, you must prevent the patient from falling forward and causing you and him/her to fall down the stairs.

If the patient loses balance backward, restrain the patient by pulling forward with one hand on the safety belt and one hand grasping the handrail. Move closer to him/her while maintaining your anterior-posterior stance. Assist the patient to regain his/her balance and to stand erect. If you are unable to maintain the patient standing, instruct the patient to release the crutches and to grasp the handrail, or instruct and assist the patient to sit on a step.

When you are positioned behind the patient and he/she loses balance forward, restrain him/her by pulling back on the safety belt while you hold the handrail or by pulling back on the safety belt and on the anterior shoulder. The patient may briefly lean backward against you to regain his/her balance and to stand

erect. If you are unable to maintain the patient standing, instruct the patient to release the crutches and grasp the handrail, or pull back on the safety belt and instruct the patient to sit on a step. Regardless of which technique you use, you must prevent the patient from falling forward and causing you and him/her to fall down the stairs.

If the patient loses balance backward, restrain the patient by gentle but firm forward pressure against the pelvis and upper thorax, or hold the handrail and prevent the patient from falling backward with your body. Assist the patient to regain his/her balance and to stand erect. If you are unable to maintain the patient standing, instruct the patient to release the crutches and to grasp the handrail, or instruct and assist him/her to sit on the step.

These same techniques can be used for both curbs and inclines.

AMBULATION FUNCTIONAL ACTIVITIES

These components of ambulation with an aid are frequently overlooked during the ambulation training program. If a patient is to be fully independent, it is important to teach him/her to move backward and sideward, to turn to the left and to the right, and to perform a 180-degree arc. These movements are necessary because they are components of basic, functional ambulation activities. The patient will need to move backward to position himself/herself to sit or to move away from a door that opens toward him/her. A sideward movement is required in narrow spaces (e.g., the area between two rows of seats in a theater or a narrow hallway or a doorway). Turning is required to change direction of movement or for positioning before sitting or performing other activities that require a change of direction. You should not assume that each patient will be able to perform these activities without being taught. Failure to teach the patient these activities may result in decreased independence or an increased risk of injury for the patient.

BACKWARD MOVEMENT

Four-Point Pattern Instruct the patient to move one ambulation aid backward and then to step back with the opposite lower extremity; then he/she moves the other ambulation aid backward and steps back with the opposite lower extremity. Continue to repeat the pattern as necessary.

Two-Point Pattern Instruct the patient to simultaneously move one ambulation aid and the opposite lower extremity backward and then to move the opposite aid and lower extremity backward simultaneously. Continue to repeat the pattern as necessary.

Three-Point Pattern Instruct the patient to start with the crutch tips lateral to but even with the toes of the shoes. He/she steps back approximately 6 inches and repositions the crutches. Continue to repeat the pattern as necessary.

An alternative, advanced technique is to instruct the patient to place the crutches approximately 6 inches behind his/her heels to form a reverse tripod. He/she steps back through the crutches and creates a forward tripod. The crutches are repositioned, and the pattern is repeated as necessary.

The first technique is a more stable method, because the crutches remain in front of the patient to preserve the forward tripod position. The second pattern should be used only with patients who have excellent balance and coordination.

Three-One–Point Pattern Instruct the patient to step back with the strongest/least affected lower extremity while maintaining the crutches in front of or even with the weakest/most affected lower extremity. Then he/she steps back with the crutches and the weakest/most affected lower extremity to place them in line with the normal foot. Continue to repeat the pattern as necessary.

An alternative, advanced technique is to instruct the patient to simultaneously move his/her crutches and the weakest/most affected lower extremity backward; then he/she steps backward with his/her normal lower extremity until it is behind the other foot and crutches. Continue to repeat the pattern as necessary.

SIDEWARD MOVEMENT

To move to the right, instruct the patient to position the left ambulation aid next to the outside of the left foot and the right aid approximately 6 to 8 inches away from the right foot. The patient steps to the right and repositions the aids to sidestep again (Fig. 8–37).

For the four-point, two-point, or three-one–point patterns, instruct the patient to position the aids as described previously to sidestep with the right foot and then with the left foot. Reposition the aid, and repeat the pattern as necessary.

For the three-point pattern, instruct the patient to position the crutches as described previously and then support his/her weight on the hands and sidestep to the right. Reposition the crutches, and repeat the pattern as necessary.

The patient is instructed to reverse the process to sidestep to the left.

TURNING MOVEMENT

The patient should be taught to turn to the left and to the right regardless of which extremities are weakest or most affected. However, the weakest/most affected lower extremity will require more protection or support when the turn is performed, and care must be taken if the patient pivots on that lower extremity. It is suggested that the patient learn to pivot on the strongest/least affected lower extremity regardless of which lower extremity is weakest/most affected, regardless of the direction of the turn, and regardless of the type of gait pattern used. The ambulation aid should be used to protect the weakest/most affected

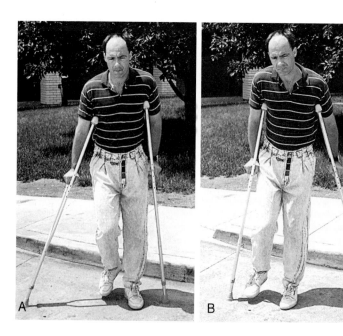

■ **FIGURE 8–37**
Sideward movement to the patient's right.

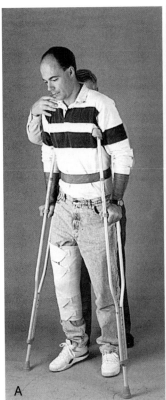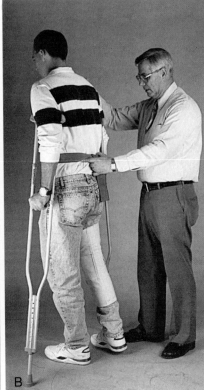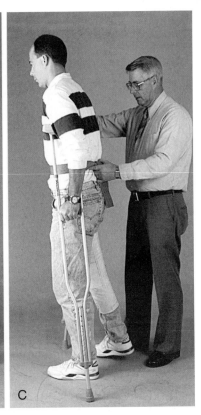

■ **FIGURE 8–38**
Guarding position for turning movement.

lower extremity and to provide stability similar to the way they are used during level-ground ambulation (Fig. 8–38). For example, the patient who uses bilateral ambulation aids or a walker to protect the right lower extremity can be taught to turn to the right by initially shifting his/her weight onto the left lower extremity. The aid and the right lower extremity are moved slightly forward and toward the right as the patient pivots toward the right on the left lower extremity. This pattern is repeated until the turn has been completed. The aid is moved in the direction of the turn to provide support and stability by maintaining the patient's COG and vertical gravity line over his/her base of support. To turn to the left, the aid and right lower extremity are moved forward and to the left as the patient pivots on the left lower extremity.

If the patient is unable to bear weight or pivot on the left lower extremity, he/she can be taught to pivot on the right lower extremity while elevating the left lower extremity from the floor and moving the aid to the left.

It will be more difficult for the patient to turn (pivot) when standing on a carpeted surface. It may be necessary to teach him/her to lift the weight-bearing foot from the carpet to initiate the turn or pivot, while supporting his/her weight on the aid and on the op-

posite lower extremity, if he/she is able to bear weight and pivot on the weaker extremity.

Encourage each patient to use caution when he/she performs a turn. This is particularly important for the elderly, poorly coordinated, or mentally confused patient. *Caution:* Turning by pivoting on a lower extremity on which a total hip replacement has been recently performed is *absolutely contraindicated*. The patient who has undergone a hip replacement must learn to pivot while bearing weight on the nonsurgical lower extremity, and he/she must avoid rotation of the pelvis or hip while bearing weight on the surgically affected lower extremity.

CURBS AND STAIRS

There are two approaches used to ascend and descend multiple steps (stairs): with the use of a handrail (bannister), and without it. It is usually desirable to initiate stair activities with the patient using a handrail to provide maximal stability and a sense of security. However, most patients should be taught to manage stairs without using a handrail, as there are apt to be instances when a handrail will not be available.

When a handrail is used, the patient should be

taught to ascend and descend with the handrail on both the left and the right side of the stairs because handrails may be located on both sides of the stairs or on only one side of the stairs in the patient's environment. For example, most stairs leading to a basement or to the second floor of a residence will have only one handrail, which could be located on either the left or right side of the stairs. If there is only one handrail and it is located on the right wall of stairs leading from the first to the second floor, it will be on the patient's right as he/she ascends the stairs but on the left as he/she descends. Therefore, it is important to have the patient ascend and descend stairs using a handrail on either side of the stairs to ensure his/her independence. The patient may develop a preference if there are two handrails available. Right-handed patients may prefer to use a handrail on the right because they can use their dominant (stronger) upper extremity on the handrail. Similarly, left-handed patients would probably prefer to use a handrail on the left. In most stair patterns in the United States, the right side is used for ascending and descending, so teaching the patient to use the right handrail will prepare him/her for that pattern.

The patient who has only one functional upper extremity and who requires a handrail for support may experience difficulty using a unilateral handrail, depending on its location and on whether he/she is ascending or descending the stairs. A patient with a nonfunctional left upper extremity and a limited functional left lower extremity but who has functional right upper and lower extremities can be used as an example. Suppose his/her home has a handrail on the left wall of the stairs leading from the second floor to the first floor. To descend the stairs, the patient must be taught to reach across the body with the right upper extremity and grasp the handrail as he/she steps down first with the left lower extremity and then steps down to the same step with the right lower extremity. An alternative method is to have the patient descend the stairs backward so that the right upper extremity will be next to the handrail. If this method is used, the patient steps down with the left lower extremity and then steps onto the same step with the right lower extremity. To ascend the stairs, the handrail will be on the patient's right side, and he/she will be able to use the right upper extremity in the conventional manner. The patient steps up with the right lower extremity and then steps onto the same step with the left lower extremity.

Now suppose the handrail is on the right side of the stairs. To descend the stairs, the patient uses his/her right upper extremity to grasp the handrail, steps down with the left lower extremity and then steps to the same step with the right lower extremity. However, to ascend the stairs, the patient must be taught to face the handrail, grasp it with the right upper extremity, step up with the right lower extremity first, and then step up onto the same step with the left lower extremity.

These examples demonstrate the need to interrelate information about the patient and his/her anticipated environment as you plan and progress through the training program.

Portable, temporary curbs or stairs can be used initially, but actual curbs and stairs should also be available for instruction and practice. Demonstrate the pattern to the patient, and reassure the patient that you will guard and protect him/her. The patient should not be challenged by a complete flight of stairs (approximately 10 to 12 steps) until he/she has practiced on a series of three to five steps or on a single curb. Patients who are non–weight bearing on one lower extremity and who have a cast or orthosis that limits the movements of the lower extremity must be guarded more carefully. You must be certain the patient has sufficient strength, balance, coordination, and endurance to perform curb and stair climbing. The patient who lacks these physical qualities may find it necessary to ascend and descend stairs by sitting and advancing one step at a time using the upper extremities and one or both lower extremities. This method is usually the least desirable and should be used only when the patient is unable to use the other methods described.

Ascending a Curb
Bilateral Canes The patient places the strongest/least affected lower extremity onto the curb and then elevates the body using the lower extremity while simultaneously raising the weakest/most affected lower extremity and both canes onto the curb. An alternative technique is to have the patient place the canes onto the step, step up with the strongest lower extremity, and then raise the weakest lower extremity onto the curb.

Unilateral Cane Instruct the patient to place the strongest/least affected lower extremity onto the curb and then elevate the body onto the curb using the strongest lower extremity while simultaneously raising the weakest/most affected lower extremity and cane onto the curb (Fig. 8–39). An alternative technique is to have the patient place the cane onto the curb simultaneously with the strongest lower extremity and then raise the weakest lower extremity onto the curb (Fig. 8–40).

Bilateral Crutches
THREE-ONE–POINT PATTERN Instruct the patient to place the strongest/least affected lower extremity onto the curb. As the patient elevates the body,

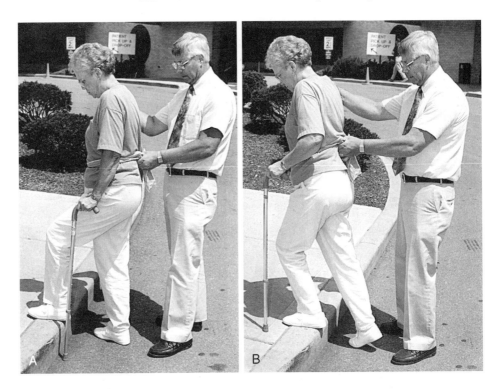

■ **FIGURE 8–39**
Guarding position for ascending a curb with a unilateral cane.

using the strongest lower extremity, he/she simultaneously raises the crutches and the weakest/most affected lower extremity onto the curb.

THREE-POINT PATTERN   Instruct the patient to place the weight-bearing lower extremity onto the curb with the affected lower extremity held in extension at the hip and knee and in external rotation at the

hip or with the knee flexed. As the patient elevates the body using the strongest lower extremity, he/she simultaneously raises the crutches onto the curb and brings the opposite lower extremity forward (see Fig. 8–33).

Standard Walker   If the curb is low (four inches or less), instruct the patient to place the walker onto

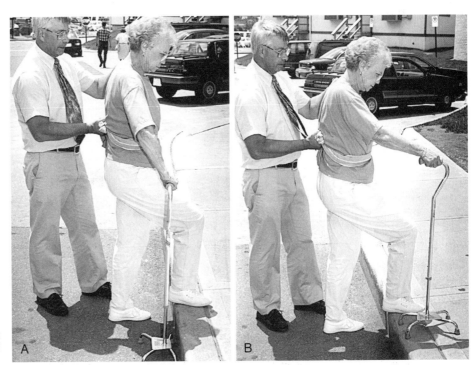

■ **FIGURE 8–40**
Guarding position for ascending a curb with a unilateral four-footed cane.

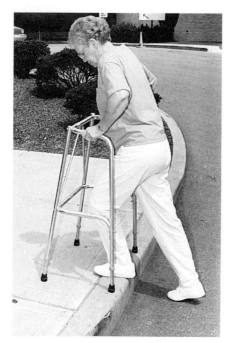

■ FIGURE 8–41
Patient ascending a curb with a walker.

the curb, place the strongest/least affected lower extremity onto the curb, and elevate the body onto the curb using the upper and lower extremities, while simultaneously raising the weakest/most affected lower extremity onto the curb (Fig. 8–41). If the curb is a standard height (6 to 8 inches), instruct the patient to turn so his/her back is toward the curb and the walker

is in front of him/her. He/she places the strongest/least affected lower extremity onto the curb and elevates the body onto the curb while simultaneously lifting the walker and other lower extremity onto the curb. Then the patient backs away from the edge of the curb before turning to move forward. Some patients may be able to ascend the curb forward using the first method described, but this may be difficult, because the walker will be too high for proper use of the upper extremities. The patient should try both methods to determine which is most efficient and safest.

Descending a Curb

Bilateral Canes Instruct the patient to simultaneously place the weakest/most affected lower extremity and both canes down onto the surface below the curb while slightly flexing the strongest/least affected hip and knee. This latter action will help to lower the patient's COG as the canes are lowered. The patient lowers the body with the strongest lower extremity and steps down with that extremity after the canes and the opposite lower extremity have been placed on the lower surface.

Unilateral Cane Instruct the patient to simultaneously step down with the weakest/most affected lower extremity and cane while flexing the strongest/least affected lower extremity slightly (Fig. 8–42*A*). The patient lowers the body with the strongest lower extremity and steps down with that extremity after the cane and opposite lower extremity have been placed on the lower surface (see Fig. 8–42*B*).

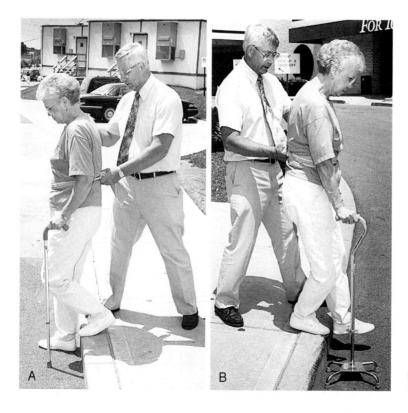

A   B

■ FIGURE 8–42
Patient descending a curb with a unilateral cane.

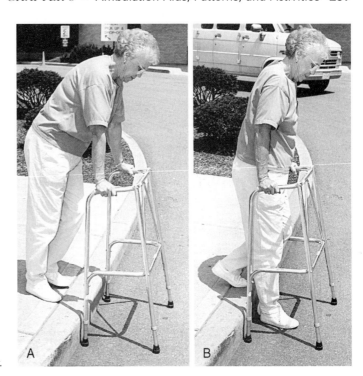

■ **FIGURE 8–43**
Patient descending a curb with a walker.

Bilateral Crutches

THREE-ONE–POINT PATTERN The same procedure described previously for bilateral canes should be taught to the patient.

THREE-POINT PATTERN Instruct the patient to place the crutches down onto the lower surface by slightly flexing the strongest hip and knee. The weakest/most affected lower extremity is positioned in front of the patient and over the edge of the curb. The patient steps down using the strongest lower extremity after the crutches are resting on the lower surface.

Standard Walker Instruct the patient to move to the edge of the curb and place the walker down onto the lower surface while flexing the strongest hip and knee slightly (Fig. 8–43*A*). The weakest/most affected lower extremity is positioned in front of the patient and over the edge of the curb. The patient moves the weakest/most affected lower extremity forward while lowering the body with the strongest/least affected lower extremity and the upper extremities and then steps down with the strongest lower extremity (see Fig. 8–43*B*).

When the patient descends a curb or stairs, it is important to teach him/her to flex the hip and knee of the supporting lower extremity as the ambulation aid is being placed onto the step below the step on which the patient stands. This technique is especially necessary for the patient using bilateral axillary crutches because it improves the patient's balance and stability. For example, if the patient does not flex the hip and knee to lower the body, the distance between the top of the axillary rest and the axilla will increase greatly when the crutches are placed down on the next step,

and the stability of the crutches will be reduced significantly. If he/she only inclines the trunk forward, his/her COG will shift forward, and his/her vertical gravity line may not remain within the base of support (BOS). In addition, the tendency for the axillary crutches to slip forward or backward is increased when the distance between the axillary rest and the axilla is excessive; this will further reduce the patient's stability. Do not overlook teaching this simple technique during the training program; the patient's safety will be improved when it is used (Procedure 8–8).

The same sequences described for the curb can be repeated to ascend and descend stairs. However, the patient should be taught initially to use a handrail when ascending or descending stairs to increase his/her stability and safety. As has been noted previously, the patient should learn to use a handrail on the right and left to ascend and descend the stairs, regardless of which lower extremity is the weakest/most affected, because he/she may be required to use a handrail on either the left or right. In addition, it is important to teach the patient to ascend and descend stairs without using a handrail to enhance his/her independence.

Modifications of the patterns used for curbs may be necessary for stairs without handrails and can be used for any ascending or descending activity.

Ascending and Descending Stairs Using a Handrail

Bilateral Canes The patient may be instructed to hold both canes in one hand and use the other hand on the handrail. An alternative method is to hold a cane in each hand, grasp the handrail and one cane si-

P R O C E D U R E   8 – 8
Independent Ascending and Descending of Stairs With Assistive Aids

For descriptive purposes, assume the right lower extremity (RLE) is the affected or weaker lower extremity when a single cane is used and when non–weight-bearing (NWB) and partial weight-bearing (PWB) crutch patterns are used.

Caution: Whenever a fixed handrail is available, the person should use it for security and stability.

I. Cane
 A. Ascending pattern
  1. The patient faces the stairs and steps up one step with the left lower extremity (LLE).
  2. He/she uses the LLE to elevate his/her body as he/she steps up with the RLE and cane simultaneously onto the step on which he/she is standing.
  3. He/she establishes his/her balance before ascending to the next step.
 B. Descending pattern
  1. The patient steps down one step with the RLE and cane simultaneously and uses the LLE to lower his/her body.
  2. He/she steps down with the LLE and establishes his/her balance before descending to the next step.
II. Crutches: NWB
 A. Ascending pattern
  1. The patient faces the stairs, stands close to them, and uses the crutches for balance and support as he/she steps up with the LLE.
  2. He/she uses the LLE to elevate his/her body as the crutches are lifted onto the step on which he/she is standing. He/she extends and externally rotates the RLE so his/her toes will not strike or become caught under the front edge of the stair tread.
  3. He/she establishes his/her balance before ascending to the next step.
 B. Descending pattern
  1. The patient stands with his/her LLE and crutches positioned toward the front portion of the stair tread; the RLE is held forward of the front edge of the stair tread so the heel will clear.
  2. He/she balances on his/her LLE and lowers his/her body by partially flexing the left hip and knee; he/she places the crutches toward the front portion of the stair tread on the step below.
  3. He/she uses the crutches for balance and support as he/she steps down with the LLE.
  4. He/she establishes his/her balance before descending to the next step.

PROCEDURE 8–8, *continued*

III. Crutches: PWB
  A. Ascending pattern
    1. The patient faces the stairs, stands close to them, and uses the crutches and RLE (PWB) for balance and support as he/she steps up with the LLE.
    2. He/she uses the LLE to elevate his/her body as he/she steps up with the RLE and lifts the crutches simultaneously onto the step on which he/she is standing.
    3. He/she establishes his/her balance before ascending to the next step.
  B. Descending pattern
    1. The patient stands with his/her feet and crutches positioned toward the front portion of the stair tread.
    2. He/she balances on the LLE and lowers his/her body by partially flexing the left hip and knee; he/she lowers the RLE and crutches simultaneously to the front portion of the stair tread on the step below.
    3. He/she uses the crutches and RLE (PWB) for balance and support as he/she steps down with the LLE onto the step on which he/she is standing.
    4. He/she establishes his/her balance before descending to the next step.

Note: *These same patterns can be used for ascending and descending a curb or other type of single elevation. When two-point and four-point patterns are used, the patient ascends the stairs leading with the stronger lower extremity followed by the other lower extremity, and then the assistive devices are lifted simultaneously or alternately. To descend the stairs, the assistive aids are lowered to the step below simultaneously or alternately, and then he/she steps down with the weaker lower extremity first, followed by the stronger lower extremity. If there is no strength difference between the lower extremities, either lower extremity may be used as the lead extremity.*

multaneously, and use the other cane as described for a curb. The cane held simultaneously with the handrail is held parallel to the direction of the handrail. The lower extremities are used in the same way described for a curb.

Unilateral Cane The patient may be instructed to hold the cane and the handrail simultaneously or to hang the cane on the forearm farthest from the handrail, on his/her belt, or in his/her pocket and to use the strong hand to grasp the handrail. He/she can grasp the handrail with one hand and use the cane in the other hand as described for ascending and descending a curb. The lower extremities are used the same way as described for ascending and descending a curb.

Bilateral Axillary Crutches Instruct the patient to place both crutches under the axilla farthest from the handrail and hold the handpieces. He/she then grasps the handrail with the hand nearest to the handrail (see Fig. 8–30*B*).

An alternative method is to have the patient place one crutch under the axilla farthest from the handrail and to hold the other crutch perpendicular to the crutch in the axilla, using the hand that grasps the crutch handpiece; the hand without the crutch grasps the handrail (Fig. 8–44).

A third method is to have the patient place one crutch under the axilla farthest from the handrail and hold the other crutch parallel with the handrail with the hand that grasps the handrail. The patient should try each of these methods to determine which is the most efficient. The lower extremities are used the same way as described for ascending and descending a curb. (*Note:* The person who uses forearm crutches can also be taught to use these techniques.)

Standard Walker *Caution:* These techniques are suggested only for the patient who has good balance, trunk control, and extremity strength. They should be performed only when a handrail is available and when all of the feet of the walker fit on the stair treads when

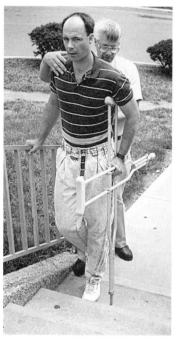

■ **FIGURE 8–44**
Patient ascending stairs with bilateral axillary crutches (alternative method).

the walker is positioned along the patient's side. You may prefer to teach these as techniques to be used for emergency situations rather than as routine techniques.

ASCENDING   Instruct the patient to face the stairs and to position the walker along the side farthest from the handrail with the closed side of the walker next to him/her. The front feet of the walker are placed one step above the step on which the patient stands; the

rear feet remain on the step on which the patient is standing (Fig. 8–45).

The patient grasps the handrail and the front handgrip or the midpoint of the horizontal bar of the walker. The patient steps up with the strongest/least affected lower extremity, elevates the body with the upper and lower extremities, and then steps up with or lifts the weaker lower extremity. The walker is advanced up one step by the patient, and the procedure is repeated. The final step at the top of the stair is performed by placing the walker on the upper surface and using it for support as the patient steps up.

DESCENDING   Instruct the patient to face the stairs and to position the walker along the side farthest from the handrail with the closed side of the walker next to him/her. The front feet of the walker are placed one step below the step on which the patient stands, and the rear feet remain on the step on which the patient is standing (Fig. 8–46).

The patient grasps the handrail and the rear handgrip or the midpoint of the horizontal bar of the walker. He/she lowers the weakest/most affected lower extremity by slightly flexing the hip and knee of the strongest lower extremity, then lowers the body using the upper and lower extremities, and steps down with the strongest lower extremity. The walker is advanced down one step, and the procedure is repeated. The patient descends the final step using the same method described to step from a curb.

Patients With Casts or Knee Immobilizers
Below-Knee Cast   To ascend stairs or a curb, the patient has several options. Each method is designed to protect the foot and lower leg immobilized by

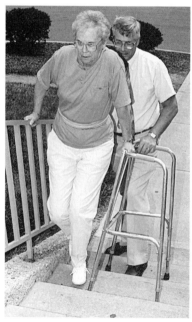

■ **FIGURE 8–45**
Patient ascending stairs with a walker.

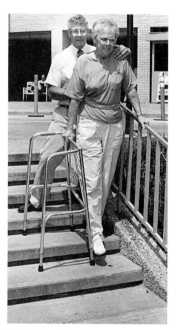

■ **FIGURE 8–46**
Patient descending stairs with a walker.

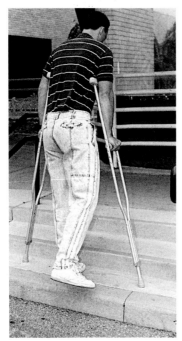

■ FIGURE 8–47
Patient independently ascending stairs using bilateral axillary crutches, three-point pattern.

the cast and to promote safety and stability for the patient.

Instruct the patient to extend the hip and flex the knee to 90 degrees, keeping the knee at 90 degrees, so his/her toes will clear the curb or the stair lip or *riser*. As an alternative, instruct the patient to extend the hip and knee and externally rotate the hip (Fig. 8–47)

or to flex the hip and knee to 90 degrees so the toes will clear the curb or the stair lip or riser. The last method does not provide as much protection to the foot and cast as the other two methods and is not recommended.

The method selected for each patient will depend on the patient's strength, balance, coordination, and, in some instances, his/her preference. The patient should try each of these methods to determine which one is the most efficient.

To descend stairs or a curb, there are several options for the patient to try.

First, the patient can flex the hip and knee to 90 degrees so the heel will clear the stair tread, and then position the lower leg in front of his/her body as he/she steps down, or the patient can partially flex the hip and maintain the knee in extension so the heel clears the stair tread (Fig. 8–48*A*). Do not teach the patient to flex the knee to 90 degrees with the hip extended because the toes are apt to contact the curb surface or stair tread as he/she steps down (see Fig. 8–48*B*).

Full-Length Cast or Knee Immobilizer To ascend stairs or a curb, the patient should extend and externally rotate the hip so the toes clear the stair lip or riser or the front of the curb as he/she steps up. The immobilized extremity will trail the body as the patient steps up.

To descend stairs or a curb, instruct the patient to partially flex the hip so the heel clears the stair tread or curb. The immobilized lower extremity remains in front of the patient and leads the body as he/she steps down.

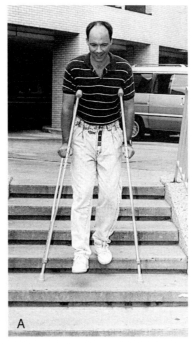
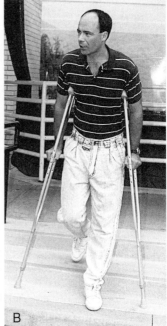

■ FIGURE 8–48
A, Proper way for a patient to descend stairs independently using crutches. *B*, Improper way.

DOORS

Patients who use ambulation aids should be taught how to manage opening and closing various types of doors. The patient should be familiar with several techniques that will assist him/her to control doors with and without self-closing devices (automatic door closers). It is likely that the patient will prefer to use only one of these techniques, but his/her independence will be enhanced if more than one method is learned and mastered.

Self-Closing Door If the door opens away from the patient, he/she approaches the door at an angle so

he/she faces the side of the door that will open (i.e., away from the hinges) (Fig. 8–49A). Instruct the patient to position himself/herself close to the door and the doorknob, latch, or crash bar; use one hand to open the door; and shift his/her weight onto the opposite crutch and lower extremity, if weight bearing is permitted on that extremity (see Fig. 8–49B). The door is opened with a quick push, and the patient returns his/her hand from the doorknob or crash bar to the crutch. The crutch nearest to the door is moved so the crutch tip engages the floor and the bottom of the door and serves as a doorstop. The door can be opened wider by repeating this procedure as the patient moves through the doorway.

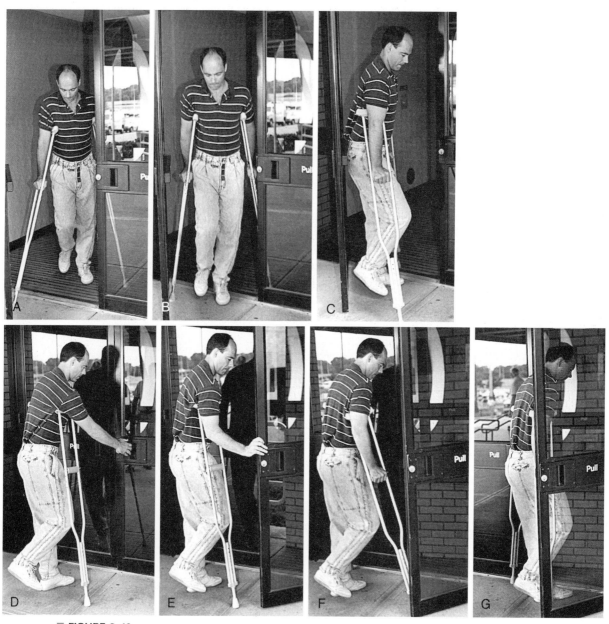

■ **FIGURE 8–49**
A through *C,* Use of bilateral axillary crutches to negotiate a self-closing door that opens away from the patient. *D* through *G,* Use of bilateral axillary crutches to negotiate a self-closing door that opens toward the patient.

The patient moves through the doorway by pushing against the door to open it farther and by repositioning the crutch tip to keep the door open. He/she must be certain that the final step through the doorway will place him/her beyond the closing arc of the door. (*Note:* If the door has a crash bar, the patient should open the door by pushing on the crash bar near to where it is attached to the door close to the door latch; this will give the patient the greatest advantage to open the door with the least expenditure of energy. Then he/she can use the crutch tip to keep the door open, or he/she may turn his/her back to the door and use the body to keep the door open while moving sideward [see Fig. 8–49C].)

Some patients may prefer to turn the back to the door and use the body to restrain the door as they move sideward through the doorway. Some patients may prefer to place both crutches under the axilla farthest from the crash bar, holding them with the corresponding hand while grasping the crash bar with the hand nearest to the crash bar. He/she may then use the crash bar as a support as he/she steps through the door. The patient must be instructed to push downward rather than outward on the bar while moving through the doorway to avoid opening the door too wide and affecting his/her base of support. He/she will need to reposition the crutches into each axilla to take the last step through the doorway.

If the door opens toward the patient, instruct the patient to approach the opening edge of the door at an angle, facing toward the hinge side of the door (see Fig. 8–49D). By being positioned at an angle to the door, the patient will be able to open the door a smaller amount than would be necessary if he/she stood directly in front of it. He/she positions himself/herself close to the door but slightly outside the area needed to open the door. He/she shifts his/her weight onto the crutch handgrip farthest from the doorknob or latch and uses the hand nearest the doorknob to open the door by quickly pulling on the doorknob and then returning the hand from the doorknob to grip the aid (see Fig. 8–49E). The crutch nearest to the open edge of the door is moved so the crutch tip engages the floor and the bottom of the door to serve as a doorstop (see Fig. 8–49F). If necessary, the door can be opened wider before the patient moves through the doorway. The patient moves through the doorway by pushing against the door and repositioning the crutch tip against the bottom of the door (see Fig. 8–49G). He/she must be certain that the final step through the doorway will place him/her beyond the door frame and the closing of the door.

The same procedures can be used for forearm crutches, canes, or a walker.

Standard Doors Instruct the patient to use the same positions and techniques previously described for a door that opens away from or toward him/her. However, the patient will have to open the door only wide enough for the crutches, canes, or walker and the patient to move through the doorway. The door does not need to be opened to its full width if the patient is taught to move through the doorway at an angle. The crutch or cane tip or the walker feet are not required to restrain the door. The patient will have to turn to close the door, and he/she may have to move sideward or backward after the door has been closed to resume the gait pattern and direction. When the door opens toward the patient, he/she will need to back up while opening the door, especially if he/she cannot approach the door at an angle toward or facing the opening edge of the door.

Ascending or Descending Ramps, Inclines, or Hills Instruct the patient to ascend a ramp, incline, or hill using techniques similar to those used to ascend a curb or stairs.

Teach the patient to advance the aid and the strongest/least affected lower extremity before advancing the weakest/most affected lower extremity; a shorter stride may be necessary (Fig. 8–50). With a full-length cast or knee *immobilizer*, the patient will have to extend and externally rotate the hip to clear the foot when ascending the ramp, incline, or hill and will have to flex the hip when descending. With a below-knee cast, that extremity should be extended at the hip and flexed at the knee when ascending. On a steep incline or hill, the patient may need to "zigzag" by moving diagonally as he/she ascends.

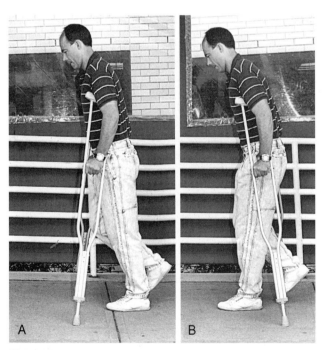

■ **FIGURE 8–50**
Patient ascending a ramp with bilateral axillary crutches, three-point pattern.

The patient is instructed to descend a ramp, incline, or hill using techniques similar to those used to descend a curb or stairs, but he/she should shorten his/her stride and placement of the ambulation aid(s) (Fig. 8–51). Instruct the patient to advance the weakest/most affected lower extremity and ambulation aid before advancing the strongest/least affected lower extremity. With a full-length cast or knee immobilizer, the patient will have to partially flex the hip to clear the foot, and thus the immobilized extremity will lead the movement. With a below-knee cast, the hip and knee should be partially flexed, with the foot positioned in front of the body to clear the foot; alternatively, the hip should be partially flexed and the knee extended to clear the foot. The lower extremity should not be allowed to trail the body. On a steep incline or hill, the patient may need to zigzag by moving diagonally as he/she descends.

Elevator Access   The patient should be taught to enter and leave the elevator in a forward position whenever possible. The ambulation aid or the patient's hand or arm can be used to activate the device that automatically prevents the door from closing, but the patient will need to determine the type of device used (e.g., photoelectric beam, pressure bar, or rubber-covered flange on the edge of the door). The patient should be taught to observe the area where the floor of the elevator and the floor of the corridor meet. There may be a space between the two surfaces, and the tip of the crutch, cane, or walker must not be

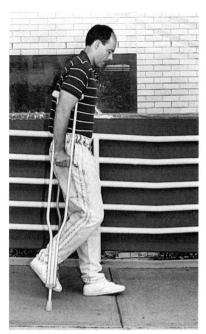

■ **FIGURE 8–51**
Patient descending a ramp with bilateral axillary crutches, three-point pattern.

placed in that space. Furthermore, when some elevator cars stop, their floor may not be level with the corridor floor; the patient should be alert for this potential hazard. After the patient is in the elevator, he/she will have to turn around to face forward in preparation to exit the car and to use the control panel.

PROCEDURE 8 – 9
Standing Transfers Into an Automobile

Independent transfer with crutches
  a. Instruct the patient to approach the passenger door at an angle; position yourself to guard him/her by standing behind and to one side.
  b. He/she reaches to open the door and opens it; he/she shifts the crutches into the hand farthest from the car.
  c. He/she places the free hand on a solid surface of the car (i.e., roof, back of the seat, dashboard, door frame) and pivots so his/her body is toward the car seat.
  d. He/she lowers his/her body onto the car seat using the upper extremities and functional lower extremity.
  e. He/she pivots and lifts the lower extremities into the car; the crutches are placed in the car.
  f. He/she closes the car door and applies the seat restraints.

Note: *For many persons, the transfer will be performed more easily if the car seat is positioned back as far as possible. This position will make it easier to place the lower extremities and crutches in the car.*

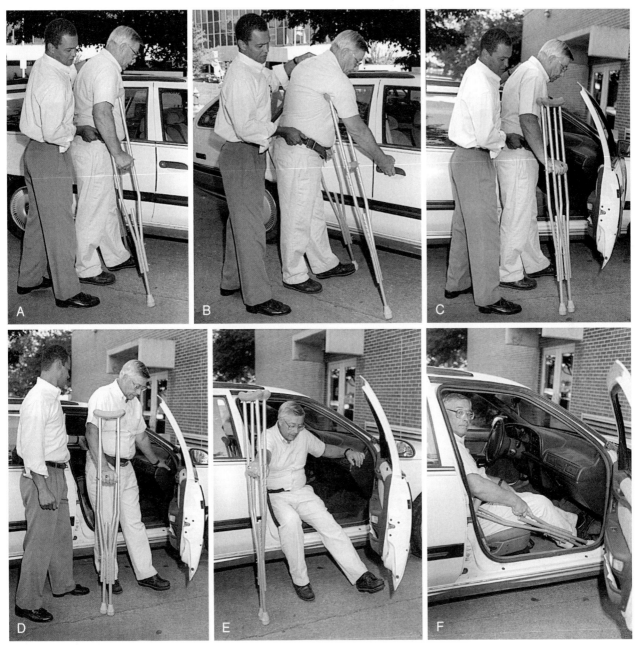

■ **FIGURE 8–52**
Transfer from crutches into a motor vehicle: *A,* The person approaches the passenger door at an angle.
B, He reaches for the door latch. *C,* The door is opened and crutches placed in one hand. *D,* The person
pivots and places the free hand on the dashboard. *E,* He lowers his body onto the car seat using the
upper extremities and uninvolved lower extremity. *F,* The lower extremities and crutches are placed in
the car.

Automobile Access Frequently, the patient will find it more convenient to enter and leave the car from the passenger side to avoid interference from the steering wheel. An automobile with two doors is usually easier for the patient to enter and exit because the door is wider, giving the patient more space in which to sit, and the access to the rear seat area is more convenient for storage of the aid (Procedure 8–9).

To enter the car, instruct the patient to approach the car door at an angle so that it opens away from him/her (Fig. 8–52A–C); open it only as far as neces-

sary to have access to the seat. He/she pivots his/her body so he/she faces away from the car interior and places both crutches in one hand; the other hand can be placed on the back of the seat or on the dash or on the door with the window rolled down (see Fig. 8–52D). He/she lowers himself/herself onto the seat and places the lower extremities and ambulation aid(s) into the car (see Fig. 8–52E,F). He/she will have to slide across the seat if he/she entered on the passenger side and will drive the automobile. The patient with a full-length cast or knee immobilizer may be more comfortable in the back seat because the extremity can be placed on the seat. If he/she plans to drive the automobile and the right lower extremity is immobilized, it can be placed on the front seat or on the floor on the passenger side of the car, or the seat can be adjusted to its most rearward position to provide more space between the front seat and the foot controls. The patient with a full-length cast or knee immobilizer on the left lower extremity will have difficulty driving the vehicle because it will be difficult to position the left lower extremity and still have access to the foot controls with the right foot.

To leave the car, the patient is instructed to open the car door, obtain the ambulation aid, and adjust his/her body so the lower extremities are placed outside the car. The patient grasps both crutches in one hand and places the other hand on the back of the seat, on the dash, or on the door frame with the window rolled down. The patient uses the upper and lower extremities to push himself/herself to stand, positions the crutches in each axilla, and steps away from the car. It may be necessary for the patient to turn to close the door and then to move backward before he/she resumes the gait pattern and direction.

TRANSFERRING TO THE FLOOR FROM CRUTCHES

There may be instances when a patient desires to sit on the floor or ground. Several methods can be taught to the patient to allow him/her to move from standing to sitting on the floor. This activity is not to be confused with a protective fall; this is an activity that the patient controls and performs independently.

If the patient is non–weight bearing on one lower extremity and uses bilateral axillary crutches, instruct him/her to drop both crutches to the floor and to balance briefly on the strongest lower extremity. He/she reaches forward toward the floor with the upper extremities while flexing the stronger lower extremity and extending and externally rotating the hip of the most affected lower extremity. The patient lowers the body using the strongest lower extremity until the hands contact the floor. He/she can kneel on the strongest knee or turn the hips and sit on the hip of the strongest lower extremity to complete the activity. Alternatively, instruct the patient to drop both crutches and to reach backward toward the floor with the upper extremities, flex the hip of the weakest/most affected lower extremity and slide the heel forward on the floor, and then flex the hip and knee of the strongest lower extremity. He/she lowers the body using the strongest lower extremity until his/her hands contact the floor, and then he/she sits

on the floor to complete the activity. Alternatively, instruct the patient to shift both crutches to the hand on the side of the weakest/most affected lower extremity and grasp both handpieces (Fig. 8–53A). He/she flexes or extends the hip of the most affected lower extremity and slides that heel forward or backward on the floor. He/she lowers the body using the strongest lower extremity and the hand holding the crutches while reaching toward the floor with the opposite upper extremity (see Fig. 8–53B,C). He/she sits on the floor to complete the activity (see Fig. 8–53D).

(*Note:* The patient can be taught all of these techniques or only one of them depending on his/her strength, coordination, balance, flexibility, and personal preference. The same techniques can be used for the patient who is able to partially bear weight on one lower extremity and fully bear weight on the other lower extremity.)

RISING FROM THE FLOOR TO STANDING

If the patient is non–weight bearing on one lower extremity and uses bilateral axillary crutches, he/she is instructed to turn so his/her hands and the foot of the strongest lower extremity are on the floor and to assume a half-kneeling position with that one lower extremity. The hip of the weakest/most affected lower extremity is extended and externally rotated. The crutches are positioned within easy reach, and the patient pushes to stand using the strongest lower extremity and the upper extremities. The patient picks up the crutches with one hand and grasps the handpieces while still in a semistanding position. He/she straightens the trunk, stands erect, and positions the crutches in each axilla to complete the activity. Alternatively, the patient turns so his/her hands and the foot of the strongest lower extremity are on the floor to assume a half-kneeling position, with the hip of the weakest/most affected lower extremity extended and externally rotated (Fig. 8–54A). The crutches are held vertically by the handpieces with the hand on the side of the weakest/most affected lower extremity (Fig. 8–54B). The patient pushes to stand using his/her strongest lower extremity and the hand on the crutch handpieces (Fig. 8–54C,D); after he/she is standing, the crutches are positioned into each axilla (see Fig. 8–53A). In a third technique, the patient sits on the floor and flexes the strongest hip and knee so the foot is flat on the floor. He/she maintains the weakest/most affected lower extremity in front of the body. The patient holds both crutches by the handpieces, using the hand on the same side as the weakest/most affected lower extremity, *or* the

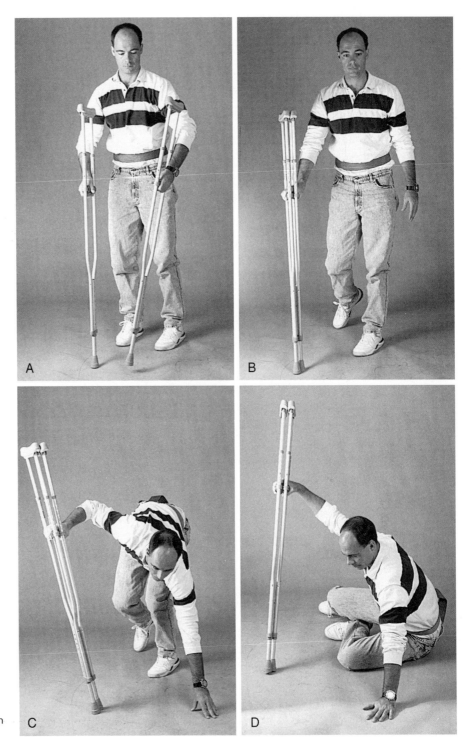

■ **FIGURE 8–53**
Patient transferring to the floor from crutches.

crutches may be placed between his/her thighs with both hands grasping the crutch handpieces. The patient pushes to stand using the strongest lower extremity and the upper extremities holding the crutches; after he/she is standing, the crutches are positioned into each axilla.

Similar methods or techniques can be used for patients who use ambulation aids other than axillary crutches. In some instances the patient may prefer to use a firm object (e.g., a table, chair, sofa, tree trunk, bench, or railing) for support and stability as he/she moves to the floor or returns to standing. However, the patient will be more independent when he/she is able to perform these activities without the use of a firm object because such an object may not be available or accessible to the patient. Special needs or techniques may have to be resolved by problem solving with the patient. There are some risks to patient safety

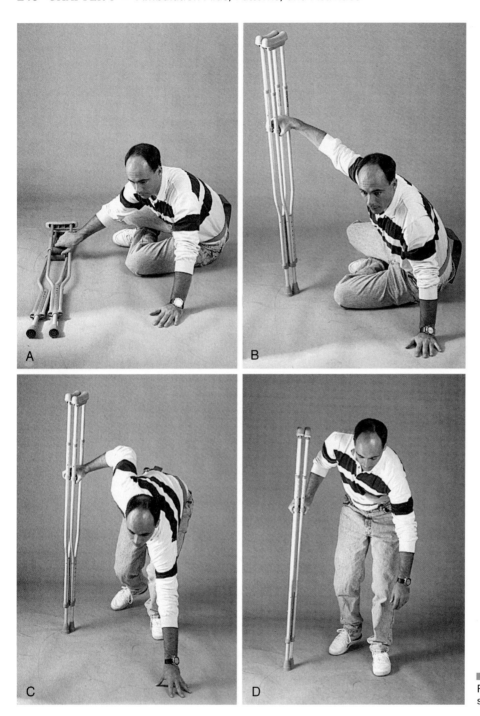

■ **FIGURE 8–54**
Patient rising from the floor to a standing position using crutches.

associated with this activity, so you must use caution and guard the patient as he/she practices these techniques.

FALLING TECHNIQUES

Backward The patient should be taught to control his/her body if a backward fall occurs. Instruct the patient to release the crutches (or other aid) and flex the trunk and head while reaching forward. The force of the fall is absorbed by the buttocks, and the patient's head is protected. It is not recommended that the patient be taught to reach backward with his/her upper extremities for protection. When this method is used, his/her head will tend to move backward and it is more likely to strike the floor or ground. This method can also produce strains or sprains of the shoulders or elbows and fractures of the wrists. *Caution:* If this activity is demonstrated or practiced, floor mats should be used to prevent injury (Fig. 8–55).

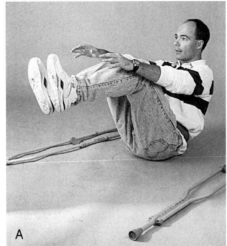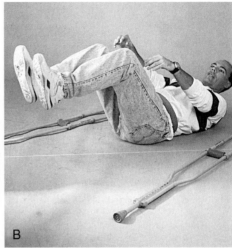

A   B

■ **FIGURE 8–55**
Technique for teaching a patient how to fall backward using crutches.

Forward   The patient should be taught to release the crutches and reach toward the floor with the upper extremities. He/she should "break" the fall with the upper extremities and lower the body to the floor. Turning the face to one side may reduce facial injuries (Procedure 8–10).

SUMMARY

Ambulation with an aid or aids can be a potentially hazardous or dangerous activity for a patient. Therefore, it is important to emphasize specific pre-

---

PROCEDURE 8-10
Protective Fall When Using Crutches

These procedures should be described and demonstrated by the caregiver before the patient attempts them; when the patient practices the activity, he/she must be guarded closely, and protective mats should be placed on the floor to prevent injury.

1. Forward fall
   a. The patient releases the crutches and quickly flips them to the side; he/she must not allow the crutches to fall to the floor in front of the body.
   b. He/she reaches forward with both upper extremities and turns the head to one side.
   c. When the hands contact the floor, he/she bends the elbows to absorb some of the force of the fall.
   d. He/she lowers the body to the floor and regains the crutches in preparation for standing using one of the techniques presented in this chapter if no serious injury has occurred.

2. Backward fall
   a. The patient releases the crutches and quickly flips them to the side; he/she must not allow the crutches to fall to the floor behind the body.
   b. He/she tucks the chin toward the chest and reaches *forward* with both upper extremities.
   c. He/she maintains a semiflexed position so the buttocks will contact the floor first.
   d. He/she regains the crutches in preparation for standing using one of the techniques presented in this chapter if no serious injury has occurred.

cautions to the patient and his/her family to promote safety.

All ambulation aids should be inspected and evaluated frequently for damage or disrepair. Nuts, adjustment buttons, tips, and handgrips must be secure and properly tightened or applied before using the aid for ambulation. The patient should be instructed to examine the equipment periodically and maintain it properly. The family and the patient should be instructed to maintain the environment of the home so it will be free of hazards that could lead to patient injury. For example, small area (throw) rugs should be removed; linoleum or tile floors should not be waxed or highly polished; smooth floor surfaces should be dry and any fluids spilled on them removed immediately; wall or grab bars should be attached to the wall studs, not to the wall board or plaster; one or two handrails may have to be added to stairs; and furniture should be arranged to provide adequate space for the patient to maneuver. Safety information can be provided in written form, and you should document your activities and the patient's performance according to the policies of the facility or agency with which you are employed or associated (Box 8–5).

Each patient must be instructed in the proper gait pattern and how to perform selected functional activities before initiating ambulation or attempting each functional activity. You must guide, encourage, and correct the patient until he/she is proficient and competent to perform the gait pattern safely. In addition, you must guard and protect the patient throughout the training sessions by using proper positioning and the safety belt. Demonstrations are helpful and usually necessary as part of the teaching-learning cycle. The family may need to be instructed how to protect or manage the patient at home.

The patient should be reminded to bear his/her body weight on the hands rather than on the axillary bar of the axillary crutch to avoid possible injury to nerves and circulatory vessels located in the floor of the axilla. The axillary bar must not be used as the primary weight-bearing surface during ambulation or when the patient is standing. Finally, inform the patient and the family how to contact you for advice or assistance after the patient has returned home. This information should be provided in writing and should include your business telephone number and the hours you are available.

■ SELF-STUDY/DISCUSSION ACTIVITIES

1. Describe the patient characteristics and abilities necessary to perform the following gait patterns: two-point, four-point, three-point, three-one–point, and modified two-point or four-point.

2. Discuss the factors you would consider when selecting each of the following ambulation aids: canes, axillary crutches, platform crutches, forearm crutches, walker, and parallel bars.

3. Outline the assessment or evaluation techniques or procedures you would perform before initiating a gait pattern that required ambulation aids or equipment. Provide a rationale for the selection of the techniques.

4. Explain how you would initially measure and confirm the fit of each ambulation aid; state the important principles related to the proper fit of the device.

5. Explain how you would instruct a patient to use a unilateral ambulation aid, and provide a rationale for your instructions.

6. Describe how you would guard a patient ambulating on a level surface or on stairs and when moving from sitting to standing and from standing to sitting.

7. Describe how you would monitor a patient's response to ambulation activities and how you would use the findings to plan the patient's treatment.

BOX 8–5

Precautions for Ambulation in the Home

1. Remove small rugs or mats that are likely to slip or slide (e.g., area or throw rugs); be extremely cautious when using a bathmat.

2. Avoid waxing floors or use a "nonskid" wax.

3. Immediately wipe fluids from noncarpeted floors.

4. Check ambulation aids frequently for cracks, loose nuts, or worn tips; clean dust and dirt on tips weekly.

5. Remove items stored on stair steps; be certain stair handrails are secure and strong.

6. Position furniture in each room to provide a 36-inch-wide unobstructed pathway, when possible.

7. Provide safety (grab) bars for the toilet, shower, and bathtub; be certain they are attached to wall studs or floor.

Chapter 9

Special Equipment and Patient Care Environments

After studying this chapter, the reader will be able to:

1 Describe the use of the equipment used for special patient needs.

2 Describe the precautions necessary when treating a patient using the equipment.

3 Understand and apply appropriate measures to resolve a patient emergency.

4 Define acronyms used to describe special patient care units (CCU, ER, ICU, MICU, NICU, OHRU, SICU).

5 Describe treatments that could be performed with a patient in a special care unit or who uses special support equipment/systems.

■ ■ ■ KEY TERMS

Alveolus: A little hollow; one of the thin-walled chambers of the lungs (pulmonary alveoli), surrounded by networks of capillaries through whose walls exchange of carbon dioxide and oxygen takes place.

Arrhythmia: Variation from the normal rhythm, especially of the heartbeat.

Arterial monitoring line (A line): A catheter inserted into an artery and attached to an electronic monitoring system to directly measure arterial blood pressure.

Catheter: A rubber, plastic, metal, or glass tube used to remove or inject fluids into a person.

Comminuted: Broken or crushed into small pieces.

Cyanosis: A bluish discoloration of the skin and mucous membranes due to excessive concentration of reduced hemoglobin in the blood.

Dialysis: The diffusion of solute molecules through a semipermeable membrane passing from the side of higher concentration to the side of lower concentration; a method sometimes used in cases of defective renal function to remove elements from the blood that are normally excreted in the urine (hemodialysis).

Electrocardiogram (ECG or EKG): A graphic record of the heart's electrical action derived by amplification of the minutely small electrical impulses normally generated by the heart.

Endotracheal tube (ETT): A hollow tube, approximately 10 inches long, with an inflatable cuff near one end that is inserted and positioned in the trachea. After the tube has been positioned, the cuff is inflated to maintain the tube's position so the patient can breathe through the tube.

Fistula: Any abnormal, tubelike passage within body tissue, usually between two internal organs or leading from an internal organ to the body surface.

Fowler's position: A position in which the head of the patient's bed is raised 18 to 20 inches above level with the knees flexed.

Gastrointestinal: Pertaining to the stomach and intestines.

Hyperventilation: Abnormally prolonged and deep breathing.

Hypoxemia: Deficient oxygenation of the blood.

Infusion: The slow therapeutic introduction of fluid other than blood into a vein.

Infusion pump (IMED, IVAC): An electronic device designed to automatically control the flow and rate of intravenous fluids into a patient.

Intravenous: Administration of fluids into a vein through the use of a steel needle or plastic catheter.

Intravenous therapy: The introduction of a fluid into a person's vein; nutrients or medications may be supplied intravenously.

Mediastinum: The mass of tissues and organs separating the sternum in front and the vertebral column behind, containing the heart and its large vessels, trachea, esophagus, thymus, lymph nodes, and other structures and tissues.

Micturition: Voiding of urine.

Monitor: An apparatus designed to observe, report, and measure a given condition or phenomenon such as blood pressure, heart rate, or respiration rate.

Myocardial infarction (MI): Necrosis of the cells of an area of the heart muscle resulting from oxygen deprivation caused by obstruction of the blood supply.

Nasogastric (NG) tube: A plastic tube usually inserted into a nostril and ending in the stomach. It can be used to remove fluid or gas from the stomach, monitor the digestive function of the stomach, administer medications or nutrients, or obtain specimens of the stomach contents.

Oximeter: A photoelectric device that measures oxygen saturation of the blood.

Patent: Open, unobstructed, or not closed.

Pneumothorax: Accumulation of air or gas in the pleural cavity resulting in collapse of the lung on the affected side.

Shunt: A passage or anastomosis between two natural vessels, especially between blood vessels.

Suprapubic: Above the pubis.

Swan-Ganz catheter: A long intravenous tube inserted into a vein (usually the basilic or subclavian vein) and terminating in the pulmonary artery. A monitor attached to the catheter measures the pulmonary artery pressure (PAP) and the pulmonary capillary wedge pressure (PCWP); it permits evaluation of cardiac function.

Tachypnea: Very rapid respirations.

Tract: A longitudinal assemblage of tissues or organs, especially a bundle of nerve fibers having a common origin, function, and termination, or a number of anatomic structures arranged in series and serving a common function.

Traction: The exertion of a pulling or distracting force to maintain a proper position of bone ends or joint to facilitate the healing process.

Trendelenburg's position: A position in which the patient lies supine with the head lower than the rest of the body.

Turning frame: An apparatus that allows a patient's position to be changed from supine to prone, and vice versa, by one person by maintaining the patient's position between two frames of the apparatus; the patient may be turned horizontally or vertically depending on the apparatus used.

Ventilator: A mechanical apparatus designed to intermittently or continuously assist or control pulmonary ventilation (breathing); also referred to as a *respirator.*

Wedge pressure: Intravascular pressure measured by a catheter inserted into the pulmonary artery (Swan-Ganz catheter) to permit indirect measurement of mean left atrial pressure.

INTRODUCTION

Many patients who occupy hospital beds are acutely ill and require extensive nursing care. The equipment and technology available to treat and monitor these patients have changed dramatically during the past 10 to 20 years. Life-supporting or life-sustaining equipment is commonplace. Patients who probably would not have survived life-threatening trauma or illness several years ago are surviving now because of advances in medical treatment and equipment. Requests for treatment of these seriously ill patients by various members of the rehabilitation team have increased, in part because medical and nursing personnel have recognized the advantages of the early application of rehabilitation techniques for these patients. Consequently, the physical therapist, respiratory therapist, and other caregivers have become integral members of this medical management team. Many of these very ill patients are initially managed in specialized nursing units listed in Box 9–1.

The initial exposure to the equipment and devices used in these units can overwhelm, intimidate, or create apprehension in an inexperienced, uninformed practitioner. In this text, descriptions of some of the frequently used equipment and devices used to treat the seriously involved patient are designed to assist the caregiver to become better prepared to treat these patients in a specialized environment. However, the caregiver should be oriented specifically to the equipment and treatment protocols in each employment setting before providing patient care. Also, information should be provided to the caregiver so that he/she will be prepared to react and will know from whom assistance can be obtained, if a patient emergency occurs.

BOX 9–1

Specialized Patient Care Units

CCU: Coronary (cardiac) care unit or critical care unit

ER: Emergency room

ICU: Intensive care unit or intermediate care unit

MICU: Medical intensive care unit

NICU: Neurologic (neuro) intensive care unit

OHRU: Open heart recovery unit

SICU: Surgical intensive care unit

ORIENTATION TO THE SPECIAL INTENSIVE CARE UNIT

A typical patient cubicle in an intensive care unit (ICU) is apt to have several types of equipment to monitor the patient's physiologic state, ventilate the patient, provide *intravenous* (IV) *therapy,* deliver oxygen, and remove fluids from the patient (i.e., suction). The patient may have IV lines, *arterial monitoring lines,* drainage tubes, oxygen being applied, or leads going from the patient to a monitor of vital signs; he/she may also be receiving respiratory support from a *ventilator* (*respirator*). After you have reviewed the medical record, take a few minutes to observe the unit and the patient before you initiate any treatment. Some patients will be alert, whereas others may be comatose or unresponsive, but most patients in specialized care units will be acutely ill or seriously traumatized.

If you are unfamiliar with the equipment applied to the patient, obtain assistance from a nurse in the unit or participate in a program designed to prepare you to treat patients who are in the unit (Figs. 9–1 and 9–2). Because the patient is acutely ill, it will be necessary to reduce the intensity of the treatment compared with the intensity you might use with less ill patients. Shorter treatment sessions, fewer exercise repetitions, and less demand for active participation by the patient may be necessary. Careful and continuous monitoring of the patient's response to treatment will be required. You can accomplish this through observation of and communication with the patient, awareness of his/her vital signs, and a comparison of his/her current responses with previous responses to the treatment. It is recommended you discuss the patient's current condition with one of the nursing personnel prior to treatment, because a patient's condition may fluctuate from hour to hour or from day to day, and you may

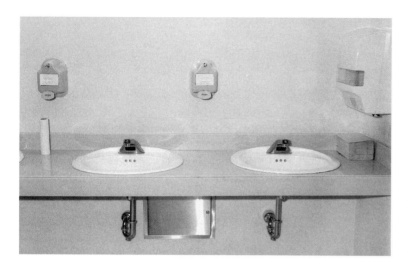

■ **FIGURE 9–1**
Handwashing area at the entrance to the intensive care unit for use by visitors before entering and when leaving the unit; water flow is activated when the hands are placed beneath the faucet spout.

not be able to rely on information obtained at your previous visit (Procedures 9–1 and 9–2).

The caregiver who treats patients in an ICU is most apt to find that his/her roles in that environment will be very similar to his/her roles in treating patients whose conditions are less acute or life threatening. The general, overall goals of treatment for patients in the ICU will be to minimize or prevent the adverse effects of inactivity and immobility and assist each person to become functionally independent.

There are several areas of care and intervention of which caregivers should be aware as they treat patients in the ICU. One area is to prevent the development of contractures through the use of passive and active exercise, proper positioning, and body alignment. In addition, the use of exercise and physical activity will be important to improve the general condition of the patient. Bed mobility training will be necessary because it is a precursor to transfer and ambulation activities; all of these are requisites for functional independence. Passive and active exercise assist to stimulate the sensory system; therefore, sensory

awareness and coordination may be enhanced through exercise. Some patients will have respiratory difficulties, and they may need to be taught how to breathe more efficiently during their recovery, even when a respiratory aid is being used. Patients with respiratory deficits or who have experienced thoracic or abdominal surgery may need to be instructed how to cough effectively. For some patients, wound care and management will be required, and the prevention of pressure ulcers will be particularly important for all caregivers. Finally, assisting the patient to cope with, adjust to, or overcome painful stimuli may be accomplished through selected exercise techniques or the use of pain-relieving electrotherapy equipment.

TYPES OF BEDS

The standard manually operated and electrically operated bed are the two most common beds used in a hospital. These beds provide support, access to care,

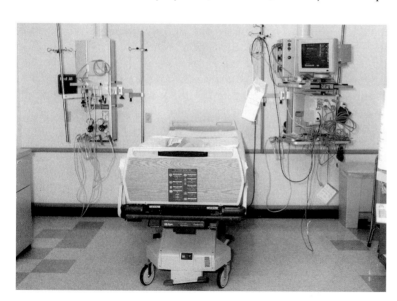

■ **FIGURE 9–2**
Typical intensive care unit patient unit or cubicle prepared for patient use.

PROCEDURE 9-1
Treating a Patient in an Intensive Care Unit

1. Review the patient's medical record before each treatment session, even when multiple sessions occur during the same day.
2. Request information about the patient's current status (i.e., physical activity level, mental capacity, or alertness) from nursing personnel.
3. Wash your hands, and apply protective garments as necessary.
4. Observe the equipment or devices used to monitor the patient for current information about his/her physiologic status.
5. Observe the type and location of the equipment or devices being used by the patient (e.g., ventilator, IV line, oxygen, urinary catheter, supplemental nutrition, suction).
6. Identify the location of all tubes, monitor lead connections, IV line connections and insertion sites, and patient-controlled analgesia; maintain all tubes and leads free of occlusion and tension.
7. Evaluate or determine the patient's present physical and mental status before initiating treatment.
8. Observe the patient and monitoring devices frequently; determine his/her response to the treatment; identify significant change in his/her condition or physiologic status.
9. Notify nursing personnel of significant change in his/her condition or physiologic status; document and record your activities and observations as necessary.

and the ability to alter the patient's position for most patients. However, the acutely ill or traumatized patient frequently requires special features not available on the standard hospital bed.

If the caregiver finds the patient's position to be inappropriate for treatment, three options are available: reschedule the treatment when the patient is positioned more appropriately, temporarily reposition the patient to permit treatment, or treat the patient as much as possible without changing his/her position. If the patient's original position is changed, the caregiver should follow the nursing policies and procedures regarding repositioning the patient. It may be necessary to request the nurse to reposition the patient or readjust the position of the bed, or it may be necessary to have a nurse present when position changes are made by the caregiver. Usually the caregiver should return the patient to his/her original position at the conclusion of the treatment session and adhere to any time schedule related to patient positioning. For example, a patient may need to follow a turning schedule and may be limited in the amount of time he/she can remain in one position. Therefore, the caregiver should be aware of and comply with any special schedule the patient is expected to follow.

Standard Adjustable Bed Most hospital beds can be adjusted using electrical controls. The controls may be located at the head or foot or on the side rail of the bed or attached to a special cord so the patient can operate them independently. The controls should be marked according to their function and can be operated by using the hand or foot. The bed can be raised and lowered in relation to the floor as a total unit, or the upper and lower components can be adjusted separately or together. On most beds, the lower portion is hinged so it can be adjusted to provide knee flexion, which in turn causes hip flexion. On some beds, the lower component will become flexed whenever the upper component is raised. This action creates hip and knee flexion, which is more comfortable for the patient and tends to help prevent him/her from sliding down in the bed. When the upper portion is raised slightly, the patient's position is referred to as *Fowler's position.* Sometimes when the bed is adjusted with the upper portion raised and the lower portion flexed, the bed is considered to be "gatched."

Most beds have some type of side rails or protective devices. Some rails are lifted upward until the locking mechanism is engaged, whereas other types are adjusted by moving them toward the upper por-

---

P R O C E D U R E   9 – 2
Precautions to Use in the Intensive Care Unit

1. Avoid occlusion or excessive tension on all tubes, monitor leads, suction units, supplemental nutrition items, and oxygen service.

2. Observe and assess the patient before, during, and after treatment; determine his/her objective and subjective response to the treatment.

3. Modify or cease treatment if he/she exhibits abnormal, unexpected, or undesired response or responses to the treatment (e.g., changes in vital signs, breathing pattern, indication of increased pain, reduced mental awareness or alertness).

4. Request assistance from nursing or respiratory service personnel if you identify changes in the function or performance of the patient support systems (e.g., IV line, monitors, ventilation, supplemental nutrition, or drainage devices).

5. Note the appearance and odor of visible wounds and wound or urine drainage; observe the general appearance of the patient.

6. Request assistance, as necessary, to adjust or move equipment or reposition the patient.

7. At the conclusion of the treatment:
   a. Be certain the patient is properly positioned.
   b. Elevate or replace side rails on the bed.
   c. Position the bedside table so it is accessible to the patient.
   d. Position other personal items so they are accessible.
   e. Inform him/her of the location of the "nurse call" device; position it so it is accessible.

---

tion of the bed until the locking mechanism is engaged. When a side rail is used for patient security, it is important to check to be certain the rail is locked securely before you leave the patient. Also, you should check to be certain you have not compressed or stretched any IV or other tubing with the side rail. Adjust the bed into the position that will allow you the best access to the patient and enable you to use proper body mechanics. Be certain to return the patient to his/her original, required, or preferred position at the conclusion of the treatment.

The patient will probably have a device that is either located on the side rail or attached to a long electrical cord that enables him/her to contact nursing personnel from the bed. At the conclusion of treatment, the caregiver should be certain the patient has access to the device and is aware of its location or position. This device may be referred to as a "call button."

Turning Frame (e.g., Stryker Wedge Frame) A *turning frame* has an anterior and a posterior frame, each of which has a canvas cover. It has a support base

that allows elevation of the head or foot ends of the frames or of the entire bed. A pivot joint allows the patient to be turned in a horizontal plane from a prone to a supine position or from a supine to a prone position by one person. A similar device is the Foster frame.

This device is indicated when skeletal stability and alignment are desired to permit a patient to be turned horizontally from prone to supine or from supine to prone; when continuous maintenance of skeletal cervical *traction*, such as Crutchfield or a similar type of skeletal traction, is desired; and when a patient must be immobilized after a spinal fracture and safe and efficient change of position from supine to prone, or vice versa, must be performed.

This equipment has several advantages. It allows access to the patient for a variety of therapeutic interventions and nursing care; it allows one person to safely and easily turn the patient from supine to prone, and vice versa; and it allows the patient to be wheeled or transported from one location to another without being removed from the frame. Furthermore, the unit can be elevated or lowered as a unit to several heights or positions, and the height of the head or foot of the frame can be changed independently. The patient can be positioned in *Trendelenburg's position* when he/she is supine or prone. The unit requires relatively little space, even when the patient is turned, and it allows cervical traction to be applied and maintained even when the patient is turned.

The equipment does have several disadvantages. The patient can be positioned only supine or prone, and patients who weigh more than 200 pounds or who are more than approximately 6 feet tall will be difficult to position on the frames. Most of the patients who exceed these limits will not be able to tolerate this device for extended periods of time. Patients are at risk of developing skin problems as a result of shear and pressure forces related to being positioned only prone or supine, and contractures may develop unless appropriate exercise and positioning techniques are used. *Note:* The development of new equipment and other technological advances in patient care have reduced the need for this piece of equipment in most hospitals in the United States, and it is rarely used currently.

Circular Turning Frame (Circ-O-Lectric Bed) The circular turning frame has an anterior and a posterior frame that are attached to two circular supports. The frames on which the patient is positioned move the patient vertically from supine to prone or from prone to supine as the circular supports rotate through 180 degrees around a short axis. The circular support frames are moved by an electric motor, and they can be stopped at any point within their half-circle range. A control switch can be operated by the patient or other persons to adjust his/her position. The patient can be positioned in Trendelenburg's position when he/she is prone or supine. The posterior patient support frame can be adjusted to provide hip and knee flexion and trunk elevation when he/she is supine so a partial sitting posture can be attained. Additional attachments can be added to the circular support frames to provide traction or immobilization for the extremities.

This equipment is indicated when skeletal stability and alignment are desired when a patient is turned vertically from supine to prone, or vice versa; when it is desired to have one person change the patient's position safely; and when frequent position changes, to relieve pressure or enhance function, are desired or necessary.

The equipment has several advantages. It allows one person to safely and easily turn the patient from supine to prone or from prone to supine or to be positioned at any point within an arc of 180 degrees, providing the patient frames are secured properly. It also allows easy access to the patient for a variety of therapeutic interventions and nursing care. The patient can be wheeled or transported from one location to another without being removed from the bed, provid-

ing the height of the doorway is sufficient (i.e., 7 feet) for the turning support frame to pass through. Additional attachments can be added to the circular support frames to provide traction or immobilization. Hip and knee flexion and a semirecumbent position can be provided, and the patient can be placed in a fully upright position so that he/she can step off the bed onto the floor.

The equipment also has several disadvantages. It requires sufficient space to allow the frames to rotate and to permit access to the patient. The compressive pressure through the axial skeleton increases as the patient is moved into a vertical position during the turning cycle. Therefore, this device is contraindicated for most patients with an unhealed, unstabilized vertebral fracture because of the vertical compressive loading that occurs to the spine during the turning process. A patient is at risk of developing skin problems as a result of the shear and pressure forces that occur as he/she is turned or rotated vertically. Some patients may experience signs or symptoms of motion sickness such as vertigo, nausea, or hypotension when being turned. *Note:* The development of new equipment and other technological advances in patient care have reduced the need for this piece of equipment in most hospitals in the United States, and it is rarely used currently.

Air-Fluidized Support Bed (Clinitron) The air-fluidized bed is a rectangular or ovoid bed that contains 1600 pounds of silicone-coated glass beads called microspheres. Heated, pressurized air flows through the beads to suspend a polyester cover that supports the patient. When set in motion, the microspheres develop the properties associated with fluids. The patient feels as if he/she is floating on a warm waterbed. Contact pressure of the patient's body against the polyester sheet is approximately 11 to 15 mm Hg.

This equipment is indicated for patients who have several infected lesions or require skin protection and whose position cannot be altered easily; patients with extensive pressure sores or at risk of developing deterioration of the skin (e.g., obese persons); patients with recent, extensive skin grafts; or patients who require prolonged immobilization (Fig. 9–3).

This piece of equipment has several advantages. It reduces the need for the application of topical medications and dressings by establishing a microclimate environment favorable for the healing process. The temperature of the air in the bed can be controlled according to the needs of the patient. There is reduced pressure on the skin, and pressure sores are less likely to develop because of the lowered pressure. Friction or shear forces to the body are reduced significantly or eliminated, and the patient can lie on his/her lesions or wounds for brief periods of time. When the unit is turned off, the polyester cover becomes a firm surface,

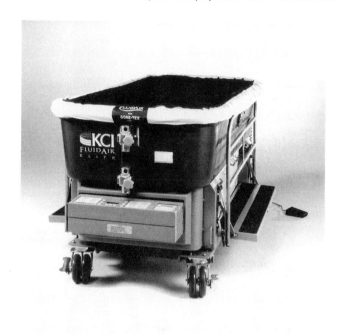

■ **FIGURE 9–3**
Air fluidization bed. [Photograph courtesy of Kinetic Concepts Incorporated (KCI).]

which may be beneficial for certain therapeutic interventions or nursing care.

The unit also has several disadvantages. The polyester cover (filter sheet) can be damaged (punctured) easily by a sharp object, and if the filter sheet is punctured, the microspheres will be expelled. Air flowing across the patient's skin may cause body fluids to evaporate more rapidly than normal, and it may be necessary to have the patient ingest small amounts of extra fluids to compensate for the fluid loss. A patient may require frequent position changes because of the tendency for fluid to pool in the lobes of the lungs, and obese or tall patients are apt to be uncomfortable on this bed. The height of the bed from the floor will probably be fixed, so it may be difficult to provide care or to transfer the patient. A draw sheet can be used to assist in positioning the patient, and a two-person sliding transfer from the bed to a stretcher can be performed with the unit turned off. Finally, this is a very expensive piece of equipment.

Post-trauma Mobility Beds (e.g., Keane, Roto-Rest)
Post-trauma mobility beds are designed to maintain a seriously injured patient in a stable position and maintain proper postural alignment through the use of adjustable bolsters. The bed oscillates from side to side, in a cradle-like motion, to reduce the amount of prolonged pressure on the patient's skin.

These beds are indicated for patients with restricted respiratory function, patients with advanced or multiple pressure sores, or patients who require stabilization and skeletal alignment after extensive trauma or as a result of severe neurologic deficits.

These beds have several advantages. The constant side-to-side motion assists in improving upper respiratory *tract* function and reduces the need to turn the patient to relieve pressure or prevent the development of pressure sores. The friction and shear forces associated with turning the patient are eliminated, and the constant motion of the bed may provide some environmental stimulation for neurologically impaired patients. Urinary stasis is reduced, and bowel function is improved as a result of the constant motion of these beds (Fig. 9–4*A,B*).

Several disadvantages have also been reported. Some patients may experience signs or symptoms of motion sickness, such as vertigo or nausea, and some patients may feel isolated from the environment as a result of a decrease in their visual orientation. Exercises and other forms of patient care may be restricted due to the bolsters and alignment supports, although some beds have ports or hatches for better access. Finally, sufficient space must be available to allow the bed to oscillate without interference from other objects. The bolsters and alignment supports must be maintained in position to provide proper stabilization and alignment. This is especially necessary for adequate support to the thorax.

Low Air Loss Therapy Bed The low air loss bed has several segmented and separated air bladders that allow the limited escape of air. The amount of air pressure in each bladder is individually controlled for each patient based on his/her size, weight, and shape, and the bed may be adjusted to several different positions (Figs. 9–5 and 9–6).

This bed is indicated for patients who require prolonged immobilization; patients who are at high risk of developing pressure sores or who have existing sores; patients whose condition requires frequent elevation of the trunk to promote proper respiratory function; and obese patients.

This bed has several advantages. It can be adjusted to accommodate the need to change the patient's position to hip and knee flexion, sitting, or a semirecumbent position. The patient's position can be altered through the use of electronically operated controls. The patient's weight is measured by sensors in the bed, and the air bladders are inflated or deflated automatically to distribute the patient's weight.

Several disadvantages have also been reported. The air bladders can be punctured or torn by sharp objects, and frequent alterations in the patient's position must be performed to prevent pressure sores. (*Note:* To be able to transfer a patient, you should lock the wheels, elevate the patient's trunk approximately 20 to 30 degrees, deflate the seat section, perform the transfer, and turn off the seat deflation control to reinflate the seat.)

The surfaces of the three beds described in this

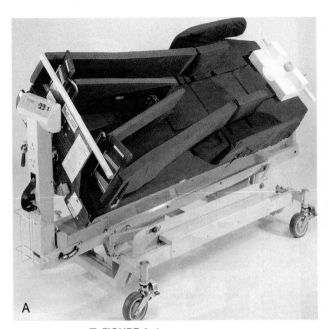
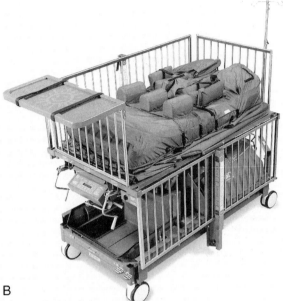

A   B

■ **FIGURE 9–4**
A, Roto-Rest bed. [Photograph courtesy of Kinetic Concepts Incorporated (KCI).] *B,* Pediatric bed.

section may not be rigid enough to allow effective performance of the chest compressions required for cardiopulmonary resuscitation (CPR). Therefore, a flat rigid wooden or plastic device must be placed beneath the patient to provide a firm solid surface before the initiation of CPR, or the person may need to be transferred to the floor. It will be easier to transfer the person when he/she is supine if a similar device is used.

LIFE SUPPORT AND MONITORING EQUIPMENT

MECHANICAL VENTILATORS

Most ventilators, also known as respirators, currently use positive pressure to move or propel gas or

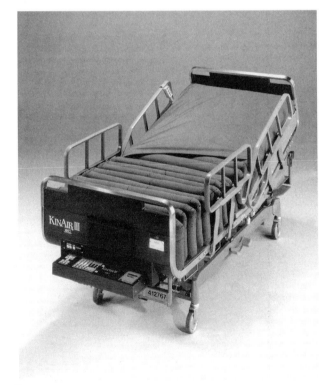

■ **FIGURE 9–5**
Air suspension bed with individual air bladders. [Photograph courtesy of Kinetic Concepts Incorporated (KCI).]

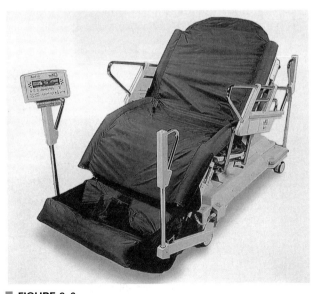

■ **FIGURE 9–6**
Air suspension bed for a heavy patient (300 to 850 lb). [Photograph courtesy of Kinetic Concepts Incorporated (KCI).]

air into the patient's lungs. The purpose of a ventilator is to maintain adequate and appropriate air exchange when normal respiration is inhibited or cannot be actively performed by the patient. A ventilator may be indicated for diseases or conditions that affect the patient's neurologic or musculoskeletal control of respiration or that interfere with the exchange of gases in the lungs. A ventilator may be used when the patient experiences apnea or when the potential for respiratory distress or failure exists.

An example of respiratory distress that may develop is adult respiratory distress syndrome (ARDS); a similar syndrome affects infants. This syndrome is potentially life threatening, and its existence must be recognized soon after it affects the patient so immediate steps can be initiated to counteract the syndrome. Some of the possible causes of ARDS are systemic shock, diffuse respiratory infection, and systemic response to sepsis or extensive trauma. Clinical signs and symptoms include dyspnea, *tachypnea, cyanosis*, and *hypoxemia*. The caregiver who treats a patient with ARDS or the infant syndrome must monitor the patient's response to activity and observe the monitoring equipment frequently to be certain his/her vital signs and arterial blood gases (ABGs) remain within acceptable ranges or limits. The person with ARDS will have a restricted respiratory capacity and will receive respiratory assistance from a ventilator. The person is likely to be intolerant of active exercise, especially resistive exercise, in the early stages of recovery, and complete recovery from ARDS may require several weeks. The syndrome is life threatening because it can cause the failure of one or more major organs such as the kidneys; therefore, early detection of the syndrome and aggressive treatment are extremely important.

TYPES OF VENTILATORS

Volume-Cycled Ventilators Volume-cycled ventilators are used primarily for patients who require long-term support. A predetermined volume of gas ("air"), dependent on the patient's needs, is delivered during the inspiratory phase of respiration, but the expiratory phase remains passive (Fig. 9–7).

This type of equipment is indicated when long-term ventilation assistance is needed, for the patient with severe chronic obstructive pulmonary disease (COPD), after thoracic surgery, and for disorders of the central nervous system and musculoskeletal disorders that affect the respiratory system, such as a cervical spinal cord injury, brain injury, amyotrophic lateral sclerosis, or poliomyelitis.

Pressure-Cycled Ventilators Pressure-cycled ventilators deliver a predetermined established maximum pressure of gas during respiration, and the inspiratory

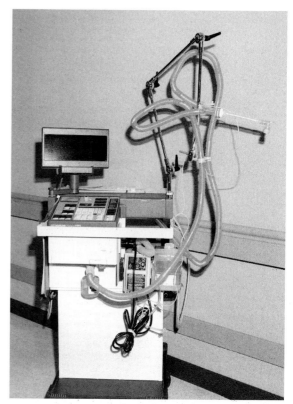

■ **FIGURE 9–7**
Ventilator with computer functions.

phase ends when that level is reached. The expiratory phase remains a passive phase. The flow rate may vary from one respiration cycle to the next.

This device is indicated when only short-term ventilation is needed in the form of intermittent positive-pressure breathing (IPPB) and for selected patients with neuromuscular or musculoskeletal distress.

Negative Pressure Device Negative pressure ventilation currently is rarely used in the management of patients with respiratory problems. The primary types are the tank respirator ("iron lung") and the chest respirator ("turtle shell"). These devices create a negative pressure in the patient's chest so the environmental air pressure exceeds the internal thoracic pressure. Because of this pressure imbalance, air enters the patient's lungs passively to provide inspiration.

MODES OF VENTILATION

Several modes by which patients can be ventilated are described in Box 9–2.

Airway Placement Usually, the gas delivered by the ventilator will be induced into the patient through a tube in one of several possible airways. The tube is referred to as an *endotracheal tube* (ETT), and when it

BOX 9–2

Modes of Ventilation

Assist Mode: The patient must develop or cause a negative pressure to "trigger" the ventilator to provide assistance to deliver gas, such as oxygen and air, to the patient.

Continuous Positive Airway Pressure (CPAP) Mode: This mode superimposes the use of PEEP (refer to the description below) on the patient's spontaneous breathing pattern. It is particularly useful to assist a patient to become weaned from the ventilator or to assist to maximize the gas exchange capabilities for an immobile, inactive patient.

Control Mode: The inspiration phase of respiration begins at timed intervals based on the patient's need for gas.

Assisted Control Mode: This mode is a combination of the previous two modes.

Intermittent Mandatory Ventilation (IMV) Mode: The patient's ventilation cycle is established so that ventilation occurs a minimum number of times per minute. This is the mode that is frequently used to begin to wean the patient from the ventilator and to develop an independent respiration pattern.

Synchronized IMV Mode: This mode allows the ventilation cycle to be coordinated with the patient's own breathing cycle.

Positive End-Expiratory Pressure (PEEP) Mode: This mode allows oxygen to be induced into the patient's lungs by maintaining positive pressure at the end of expiration which increases the alveolar surface area able to absorb the gas induced by the ventilator and leads to maximal alveolar ventilation. PEEP helps to expand and maintain the *alveoli*, that would normally close at the end of expiration, *patent*.

is in place, the patient is considered to be intubated. The possible locations for an ETT are in the oral pharyngeal, nasal pharyngeal, oral esophageal, nasal endotracheal, or oral endotracheal airway. Other means of insertion of the tube include tracheostomy or laryngostomy. Each of these artificial airways provides a clear airway through the patient's nasal, oral, or other passageways to the lungs. The ETT allows suction of the bronchial tree, but insertion of the ETT will restrict the patient from talking. When the ETT is removed, the patient will probably complain of throat discomfort, and his/her voice is apt to be distorted for a short period of time. The caregiver must avoid dis-

turbing or accidentally disconnecting the tube of the ventilator from the ETT and bending, kinking, or occluding the connector tubing. You should be certain the tubing is not obstructed by the weight of one of the patient's extremities or trapped under the bed rail.

The patient who uses a ventilator can participate in various types of exercise and other bedside activities, including sitting and ambulation. The patient must be informed of the activity, and the caregiver must be certain that the tubing is sufficiently long to allow the physical activity to be performed. Because the patient will have difficulty communicating orally, questions that can be answered with head nods or other nonverbal means should be asked. The patient's response to the activity must be monitored closely by the caregiver, and undue stress to the patient should be avoided. A patient using a ventilator probably will not tolerate exercise as well as other patients, so you should be cautious when you treat him/her. You should monitor his/her vital signs and observe him/her for signs of respiratory distress such as a change in the respiration pattern, syncope, or cyanosis.

The ventilator has an auditory and visual alarm that will be activated by various stimuli such as a disconnected tube, coughing by the patient, movement of the tubing, or a change in the respiratory pattern or needs of the patient. During orientation to the special care unit, the caregiver should be instructed how to determine the cause of the alarm and how to return the system to normal function. If this educational program is not provided, the caregiver should know how to obtain assistance from a nurse or respiratory therapist in the unit. The caregiver should be alert for signs or symptoms of respiratory or cardiopulmonary distress exhibited by the patient, such as dyspnea, tachycardia, *arrhythmia*, or *hyperventilation*.

The caregiver should become familiar with the various types of ventilators and modes of ventilation prior to initiating treatment on any patient. This can be accomplished through one or more inservice orientation programs.

MONITORS

The patient who requires special care may have his/her physiologic status monitored by various pieces of equipment. Common monitoring parameters include cardiac-vital signs, ABGs, intracranial pressure, pulmonary artery pressure (PAP), central venous pressure (CVP), and arterial pressure (A line) monitoring equipment. Exercise can be performed by patients who are being monitored, provided care is taken to avoid disruption of the equipment. Many of these units have an auditory and visual signal that may be activated by a change in the patient's condition, a change in the function of the equipment, or a change

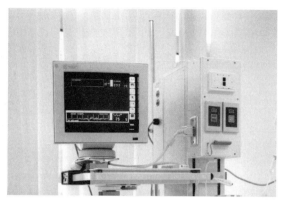

■ **FIGURE 9–8**
Patient monitor located in the patient's unit; heart rate, temperature, respiration rate, electrocardiogram patterns, and blood gases can be displayed separately or simultaneously.

in the patient's position. In some instances it will be necessary for a nurse to evaluate and correct the cause of the alarm, but in other instances, the caregiver may be able to correct the cause safely. For example, cease exercise and allow the patient to rest so his/her physiologic state returns to an acceptable level.

The caregiver should recognize that the patient's condition is most likely to be unstable, and caution should be used to avoid causing stress for the patient. Orientation to the purpose and function of the monitoring equipment and devices is recommended for persons who will treat the patient to whom the equipment is attached. *Caution:* Be certain you understand which parameters the various channels on the monitor are measuring or reporting at a given time and which channels are active. The channels can be changed to monitor different parameters at different times or they can be deactivated. Therefore, it is important that the caregiver knows which of the patient's physiologic responses are being monitored when treatment is being provided.

Vital Signs Monitor (e.g., Electrocardiogram [EKG or ECG]) The *electrocardiogram* monitors the patient's heart rate, blood pressure, and respiration rate (Fig. 9–8). Acceptable or safe parameters or ranges for the three physiologic indicators can be set in the unit. An alarm is activated when the upper or lower limits of the ranges are exceeded or when the unit malfunctions. A graphic and a digital display of the values are apparent on the monitor screen so the caregiver can observe the effects of the exercise and the patient's responses to activity (Fig. 9–9).

Oximeter This photoelectric device is used to measure the oxygen saturation (SaO_2) of the patient's blood by recording the different modulations of a transmitted beam of light by reduced hemoglobin and oxyhemoglobin as seen during the pulse. Usually, the *oximeter* will be positioned on or attached to a

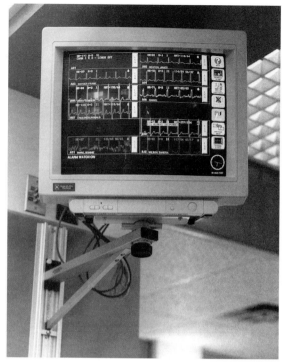

■ **FIGURE 9–9**
Patient monitor located in nurses' unit in intensive care unit; several patients can be monitored simultaneously.

patient's finger, and it will measure and report his/her pulse rate as well as the percentage of oxygen saturation of his/her hemoglobin (blood) (Fig. 9–10).

Pulmonary Artery Catheter (PAC) (e.g., Swan-Ganz Catheter) The *Swan-Ganz catheter* is a long, plastic, intravenous tube that can be inserted into the internal jugular or the femoral vein, guided into the basilic or subclavian vein, and then passed into the pulmonary artery. This *catheter* is used to provide accurate and continuous measurements of PAPs and will detect

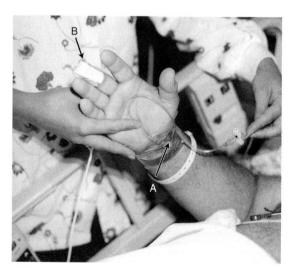

■ **FIGURE 9–10**
This person has an *(A)* arterial line inserted at the wrist with *(B)* an oximeter on the middle finger.

even very subtle changes in the patient's cardiovascular system, including responses to medications, stress, and exercise.

This device is indicated when measurements of right atrial pressure, PAP, and pulmonary capillary *wedge pressure* (PCWP) are desired. Readings are performed frequently; the monitor screen will show a rolling wave form, and a digital reading of the various values will appear. Normal values are right atrial pressure, 0 to 4 mm Hg; PAP, 20 to 30 mm Hg systolic and 10 to 15 mm Hg diastolic; PCWP, 4 to 12 mm Hg.

Exercise can be performed with the PAC in place, but it may be necessary to limit the exercise because of the location of the catheter's insertion. For example, if the catheter is inserted into the subclavian vein, shoulder flexion should be avoided and shoulder motions restricted. Similar restrictions in hip flexion and abduction exist for a femoral vein insertion. Some complications associated with this catheter are pulmonary artery vascular damage, damage to intracardial structures, cardiac dysrhythmias, endocarditis, and sepsis (infection).

Intracranial Pressure (ICP) Monitor The ICP monitor measures the pressure exerted against the skull by brain tissue, blood, or cerebrospinal fluid (CSF). It is used for patients who have experienced a closed head injury, cerebral hemorrhage, brain tumor, or an overproduction of CSF. Normal ICP pressure is 4 to 15 mm Hg, but a fluctuation of as much as 20 mm Hg can occur from a variety of routine activities.

This device is indicated to monitor ICP easily, to quantitate the degree of abnormal pressure, to properly initiate treatment, and to evaluate the results of treatment. Some of the complications associated with this device are sepsis, hemorrhage, and seizures.

Types of ICP Monitoring Devices

VENTRICULAR CATHETER The ventricular catheter is inserted into a lateral ventricle of the brain through a hole drilled in the skull. This is a very accurate method to monitor the ICP and allows withdrawal of CSF.

SUBARACHNOID SCREW A screw is inserted into the subarachnoid space through a small hole drilled in the skull. This device also permits accurate measurement of the ICP but does not permit withdrawal of CSF.

EPIDURAL SENSOR A sensor plate can be placed in the epidural space, but this has proved to be a relatively inaccurate measurement device and has poor reliability. Therefore, this device is rarely used.

Minimal physical activities can be performed when these devices are in place, but activities that would cause a rapid increase in ICP, such as isometric exercises and the Valsalva maneuver, should be avoided. The patient should be positioned to avoid neck flexion, hip flexion greater than 90 degrees, and

lying in a prone position. The patient's head should not be lowered more than 15 degrees below horizontal. As with other devices that use plastic tubing, care must be taken to avoid disruption, disconnection, or occlusion of the tube.

Central Venous Pressure Catheter The CVP catheter is a plastic intravenous tube used to measure pressures in the right atrium or the superior vena cava. It measures the pressure associated with the filling of the right ventricle (i.e., the diastolic pressure). Such measurement is imprecise and may be misleading regarding the function of the right ventricle. Precautions similar to those expressed previously for other catheters also apply when a CVP line is in place. Potential complications are similar to those listed for the PAC.

Arterial Line (A Line) The A line is a catheter that is inserted into an artery, typically the radial, dorsal pedal, axillary, brachial, or femoral artery. The A line is used to continuously measure blood pressure or to obtain blood samples without repeated needle punctures, and it usually provides accurate measurements. Potential complications include sepsis, hemorrhage, development of a *fistula* or aneurysm, ischemia, or arterial necrosis.

Exercise can be performed with an A line in place, providing the precautions described previously, especially those related to disruption of the catheter, disturbance of the inserted needle, occlusion of the line, or disconnection of the line from the inserted cannula are followed (Fig 9–10).

Indwelling Right Atrial Catheter (e.g., Hickman) The right atrial catheter is inserted through the cephalic or internal jugular vein and passes through the superior vena cava into the right atrium. This device allows administration of medications, removal of blood for testing, measurement of CVP, and hyperalimentation. It can be used with patients who will receive a bone marrow transplant or who have experienced severe trauma. Some potential complications associated with this device are sepsis and blood clots.

Exercise should be performed with care, and precautions similar to those described previously for other catheters should be followed (Fig. 9–11).

REFERENCE LABORATORY VALUES

Reference laboratory values are important because they provide baseline values with which a patient's laboratory findings can be compared. Depending on his/her diagnosis, physical and mental condition, and institutional or physician guidelines or protocols, the approach to care and treatment will be adjusted for each individual. Persons with the same or

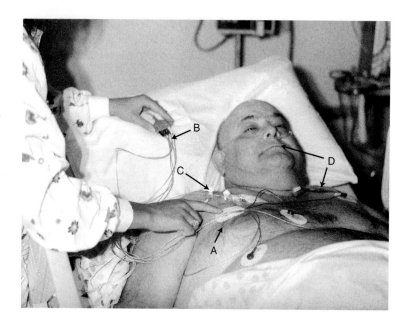

■ FIGURE 9–11
A, The nurse is pointing to one monitor lead. *B,* She holds the lead connection to the monitor. *C,* Immediately above her finger is a central line. *D,* Note the nasal cannula for supplemental oxygen.

similar diagnosis may require very different approaches to care because of differences in their physical responses to the disease, trauma, or condition that they have experienced.

Cardiac status can be determined by examination of the cardiac enzyme levels in the blood after an acute *myocardial infarction* (MI). When an MI occurs, intercellular enzymes are released into the person's blood. The enzyme creatine kinase (CK) and especially the enzyme found primarily in cardiac muscle, CK-MB, when they are present in the blood, indicate an acute MI has occurred. These increased values usually return to normal levels within 2 days after the MI. The caregiver must use caution when treating the individual, and he/she should be certain to closely observe the patient's vital signs as they appear on the cardiac monitor. The patient can receive basic care and participate in physical activities providing his/her vital signs, blood chemistry, ABGs, and physical appearance remain within acceptable ranges. Adverse responses to activity such as chest pain, fatigue, hypotension, or cardiac dysrhythmia are indicators the treatment may need to be modified, altered, or discontinued.

ABG analysis provides information about the oxygenation level of the blood. A pulse oximeter, often positioned on a fingertip or ear lobe, is used to measure the pulse rate and the percentage of oxygen saturation in the blood. Refer to Table 9–1 for ABG values and ranges.

During exercise or physical activity, a minimum of 90% saturation should be maintained to avoid hypoxemia and possible respiratory dysfunction. If supplemental oxygen is being provided for the patient, it should remain in place during the treatment. If the oxygen saturation falls below 90% and remains there, the treatment should be discontinued, and

consideration should be given to altering or modifying the treatment in the future. Changes in the individual's respiration rate or pattern may occur due to a reduced oxygen saturation level as he/she exercises. If hyperventilation occurs, the person may benefit from relaxation techniques such as abdominal-diaphragmatic or pursed lip breathing. If hypoventilation occurs, the person may benefit from deep breathing techniques and an upright, trunk-supported position.

Blood chemistry analysis provides information about an individual's red blood cell (RBC) and white blood cell (WBC) count, hemoglobin (Hgb), and hematocrit (Hct). The WBC, also known as a leukocyte, is one of the body's defense mechanisms for fighting acute or chronic disease or infection. An increased WBC count may indicate the presence of bacterial infection, leukemia, neoplasm, allergic reaction, inflammation, or tissue necrosis. A decreased WBC count may indicate bone marrow deficiency or infection with human immunodeficiency virus, or it may be due to radiation or chemotherapy treatments. A person with a decreased WBC count due to an immunosuppressed condition must be monitored carefully, and the caregiver must be certain to perform thorough hand washing, apply protective garments, and follow treatment precautions before treating him/her to reduce the possibility of cross-contamination. Depending on the diagnosis and the individual's physical condition, treatment activities may need to be modified, altered, or discontinued according to his/her response to the treatments, and frequent rest periods may be necessary.

Because they are bound to the hemoglobin contained in the cell, the RBCs transport oxygen to tissue cells throughout the body. Anemia occurs when the RBC count is decreased significantly, and polycythemia occurs when the RBC count is increased significantly. A patient with either of these conditions may participate in physical activity providing institutional and physician guidelines or protocols are followed and his/her response to the activity is monitored frequently and consistently.

The Hct is used to measure the volume percentage of packed RBCs in a sample of whole blood. The Hct is particularly important in the diagnosis of polycythemia or anemia. Persons with anemia will not tolerate vigorous physical activity, and their vital signs should be monitored frequently and consistently.

The Hgb is the protein contained in the RBC that transports oxygen in the blood; it is frequently referred to as oxyhemoglobin. Anemia, trauma, surgery, or dietary iron deficiency may cause a decrease in the Hgb. A person with a low Hgb will have a reduced tolerance to physical activity and will require frequent rest periods. Persons whose Hgb is less than 8 g/dl should not receive or participate in treatment requiring physical activity.

The caregiver who provides treatment in an ICU (or CCU) should become familiar with the reference values of various laboratory tests to understand the implications for treatment when abnormal values are identified. The level of activity that is appropriate or suitable for a given patient can be established by the caregiver to assist the patient to attain his/her maximal function effectively and without jeopardizing his/her recovery (Table 9–1).

FEEDING DEVICES

It may be necessary to provide nutrition for a patient who is unable to feed himself/herself independently or who is unable to chew, swallow, or ingest food.

Nasogastric (NG) Tube   The *nasogastric tube* is a plastic tube inserted through a nostril that eventually terminates in the patient's stomach. Purposes or uses of the NG tube include to (1) remove fluid or gas from the stomach and *gastrointestinal* (GI) tract, (2) evaluate digestive function and activity in the GI tract, (3) administer medications directly into the GI tract, (4) provide a means to feed the patient, (5) allow treatment to the upper portion of the GI tract, and (6) obtain gastric specimens. Some patients will complain of a sore throat or may have an increased gag reflex as a result of the tube. The patient will not be able to eat food or drink fluids through his/her mouth while the NG tube is in place. Exercise can be performed with the NG tube in place, but movement of the patient's head and neck should be avoided, especially flexion or forward bending.

Table 9–1 REFERENCE LABORATORY VALUES	
Arterial Blood Gases (ABGs)	
pH	7.35–7.45
$PaCO_2$	35–45 mm Hg
HCO_2	22–26 mEq/L
PaO_2	80–100 mm Hg
O_2Sat. (SaO_2)	95–98%

pH = acid-base status: <7.35 = acidosis; >7.45 = alkalosis
$PaCO_2$ = Partial pressure of carbon dioxide dissolved in arterial blood; influenced by pulmonary function
HCO_2 = Amount of alkaline substance dissolved in arterial blood; influenced by metabolic changes primarily
PaO_2 = Partial pressure of oxygen dissolved in arterial blood; influenced by pulmonary function
O_2 Sat. = Oxyhemoglobin saturation or percentage of oxygen carried by hemoglobin

Selected Blood Chemistry Values

Red blood cells (RBCs)	$4.6–6.2 \times 10^{12}$/L (male count)
	$4.2–5.4 \times 10^{12}$/L (female count)
White blood cells (WBCs)	$4.3–10.8 \times 10^{9}$/L (count)
Hemoglobin (Hgb)	14–18 g/dl (male)
	13–16 g/dl (female)
Hematocrit (Hct)	40–54 ml/dl (male)
	37–48 ml/dl (female)
Potassium (K^+)	3.5–5.0 mEq/L
Glucose	70–115 mg/dl
Platelet	$150–450 \times 10^{6}$/L (count)
Sodium (Na^+)	135–145 mEq/L
Serum creatinine	0.6–1.5 mg/dl (male)
	0.5–1.0 mg/dl (female)
Creatine kinase (CK)–total	25–225 μl/L
CK-MB isoenzyme (heart related)	0–5.9 ml/L
CK-MM isoenzyme (muscle related)	5–70 μl/L

Reference values may vary depending on the method used to obtain them or the source that reports them; many are gender or age dependent. The reference values, also referred to as "normal values," used for this table were obtained from the *Encyclopedia and Dictionary of Medicine, Nursing, and Allied Health, Fifth Edition*, Philadelphia, W.B. Saunders, 1992, except the creatine kinase values. Those values were obtained from *Laboratory Values in the Intensive Care Unit, Acute Care Perspectives*, The Newsletter of Acute Care/Hospital Clinical Practice Section–APTA, Winter 1995.

Gastric Tube (G Tube)   The G tube is a plastic tube that is inserted directly into the stomach through an incision in the patient's abdomen. Many of the purposes described for the NG tube also apply to the G tube.

Exercise can be performed providing the caregiver is aware of the presence of the G tube and avoids removing the tube.

Intravenous Feeding, Total Parenteral Nutrition (TPN), or Hyperalimentation Devices   Intravenous feeding techniques permit *infusion* of large amounts of nutrients that are needed to promote tissue growth. They also are a means to achieve an appropriate metabolic state in patients who are unable to, should not, or refuse to eat.

A catheter is inserted directly into the subclavian vein or sometimes into the jugular or another vein and then passed into the subclavian vein. The catheter

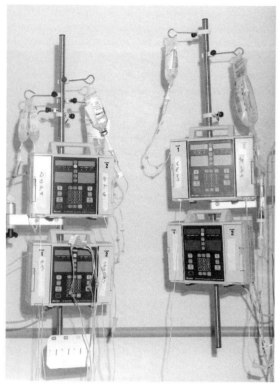

■ **FIGURE 9–12**
Multiple intravenous line systems with solutions in position for infusion.

may be connected to a semipermanently fixed cannula or sutured at the point of insertion. The caregiver should carefully observe the various connections to be certain they are secure before and after exercise. A disrupted or loose connection may result in the development of an air embolus, which could be life threatening to the patient.

Usually, the system will include an *infusion pump*, which will administer fluids and nutrients at a preselected, constant flow rate. An audible alarm will be activated if the system becomes unbalanced or when the fluid source is empty.

Exercise can be performed providing the caregiver does not disrupt, disconnect, or occlude the tubing and cause undue stress to the infusion site. Motions of the shoulder on the side of the infusion site may be restricted, especially abduction and flexion.

Intravenous (IV) Infusion Lines   IV lines are used to infuse fluids, nutrients, electrolytes, and medications; to obtain venous blood samples; and to insert catheters into the central circulatory system to monitor the physiologic condition of the patient, especially the cardiopulmonary system (Fig. 9–12).

The components of the IV system usually consist of the solution or fluid container, which may be a bottle or plastic bag; a device to measure the number of drops of fluid administered per minute; plastic tubing; a roller clamp to control the rate of the flow of

fluid; and a needle to enter the vein. Some IV systems include an infusion pump, which provides a constant, preselected fluid flow rate. Refer to Box 9–3 for a listing of commonly used IV infusion sites.

Most IV insertions are made into superficial veins. Various sizes and types of needles or catheters are used depending on the purpose of the IV therapy, infusion site, need for prolonged therapy, and site availability.

Possible complications associated with the IV administration include infiltration of fluid into the subcutaneous tissue, phlebitis, cellulitis, thrombosis, local hematoma, sepsis, pulmonary thromboembolus, air embolus, or a catheter fragment embolus. The caregiver should use caution to avoid disruption, disconnection, or occlusion of the tubing; stress to the infusion site; and interruption of circulatory flow. The infusion site should remain dry, the needle should remain secure and immobile in the vein, and no restraint should be placed above the infusion site. (For example, avoid applying a blood pressure cuff above the infusion site.) The caregiver should observe the infusion site for signs of infiltration of the fluid into the subcutaneous tissue (e.g., edema, complaint of site discomfort by the patient, reduced flow of fluid, or infection). Observe the total system to be certain it is functioning properly when you begin and when you end the treatment (Box 9–4).

Exercise can be performed, but disruption, disconnection, occlusion, or overstretching of the tubing must be avoided. If the infusion site is in the antecubital area, the elbow should not be flexed. The patient who ambulates with an IV line in place should be instructed to grasp the IV line support pole so the infusion site will be at heart level. If the extremity with the infusion site remains in a dependent position, blood flow may be affected, resulting in retrograde flow of blood into the IV line tubing. Similar procedures to maintain the infusion site in proper position should be

---

BOX 9–3

Common Intravenous Infusion Sites

Upper extremity
  Metacarpal and dorsal venous plexus of the hand
  Basilic, cephalic, and antecubital veins
Lower extremity
  Dorsal venous plexus and medial, lateral, marginal veins of the foot
  Saphenous and femoral veins
Head
  Superficial scalp veins (often selected for use with infants and the elderly)

Complications of Intravenous Therapy

Infiltration
Signs and symptoms: cool skin around the site; swelling around the site; swelling of the limb; sluggish flow rate.

Phlebitis
Signs and symptoms: pain in limb; erythema; edema with induration; streak formation.

Thrombophlebitis
Signs and symptoms: painful IV site; erythema; edema with induration; sluggish flow rate.

Air Embolism
Signs and symptoms: decrease or drop in blood pressure; weak, rapid pulse; cyanosis; loss of consciousness; increase or rise in central venous pressure.

Infection of Venipuncture Site
Signs and symptoms: swelling and soreness at the site; foul-smelling discharge.

Systemic Infection
Signs and symptoms: sudden rise in temperature and pulse rate; chills and shaking; changes in blood pressure.

Allergic Reaction
Signs and symptoms: fever; swelling or generalized edema; itching or rash; respiratory distress, especially shortness of breath.

followed when the patient is treated while in bed or on a treatment table or mat platform. Activities that require the infusion site to be elevated above the level of the heart for a prolonged period of time should be avoided so the proper direction of the flow of the IV fluid will be maintained.

Problems related to the IV system that develop as you treat the patient should be made known to nursing personnel. Unless the caregiver has been specifically instructed and trained to adjust, modify, alter, or otherwise correct the IV system, he/she should request a qualified person to correct any problems that develop during the treatment. However, simple procedures such as straightening the tubing or removing an object that is occluding the tubing should be performed by the caregiver.

URINARY CATHETERS

A urinary catheter can be applied internally (termed an "indwelling catheter") or externally. The external urinary catheter is successful only for male patients. A catheter inserted through the urethra and into the bladder is an internal catheter. A condom applied externally to the penis of a male patient with a drainage tube attached to it is an external catheter. No practical, acceptable, or effective external catheter has been developed for female patients.

A urinary catheter is used to remove urine from the bladder when the patient is unable to satisfactorily control its retention or release. This lack of control may be due to a spinal cord injury, a disease such as multiple sclerosis, or the physiologic changes associated with old age. Any form of trauma, disease, condition, or disorder that affects the neuromuscular control of the bladder sphincter may necessitate the use of a urinary catheter. The catheter may be used temporarily or for a prolonged period of time, even for the remainder of the patient's life.

Urinary catheters are used to remove urine from the bladder so it can be drained through plastic tubing into a collection bag, bottle, or urinal. Urinary catheters are used for a patient who has lost his/her voluntary control of *micturition*. Many patients require the use of a catheter, and it is not unusual for a caregiver to treat a patient with a catheter. Some common complications associated with the use of a catheter are infection of the urinary tract or bladder, development of a urethral fistula, formation of bladder calculi as a result of urinary stasis, and kidney failure. The patient with a spinal cord injury above the T6 cord level may experience autonomic hyperreflexia caused by urine retention. This condition is described in Chapter 11.

Exercises to the lower extremities can be performed by a patient with a catheter provided the caregiver avoids disruption, disconnection, stretching, or occlusion of the drainage tube. You should determine how much free tubing is available before initiating exercise to avoid causing excessive tension on the tubing or the catheter. Urine drains into the collection bag as a result of the effect of gravity; therefore, the bag should not be positioned above the level of the bladder for more than a few minutes. The bag should not be placed in the patient's lap when he/she is transported by wheelchair or on the lower abdomen when he/she is lying on a wheeled stretcher. Furthermore, the bag and tubing should be positioned and secured to minimize the possibility that the bag or the tubing will be pulled or snagged, and thus it is positioned below the level of the bladder when the patient is being transported. When the patient ambulates, the bag should be positioned and maintained below the level of the bladder so it will not interfere with gait or ambulation activities.

It may be difficult to provide an adequate position to promote drainage when the patient receives hydrotherapy in an immersion tank or sit-in whirlpool. In such cases, the bag can be positioned below the level of the bladder, but the tubing will probably have to be elevated over the edge of the tank or whirlpool before it can be directed downward to the bag. This position of the tubing may prevent urine from draining because it will have to drain upward, or against the force of gravity. You should drain any urine in the tubing into the bag before the patient is placed in the water to assist with the future drainage. The bag must not be immersed in the water. At some institutions, treatment protocols may permit clamping of the tubing or catheter before the patient is immersed so the bag can be removed for the length of the treatment. However, the flow of urine should not be occluded for an extended period of time and should not be occluded frequently to avoid the complications associated with the stasis of urine in the bladder.

The caregiver should observe the color of the urine and be alert for unusual odors associated with the urine or the urinary system. Foul-smelling urine; cloudy, dark urine; or urine with blood in it (hematuria) should be reported to a physician or nurse. You should also observe the flow and amount of urine in the bag. Any reduced flow or decreased production of urine should be reported. The caregiver should document and verbally report his/her observations of abnormal urine appearance or production promptly so that proper treatment can be initiated.

Infection can be a major complication for the person who uses a catheter, particularly if it is an indwelling catheter. All personnel who are involved with the patient should maintain cleanliness when treatment is provided. Precautions must be used when replacing any tubing that has been disengaged from the catheter or the collection bag, when replacing the bag, and when the catheter is inserted into the bladder. Many times it is safer to allow nursing personnel to replace or reconnect the tubing rather than reconnecting it with improper technique. Treatment settings that routinely treat patients with catheters have specific protocols for the care of the tubing and collection bag and the insertion and removal of the catheter. It is very important that infection be prevented from developing in the urinary system. Therefore, strict adherence to the principles of medical and surgical asepsis are necessary by all personnel.

Foley Catheter The Foley type of indwelling catheter is held in place in the bladder by a small balloon that is inflated with air, water, or sterile saline solution. The catheter has two or three tubes or channels in it. The main channel allows the urine to drain, and the other channels are used to inflate the balloon and irrigate the bladder. To remove the catheter, the balloon is deflated, and the catheter is withdrawn.

External Catheter The external catheter (condom) is applied over the shaft of the penis and is held in place by an adhesive applied to the skin or by a padded strap or tape encircling the proximal shaft of the penis. *Caution:* The tape or strap must not be applied too tightly to avoid occlusion of the urethra or the blood supply of the penis.

Suprapubic Catheter Another type of urinary catheter that may be encountered is a *suprapubic* catheter. This catheter is inserted directly into the bladder through incisions in the lower abdomen and the bladder. The catheter may be held in place by adhesive tape, but care should be used to avoid its removal.

OXYGEN THERAPY SYSTEMS

Oxygen delivery may be required for a variety of conditions, including after surgery, respiratory diseases, after myocardial infarction and other cardiac problems, or inadequate lung function. The purpose of oxygen therapy is to provide and maintain an adequate amount of oxygen in the patient's blood in response to the patient's needs when the patient is unable to provide an adequate amount independently. There are several devices or modes that can be used to deliver the oxygen, and the selection of the specific device will depend on the patient's condition or illness and his/her functional respiratory capabilities. Regardless of how it is delivered, the oxygen should be humidified to reduce its drying effect on the respiratory mucous membranes.

MODES OF DELIVERY

Nasal Cannula The nasal cannula has two plastic prongs (or points or tips) that are inserted into the patient's nostrils. The points are joined by a plastic connector that rests below the nose on the patient's upper lip. This mode is used most frequently for patients who require low to moderate concentrations of oxygen.

Oronasal Mask The oronasal mask is a triangular plastic device with small vent holes in it for exhaled air; it covers the patient's nose and mouth. It is used for short periods of time when moderate concentrations of oxygen are desired, such as to begin to wean a postsurgical patient from long-term therapy or higher concentrations of oxygen, or as a temporary approach until a decision is made regarding a permanent form of oxygen delivery.

Nasal Catheter A catheter can be inserted through the nasal passage to the nasopharyngeal junction, which is located just below the level of the soft palate. The uses of this catheter are similar to those described for the nasal cannula.

Tent   Occasionally a tentlike device that encloses the patient's trunk and head may be used, especially if the patient is restless, uncooperative, or extremely ill. The edges of the tent must be sealed to prevent the loss of oxygen; this may require frequent and repeated monitoring of the system by nursing personnel.

Tracheostomy Mask or Catheter   Some patients may have a temporary or permanent tracheostomy through which oxygen can be administered by a mask placed over the stoma or by a catheter inserted into the stoma.

In the hospital setting, oxygen is obtained from a wall unit when the patient is in bed or from an oxygen cylinder that accompanies the patient when he/she is out of the room. The oxygen in the cylinder, or tank, is compressed or pressurized, and there is a regulator on the tank to control the administration of the oxygen to the patient. The rate of flow, in liters per minute, will be determined by a physician and is delivered and maintained by proper adjustment of the regulator valve.

Caution: Oxygen supports combustion, so care must be used to prevent a fire or explosion. Excessive heat, such as a flame, spark, radiator, or even high room temperature, must be avoided. When not in use, the cylinder should be stored in a temperate, dry, and well-ventilated area and should be handled with care to avoid damage to the regulator or to the cylinder itself to prevent rapid release of the compressed gas. Cylinders should be transported on a wheeled carrier or on a wheeled pushcart for larger cylinders. Care should be used to avoid dropping or tipping the tank onto the floor to prevent damage to the tank or the control device. When a patient who is receiving oxygen therapy ambulates, the cylinder should accompany the patient in a wheeled carrier or should be carried by another person.

Precautions to be considered when treating the patient who is receiving oxygen include avoiding disruption, disconnection, or occlusion of the tubing; maintaining the prescribed flow rate; and maintaining a free flow of oxygen. In addition, you should be alert for signs or symptoms of respiratory distress exhibited by the patient. If the patient complains of dyspnea or shortness of breath or cramping in the calf muscles or exhibits cyanosis of the nail beds or lips, he/she may be experiencing respiratory or circulatory distress. Exercise or physical activity should cease, the oxygen delivery system should be evaluated for improper function, and qualified personnel may need to be contacted for assistance. The patient may obtain symptomatic relief by standing and partially flexing the trunk, using the upper extremities placed on a firm object for support. Do not place the patient supine; instead, allow him/her to lean forward slightly if he/she is seated. He/she

may rest with the forearms on the thighs, on the chair armrests, or on a firm table to relieve his/her symptoms. The prescribed flow rate *must not* be altered when the patient performs exercise. Complications can develop if the patient receives an overdose of oxygen. Careful monitoring of the patient's response to the exercise or activity must be performed to avoid or quickly identify an adverse response and to provide appropriate emergency care.

CHEST DRAINAGE SYSTEMS

Chest drainage tubes may be used to remove air, blood, purulent matter, or other undesirable material from the patient's chest or pleural cavity. These tubes are inserted through an incision in the chest and may be connected to a mechanical or gravity-based suction system. There are three types of chest tube bottle systems, and these use one, two, or three bottles. The one- and two-bottle systems function by gravity, whereas the three-bottle system and the commercially available disposable systems use a pump to create suction.

The chest tubes will be inserted in different locations depending on the type of drainage desired. Tubes that are placed in the anterior or lateral chest wall promote the removal of air (e.g., to treat a *pneumothorax*), tubes placed inferiorly and posteriorly promote the removal of fluids and blood, and a *mediastinal* tube is used to drain blood and fluid, which may be necessary after open chest or heart surgery. The drainage tubes usually will be maintained securely in place with adherent dressings, but care should be used to avoid pulling on them or the connecting tubing. Additional precautions are avoiding disruption, disconnection, or occlusion of the tubing; observing the color of the drainage; observing the system for proper function; and monitoring the patient's response to exercise or activity. For the patient who ambulates, the collection bottles should be kept below the level of the location of the inserted tube (Fig. 9–13).

OSTOMY DEVICES

An ostomy is a surgically produced opening to allow the elimination of urine or feces. More specifically, an enterostomy is the result of a surgical procedure that produces an artificial stoma into the small intestine through an incision in the abdominal wall. The ileostomy and colostomy are types of enterostomy. The stoma is covered with a plastic bag or pouch to collect waste. Most patients will find it necessary to have the collection bag in place at all times, particularly if the waste is more liquid than solid. The location of the os-

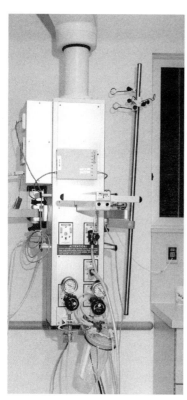

■ **FIGURE 9–13**
Suction equipment.

tomy will affect the need for and the extent to which the patient will use the collection bag or pouch.

There are three primary types of collecting devices for the patient with an ostomy; they are designated by the way they are attached to the patient. The bag may be a two-piece pouch that attaches to a skin barrier that adheres to the patient's skin with an adhesive; a one-piece pouch attached to a skin barrier; or an adhesive-backed pouch that adheres to a separate skin barrier. The pouch may be disposable or reusable. Components of the system include an odor-proof plastic pouch, a skin barrier, a filter for gas release, and a means to attach the pouch to the skin barrier or the skin barrier to the skin, such as an adhesive seal or belt tabs.

The caregiver should be aware that the patient has an ostomy, and excessive stress to the attachment of the pouch should be avoided during treatment. Most patients can be treated with minimal concern for the development of complications or the need to restrict exercise or activity. The patient with a recent ostomy may be sensitive to and concerned about whether the system will function properly. The caregiver should avoid activities that may cause the patient to experience a socially embarrassing event (e.g., leakage of waste or intestinal gas). Usually, it is desirable to schedule the patient's treatment after the pouch has been emptied or to coordinate it with the patient's bowel habits.

TRACTION

Traction applied to an extremity can be used to align fracture segments, distend soft tissue, reduce muscle spasm or contractures, and immobilize the patient. It may be applied to the skin or to a skeletal structure, and it may be applied constantly or intermittently. Skin traction must be applied with low weights because of the intolerance of the skin and soft tissue to excessive force. Skeletal traction is applied through a pin or wire inserted into bone to which traction ropes and weights are attached. Skeletal traction is used to position, immobilize, and align fracture segments to promote their proper healing.

TYPES OF SKELETAL TRACTION

Balanced Suspension Traction Balanced suspension traction is used primarily to treat displaced or *comminuted* femoral fractures. A splint under the femur (Thomas splint) and one under the leg (Pearson attachment) are used to balance and suspend the extremity. A pin or wire such as a Kirschner wire or Steinmann pin is inserted through the tibia to provide traction to the distal femoral segment. Because of this arrangement, the traction will remain "balanced" even when the patient moves in bed. Exercises can be performed to the noninjured extremities, and ankle movements can be performed on the injured extremity. This type of traction requires prolonged immobilization of the patient, which can lead to secondary complications such as contractures, pressure sores, and sepsis. The more recent use of internal or external fixation devices has reduced the need for this type of traction and enhanced the functional recovery of the patient.

Skull Traction Skull traction is applied by tongs (Crutchfield, Gardner-Wells, Vinke, or Barton tongs) positioned into small holes drilled in the outer layer of the patient's skull. The traction is applied through a rope–weight arrangement and is used for patients with a fracture or dislocation of one or more cervical vertebrae.

Exercise of the extremities can be performed, but care should be used when movement of the shoulder is attempted or when the muscles that attach to the cervical vertebrae are contracted to avoid stress to the fracture site and to the corresponding nerve roots of that area.

Precautions to be aware of when treating the patient who has skeletal traction are to (1) be certain the traction weights hang freely after the patient has been repositioned; (2) avoid removal or release of any traction weight during treatment; (3) avoid bumping the weights, as that will create motion through the rope to

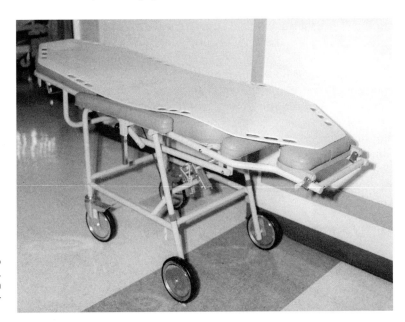

■ FIGURE 9–14
The flexible plastic item on the gurney is used to transfer a supine patient to or from a bed or gurney. It is positioned under the patient so the patient can be transferred by sliding the plastic from one surface to the other.

the fracture site; and (4) note the condition of the site of the pin. Look for bleeding, skin disruption, drainage, or signs of inflammation at the site of the pin insertion. Any unusual observations should be documented and reported promptly.

External Fixation External fixation is a form of stabilization and traction that uses a variety of frames applied externally to the patient's extremity (e.g., Haynes, Hoffmann, halo, or Anderson devices). These frames hold pins that have been inserted into the bone fragments of a severe fracture to maintain the fracture in alignment. This form of fixation allows earlier and greater mobility for the patient while providing excellent alignment and stabilization of the fracture segments. Ambulation on both lower extremities and exercise of the noninjured extremities or areas of the body can be performed, although weight bearing on the involved extremity may be contraindicated or limited. This form of fixation is particularly beneficial for a comminuted, an extensive open, or an infected open fracture or when bone grafts are involved. Be careful to avoid excess stress to the exposed frame and pins, and observe the pin sites for evidence of adverse reactions to the pins (e.g., infection, bone deterioration).

Internal Fixation This method of treatment uses hardware applied to or within bone to maintain its alignment and stability following fracture reduction. The hardware includes transfixation screws, bone plates, wires, nails, and intramedullary rods. The technique usually provides a shorter period of immobilization, stable fracture site, maintenance of local circulation, and more rapid return to functional activities.

Depending on the location and type of fracture, the hardware used to fixate the fracture, and the patient's general condition, the treatment procedures se-

lected will vary. Early active or passive mobilization of the joints proximal and distal to the fracture should be initiated. Isometric exercise of the muscles that cross the fracture and that are immobilized (e.g., in a cast) can be done to maintain muscle tone, local circulation, and muscle awareness. Active and active resistive exercise for the muscles and joints of the noninvolved extremities should be performed to maintain or improve range-of-motion and strength.

Ambulation following fracture in a lower extremity can usually be performed within a few days after the fracture has been reduced and fixated. The amount or type of weight bearing depends on the location of the fracture, the type of fixation device, the general condition of the patient, and the desires of the surgeon.

Caution may be necessary to protect the fracture site and soft tissue incision, if an open reduction was performed, until healing occurs. The surgical open reduction of the fracture has the potential for wound infection, which is a disadvantage of this procedure (Fig. 9–14).

PATIENT-CONTROLLED ANALGESIA (PCA)

The patient-controlled analgesia system allows the patient to self-administer a small predetermined dose of pain medication intravenously on demand, as frequently as every 6 minutes. A reservoir of the medication is connected by tubing to an IV line and to a small control module or pump, which the patient wears on his/her wrist. When medication is desired, the patient presses a button on the control module; the medication moves to a small area in the control module and then passes through tubing into the IV line. The unit will not deliver more medication than the premeasured dose each time the patient activates the button. In addition, the patient cannot receive the medication more frequently than every 6 minutes. The number of requests the patient has made and the number of doses the unit has delivered are recorded by the unit and are available for review. This device should not interfere with the patient's exercise program or other activities. However, the precautions outlined for IV lines should be followed.

DIALYSIS THERAPY

Dialysis is used for patients who experience acute or chronic renal failure. The objectives of dialysis are to prevent infection, restore the normal level of fluids and electrolytes, control the acid-base balance, remove waste and toxic material, and assist in or replace normal renal function. Dialysis can be performed through a peritoneal tube, which is inserted through an abdominal incision, or through a prosthetic *shunt* implanted in the patient's forearm.

Exercise and activity can be performed safely, but excessive activity involving the area of the shunt and application of any occlusive item, such as a blood pressure cuff, or restraint to the upper arm of the extremity containing the shunt, should be avoided. Care should be taken to avoid pulling on the peritoneal tube or the tubing attached to it and to avoid occluding the drainage tubing.

SUMMARY

Many times it is necessary to treat a patient who is very ill or whose condition requires highly specialized care or the use of a variety of devices and equipment to maintain his/her life. These patients should be treated with caution and frequent monitoring. A patient who uses any of the devices, systems, or procedures described in this chapter should be evaluated and his/her response to treatment should be documented at the conclusion of each treatment session. Any complications or problems encountered or any deviations from the expected treatment results should be noted. Serious or unusual adverse patient responses to treatment should be discussed directly with an appropriate person such as a physician or nurse. Remember that many of these patients are acutely ill and probably will not tolerate exercise or physical activity as easily as less ill patients would. You are encouraged to proceed carefully by maintaining the program within the functional and physiologic capacities of each patient.

■ SELF-STUDY/DISCUSSION ACTIVITIES

1. Describe how you might alter or modify your treatment plan and program to accommodate the types of patient conditions presented in this chapter.

2. Explain the immediate and long-term actions you would perform if the patient exhibited adverse responses to the treatment he/she received.

3. Define the following: IV line, SICU, CCU, A line, NG tube, skeletal traction, external fixation, TPN or hyperalimentation, and ventilator. (Select other acronyms or terms and define them also.)

4. Outline the components you believe should be included in a program designed to orient or familiarize a therapist with the equipment, environment, and patient therapy devices that are apt to be encountered in an ICU.

Chapter 10

Approaches to Infection Control and Wound Care

After studying this chapter, the reader will be able to:

1. Define asepsis, medical asepsis, surgical asepsis, and contamination.

2. Describe and perform proper techniques of hand washing for clean and sterile situations.

3. Describe and perform the proper application and removal of protective garments for clean and sterile (e.g., strict isolation, respiratory isolation, and protective isolation) situations.

4. Describe and demonstrate how to establish and maintain a sterile field.

5. Describe the functions of a dressing and a bandage.

6. Describe and demonstrate the proper application and removal of a dressing.

7. Describe and demonstrate the proper application and removal of a bandage that is used to cover a dressing.

8. Explain the concept, use, and value of universal precautions.

9. Describe the principles and function associated with graduated compression garments and how to measure an upper and lower extremity for a garment.

■ ■ ■ KEY TERMS

AIDS: Acronym for acquired immune deficiency syndrome, which is caused by the human immunodeficiency virus (HIV).

Asepsis: Absence of microorganisms that produce disease; the prevention of infection by maintaining a sterile condition.

Autolysis: The disintegration of cells or tissues by the enzymes of the body or cellular components in wound fluid.

Contamination: When something is rendered unclean or unsterile; an item, surface, or field is considered to be contaminated whenever it has come in contact with anything that is not sterile.

Debridement: The removal of devitalized tissues from or adjacent to a traumatic or infected lesion to expose healthy tissue.

Decontamination: The use of physical or chemical means to remove, inactivate, or destroy bloodborne pathogens on a surface or item to the point where they are no longer capable of transmitting infectious particles and the surface or item is rendered safe for handling, use, or disposal.

Disinfection: The destruction or removal of pathogenic organisms but not necessarily their spores.

Epithelialization: Healing by the growth of epithelium over a denuded surface.

Erythema: Redness of the skin caused by congestion of the capillaries in the lower layers of the skin.

Eschar: A dry scab; devitalized tissue.

Exudate: A fluid with a high composition of protein and cellular debris that has escaped from blood vessels and is deposited in tissues or on tissue surfaces.

Granulation: Any granular material on the surface of a tissue, membrane, or organ.

Hepatitis: Inflammation of the liver.

Induration: The quality of being hard; abnormal firmness of tissue with a definite margin.

Infection: The production of a disease or harmful condition by the entrance of disease-producing germs into an organism.

Isolation: Separation from others.

Maceration: The softening of a solid or tissue by soaking.

Medical asepsis: Practices that help to reduce the number and spread of microorganisms.

Microorganism: A tiny living animal or plant that can cause disease.

Necrosis: The morphological changes indicative of cell death.

Nosocomial: Pertaining to or originating in a hospital.

Pathogen: A microorganism that produces disease.

Sepsis: The presence of pathogenic microorganisms or their toxins in the blood or tissues.

Slough: A mass of dead tissue in, or cast out from, living tissue.

Spore: A hard, thick-walled capsule formed by some bacteria that contains only the essential parts of the protoplasm of the bacterial cell.

Sterile: Containing no microorganisms; free from germs.

Sterilization: A process by which all microorganisms, including spores, are destroyed.

Surgical asepsis: Practices that render and keep objects and areas free of all microorganisms.

Ulcer: A local defect or excavation of the surface of an organ or tissue produced by sloughing of necrotic inflammatory tissue.

Wound: A bodily injury caused by physical means, with disruption of the normal continuity of structures.

INTRODUCTION

The caregiver may be required to interact with patients who require care of open wounds or whose condition requires the use of medical or surgical aseptic techniques. You must remember that *microorganisms* are present on the skin, in the air, in patient *wounds,* and throughout the environment. Be aware of the process of *contamination* and *infection* so you, the patient, and other persons or objects can be protected from pathogenic microorganisms. This protection can be enhanced by the interruption of the cycle of infection.

Microorganisms move or are "communicated" or transmitted from place to place by various means, and they are part of a cycle. When this cycle is interrupted, the microorganism cannot grow, spread, and cause disease. This cyclic process includes a place where the microorganisms can grow and reproduce (i.e., a host or reservoir). Examples of hosts are animals and human beings.

The microorganisms require a means by which they can leave the host (i.e., exit the reservoir). Examples are a person's nose, mouth, throat, ear, eye, intestinal tract, urinary tract, multiple body fluids (especially blood), and wounds. Transmission of microorganisms from one person to another (i.e., a vehicle of transmission) is necessary to spread the infection. Examples are the air, droplets of water (by a cough or

Cycle of Cross-Contamination and Infection

1. Reservoir for organism/host:
   Person with staphylococcal infection

   ↓

2. Method of exit for the organism:
   Draining wound

   ↓

3. Method of transmission of the organism:
   Soiled dressings, exudate from the wound, soiled linen

   ↓

4. Method of entry of the organism into a new host:
   Cut, abrasion, cuticle tear, or any break in the skin

   ↓

5. Susceptible host:
   Person with low or limited systemic resistance to the organism

   ↓

6. Infection develops in new host

Barriers to interrupt the cycle include proper disposal of dressings and linen and use of universal precautions, protective clothing, gloves, and proper hand-washing techniques.

sneeze), hands, equipment or mat pads, instruments (needles, scalpels, thermometers), eating utensils, linens, and body fluids such as blood, semen, saliva, and vaginal secretions.

To infect another person, the microorganism must be able to enter that person (i.e., it must have a portal of entry). Examples of such portals are a break in the person's skin barrier; mucous membranes, mouth, nose, and ears; and the genitourinary tract. Finally, the person who receives the microorganisms must be susceptible to them (i.e., a susceptible host). An example of a susceptible host is a person whose body systems cannot destroy, repel, remove, or ward off the microorganisms (Box 10–1).

Some microorganisms are more difficult to destroy than others, and medications (i.e., antibiotics) designed to kill or reduce the number of microorganisms are necessary to augment the protective actions of the body's systems. Some pathogens are totally resistant to medications or actions taken to reduce their numbers or prevent their growth. For example, to date, no effective treatment (medication or vaccine) has been found to destroy or effectively reduce the human immunodeficiency virus (HIV) associated with *acquired immune deficiency syndrome* (AIDS).

Most microorganisms grow or proliferate best in a dark, warm, moist environment, and they are less likely to grow when they are exposed to a light, cool, dry, or extremely hot environment. Therefore, steam, gas, ultraviolet rays, and dry heat are frequently used to sterilize contaminated objects. Some microorganisms require oxygen to support their growth, whereas others do not; some produce cells that are called *spores*. Because of the thick, hard walls of the spore that protects the cell, spores are very difficult to destroy, especially when they are located deep in a wound.

The caregiver has the responsibility to interrupt or establish barriers to the infection cycle at any stage of the process. Some barriers to infection are the use of proper hand-washing techniques, the wearing of gloves and other protective clothing, the proper removal and disposal of a contaminated dressing or bandage, and being aware of *isolation* techniques. In most instances it will not be possible nor will the objective be to completely eliminate all *pathogens* from an area or object. The purpose of *medical asepsis* is to reduce the number of pathogens in an area so their concentration, influence, or capacity to create an infection is reduced by a person's immune system or by the use of medications designed to kill the remaining pathogenic microorganisms.

PRINCIPLES AND CONCEPTS

A caregiver may become involved in the management of wounds, with patients who have a transmissible infection, or with patients who must be protected from the environment to avoid becoming infected. Therefore, he/she must understand how to protect the patient, other persons, and himself/herself from becoming contaminated or infected.

There are two types of isolation used; these rely on the concepts of medical and *surgical asepsis*. The primary purpose of each technique is to protect persons or objects from becoming contaminated or infected by pathogenic microorganisms. It is important that the caregiver understand the difference between the two techniques so he/she can deliver quality care and safely apply therapeutic procedures or activities.

Techniques of medical asepsis are designed to keep pathogens confined to a specific area, object, or person. Medical asepsis may involve isolation of a patient to protect health care workers, other patients, and other persons from the pathogenic microorganisms associated with the patient. For example, patients with tuberculosis, *hepatitis*, a staphylococcal or streptococcal infection, or another communicable or transmissible disease may be isolated in a private room. Specific care must be taken by persons who have contact with the patient—including contact with his/her soiled dressings or articles of clothing—to reduce the possibility of becoming infected. The use of protective clothing by the caregiver will be necessary to protect the caregiver from the patient. Extreme care must be used when you remove protective clothing after treating a patient who is in isolation to reduce cross-contamination from the patient. This is referred to as a "clean approach."

Pathogens can be transmitted by coughing and sneezing and through body fluids such as tears, perspiration, urine, blood, semen, vaginal secretions, mucus, vomitus, and feces. The body has several means to provide barriers to pathogens or to rid the body of them. The primary barrier is the skin when it is intact. The skin is relatively impermeable to the absorption of external substances and to the loss of many body fluids. Cilia in the respiratory tract assist in filtering and trapping microorganisms to prevent them from entering deeply into the body. When these natural barriers are disrupted, protection is reduced and the possibility of becoming infected is increased. Therefore, when treating someone who has an infection or who is more apt to become infected, it is imperative to establish barriers other than the body's natural ones.

In the treatment area, general cleanliness of equipment, floors, and restrooms and proper control of heat, light, and air are important considerations. Proper disposal of soiled linen, gowns, protective garments (gloves, caps, and masks), dressing material, bandages, and other disposable items also is important. The use of appropriate techniques to maintain at least medical asepsis should be followed, especially hand-washing activities. Each employee should understand and adhere to practices and procedures that can be used to protect a specific patient, other patients, other persons such as visitors or employees, and the employee from infection or contamination.

HAND-WASHING TECHNIQUES

Before and after providing patient care, WASH YOUR HANDS. This relatively simple activity is the most effective means to reduce cross-contamination

and the spread of many pathogens from one person to another. Hand washing must become a habit for every health care worker for his/her protection and the protection of others, especially the patient.

Remember that faucet handles, towel dispensers, soap bars, and the edges and basins of sinks are all considered contaminated. Avoid touching any of these items with your hands during the hand-washing process; liquid soap that can be obtained from a hand- or foot-operated dispenser is recommended. In addition, water that splashes from the sink will contaminate your clothing. Jewelry, especially rings and bracelets, with stones or indentations should be removed before washing your hands and should not be replaced until treatment has been completed. These items can harbor pathogens and cannot be cleaned satisfactorily with soap and water. Your hands will have the greatest protection from cross-contamination if access to the faucet and the water temperature controls can be accomplished with leg or foot controls. When it is necessary to use your hands to turn the water supply on and off, use a dry paper towel as a barrier between your hand and the faucet handle.

When liquid soap is used and is dispensed by a foot control or contained in an individual, one-time-use brush, greater protection against cross-contamination will be provided. Using a bar of soap that has been used by other persons increases the possibility of cross-contamination and should be avoided whenever possible. A suggested solution to this situation is to substitute liquid soap dispensers for bar soap. If these dispensers are operated by hand, the area you touch to release the soap or detergent should be considered contaminated. For self-protection, use a dry towel to operate the dispenser.

Be certain to properly care for your hands by washing them with water that is warm, not hot or cold. Dry your hands completely after each washing, apply a skin moisturizer occasionally during the day, and be cautious when you have torn cuticles, skin irritations, and other skin lesions.

Hand washing is used to remove or reduce the number of pathogenic microorganisms on the skin of your hands, wrists, and forearms. Many of these microorganisms may not be troublesome or dangerous to the person with an intact and fully functioning immune system and whose other barriers to infection function normally. However, these same microorganisms may produce an infection in a patient when they enter a wound, when the patient's immune system has been disrupted, or when the patient's condition is a debilitating one. The caregiver may transmit pathogenic microorganisms obtained from one patient to another patient with his/her hands, causing an infection to develop in the second patient. This is one example of how a *nosocomial* infection can be transmitted. Other methods include soiled linen or clothing; air movement or circulation; improperly cleansed eating utensils, instruments, or equipment; and through moisture droplets.

Friction is a very important component of hand washing and is used to cleanse the creases and wrinkles of the fingers and loosen soil and pathogens that have collected on the skin. The use of a brush to cleanse the wrinkles and creases of your knuckles is recommended before treating a patient who is highly susceptible to infection and as a part of surgical asepsis.

Various types of soap or detergent may be used as a cleanser. In some settings an antimicrobial or germicidal agent may be added to the cleansing medium, but these additives may produce an allergic skin reaction on some people's hands. The lather that is produced by the cleansing medium helps to lift the soil and microorganisms from the skin and hold them in the lather so they will be removed when you rinse your hands.

The principle regarding hand washing is to wash your hands before and immediately after treatment of a patient. The more likely it is that the patient is contaminated or has an infection, the more important it is that you wash your hands before and after providing treatment. When you are required to expose a wound or change a dressing, you should apply gloves after you wash your hands and then wash your hands after the gloves are removed. You should also avoid placing your fingers in your nose, eyes, ears, or mouth after patient care, and it is also important that you perform hand washing after toileting.

There are several techniques that can be used to wash your hands. Regardless of the method you use, it is important to cleanse your hands thoroughly and frequently (Procedures 10–1 and 10–2). *Caution:* Avoid touching any potentially contaminated surface during or at the conclusion of the hand-washing process. If gloves or other protective clothing is to be applied, it should be applied at this time.

ISOLATION SYSTEMS

Two primary isolation systems have been described in the literature: System A, category-specific isolation precautions; and System B, disease-specific isolation precautions. These systems rely on the concepts and principles associated with medical and surgical asepsis to protect a person or object from becoming contaminated or infected by transmissible pathogens.

Generally a patient may be isolated from other patients and the hospital environment because he/she has a transmissible disease. Therefore, the patient is isolated by being placed in a room either alone or with one or more patients with the same disease to reduce the opportunity for the disease or infection to be transmitted to others. When a patient is placed in isolation, a variety of methods or techniques, designed to reduce or prevent the transmission of the disease or infection, will have to be followed by any person who enters the patient's environment. These methods and techniques will include, at the very least, judicious hand washing before and after contact with the patient. In addition, other barriers to transmission, such as wearing a cap, mask, gown, or gloves, will be required before the person enters the patient's room. The type, amount, and sequence of application of the garments needed to be worn will depend on the type of disease or infection, its mode of transmission, and the amount of contact the person has with the patient.

P R O C E D U R E 1 0 – 1
Hand Washing for Medical Asepsis

1. Remove all jewelry (an exception may be made for a smooth, band-type ring); approach the wash area, but avoid touching the sink and other nearby objects with your clothing or hands.
2. Turn on the water and mix it to a warm temperature to allow the soap to lather easily and to cause the least harm to your skin.
3. Wet your wrists and hands with your fingers directed downward, but do not touch the sink rim or basin.
4. Apply the soap and begin to wash your hands using friction and rotatory or rubbing motions (Fig. 10–1A,B).

continued

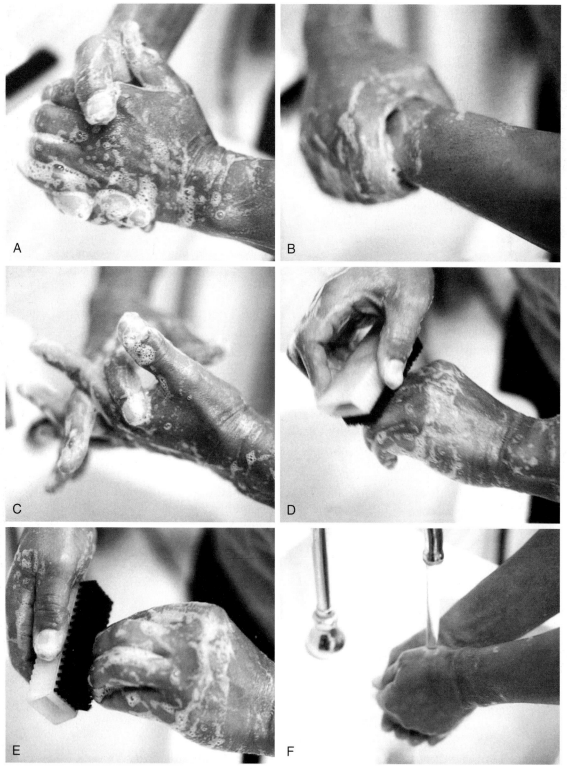

■ **FIGURE 10–1**
Hand washing for medical asepsis.

PROCEDURE 10–1, *continued*

5. Wash for at least 30 seconds; wash longer if you have treated a patient known to have an infection.
   a. Wash the palm and dorsum of each hand at least 10 seconds each, using friction and rotary motions.
   b. Interlace your fingers and wash between them for at least 10 seconds, being certain to wash the web or interspace between each finger (see Fig. 10–1C).
   c. Use a soft brush to wash the creases of each finger and its cuticle and under the fingernails; or you may use a pointed, disposable wood probe ("orange stick") to clean under each fingernail, discarding the probe after use (see Fig. 10–1D,E).
   d. Wash your wrist and the lower 2 to 3 inches of your distal forearm using friction and rotary motions.

6. Rinse your hands from the wrist to the fingers with the fingers directed downward, but do not rinse the area of skin proximal to where it was washed. If you have just treated a patient or removed a dressing from a patient with a known infection, wash your wrist and lower forearm again for 30 seconds and rinse as described previously; repeat steps 4 through 7 for a total of approximately 60 seconds, and do a final rinse as described previously (see Fig. 10–1F).

7. Dry your hands thoroughly with a disposable towel. (The towel may be paper or cloth but must be disposed of after use.) The water should continue to flow from the tap as you dry your hands. Use a dry paper or cloth towel to turn off a hand-operated faucet, and then discard all towels in an appropriate container.

P R O C E D U R E   1 0 – 2
Hand Washing for Surgical Asepsis

1. Remove all jewelry from your hands, neck, and ears, and approach the wash area with your arms exposed to approximately 3 inches above the elbow. Avoid touching the sink and other nearby objects with your clothing or hands.

2. Turn on the water and mix it to a warm temperature; follow the directions given previously for turning on the water if the faucet is hand operated.

3. Wet your hands and apply the soap or detergent according to the previous directions.

4. Wash your hands as outlined for medical asepsis, except you will have to wash your entire forearm to approximately 3 inches above your elbow. This process will require approximately 7 minutes (Fig. 10–2A).

5. Rinse your hands by holding them with your fingers upward so that the rinse water flows from a clean to an unclean area (i.e., from your fingers to your elbows). Do not allow your hands, forearms, or upper arms to contact the sink or your body (see Fig. 10–2B).

6. Clean your fingernails, cuticles, and skin creases with a brush using vigorous strokes; you may use a pointed, disposable wood probe ("orange stick") to clean under each fingernail, discarding the probe after use.

continued

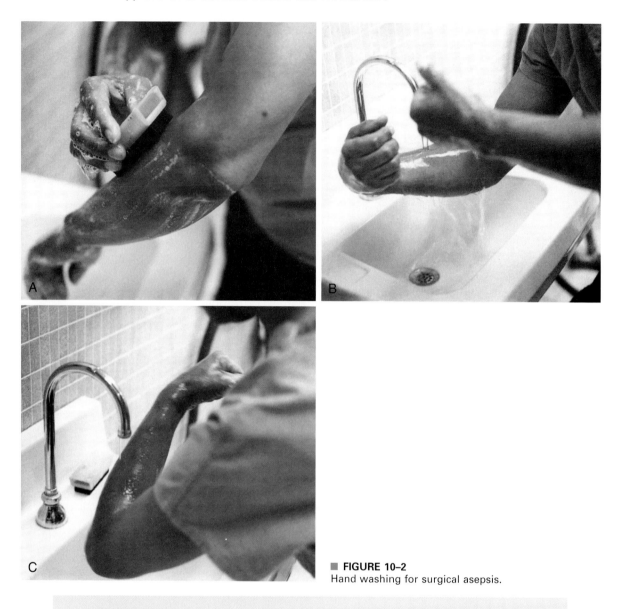

■ **FIGURE 10–2**
Hand washing for surgical asepsis.

PROCEDURE 10-2, *continued*

7. Perform a final rinse with your hands directed upward (see Fig. 10–2*C*).

8. Dry your hands, forearms, and distal upper arms thoroughly using a sterile towel or air dryer. Avoid contact between the towel and your clothing and between your washed skin and your clothing or other nonsterile areas. Wrap your hands and forearms in a dry, sterile towel prior to applying protective clothing or gloves; hold your hands above waist level and slightly away from your body until you initiate your treatment or patient care activities.

The following seven isolation categories can be designated in the category-specific isolation system:

Strict isolation

Contact isolation

Respiratory isolation

Tuberculosis (AFB) isolation

Enteric precautions

Drainage/secretion precautions

Blood/body fluid precautions

The requirements for the amount and type of protection required for each category are listed on a color-coded card. This card is placed on or next to the door of the patient's room, and a copy may be placed with the medical record. The strict isolation and respiratory isolation requirements are shown in Boxes 10–2 and 10–3.

BOX 10–2

Strict Isolation*

Visitors: Report to Nurses' Station Before Entering Room

1. Masks are indicated for all persons entering the room.
2. Gowns are indicated for all persons entering the room.
3. Gloves are indicated for all persons entering the room.
4. HANDS MUST BE WASHED AFTER TOUCHING THE PATIENT OR POTENTIALLY CONTAMINATED ARTICLES AND BEFORE TAKING CARE OF ANOTHER PATIENT.
5. Articles contaminated with infective material should be discarded or bagged and labeled before being sent for decontamination and reprocessing.

*Card will be color-coded yellow.

BOX 10–3

Respiratory Isolation*

Visitors: Report to Nurses' Station Before Entering Room

1. Masks are indicated for those who come close to the patient.
2. Gowns are not indicated.
3. Gloves are not indicated.
4. HANDS MUST BE WASHED AFTER TOUCHING THE PATIENT OR POTENTIALLY CONTAMINATED ARTICLES AND BEFORE TAKING CARE OF ANOTHER PATIENT.
5. Articles contaminated with infective material should be discarded or bagged and labeled before being sent for decontamination and reprocessing.

*Card will be color-coded blue.

When the disease-specific isolation system is used, each disease is considered individually, and only the specific precautions required for that disease apply. Some hospitals have decided to use only the strict isolation and respiratory isolation categories because they believe the precautions needed for all diseases or infections are contained in one or the other category. It is important for the caregiver to know of and understand the isolation system or the approach used in his/her facility so the requirements and means of protection can be properly used. It is quite important that protective garments be removed carefully and in the proper sequence after the treatment of a patient with a transmissible disease or infection. The sequence and method of removal are described later.

Occasionally, the term "protective isolation" may be used to designate a patient whose condition or disease places him/her at a high risk of becoming infected through contact with another person. A patient with extensive burns, a compromised immune system, or a systemic infection is an example of a patient who may require protective isolation. If this isolation approach is used, it may be necessary for any person who enters the patient's room to carefully apply protective garments to reduce or prevent the transmission of pathogens to the patient. The sequence and method for applying protective garments are usually more important than the sequence used to remove them when treating the patient in protective isolation. The sequence and method of application are described later.

APPLICATION OF PROTECTIVE GARMENTS

The caregiver may have to protect himself/herself from the patient, or the patient may have to be protected from the caregiver. In either situation, it is likely that protective clothing will be required. This section will describe a method that can be used to apply clothing before treating a patient who has been placed in protective isolation (Procedure 10–3) and a method that can be used to remove clothing after treating a patient who has been placed in isolation (Procedure 10–4). In the first situation, the application sequence is extremely important, but the removal sequence is relatively unimportant. In the second situation, the application sequence is relatively unimportant, but the removal sequence is extremely important.

Each facility or nursing unit will have its own specific protocols related to the application and removal of protective clothing. The information in this chapter is sufficient to allow a caregiver to satisfactorily protect himself/herself or the patient, but it may not be as complete or specific as individual facility protocols. Therefore, the caregiver should become familiar with the established protocols at the facility where he/she provides patient care.

After treating the patient in protective isolation, your gloves and clothing can be removed in any sequence because there is very little danger that you will become contaminated from a noninfectious patient. However, you should wash your hands after removing the gloves and clothing and avoid contact between your hands and your eyes, ears, nostrils, and mouth until you have washed your hands thoroughly.

Text continued on page 289

PROCEDURE 10-3
Clothing Application for Protective Isolation

1. Wash your hands as described previously for medical asepsis.

2. Apply a cap, but avoid touching your hair as much as possible. Include all of your hair in the cap and, if possible, cover your ears (Fig. 10–3A,B).

3. Apply a mask, handling it by its ties or edges. Position the metal or plastic band of the mask over your nose, or center the dome type mask over your nose and mouth. Gently open the mask so that its bottom edge fits over your chin. Tie the upper ties snugly behind your head and above your ears; tie the lower ties snugly behind your neck. Avoid touching your neck or cap as you tie the mask. (*Note:* In some settings it may be preferred to apply the mask before the cap) (see Fig. 10–3C–E).

4. Open the outer package of a sterile disposable gown and the sterile gloves and place them on a table or counter in a sterile field at the approximate height of your waist. The inner cover of the gloves should remain closed (see Fig. 10–3F–H).

5. Wash your hands as described previously for surgical asepsis. (The medical asepsis technique may be acceptable for certain specific protocols.) Dry your hands thoroughly, and avoid touching your clothing or other objects with the washed areas of your skin.

6. Grasp the center of the gown with one hand, pick it up, and allow it to unfold without touching your body, clothing, or any other object. The gown will be folded inside out, and you should avoid touching the outside of the gown (see Fig. 10–3I).

7. Gently shake the gown so that it opens fully, and insert your left or right hand and arm into the left or right sleeve; DO NOT ALLOW YOUR HAND TO EXTEND THROUGH THE GOWN CUFF; in this way a closed-glove technique can be used. Insert your other arm into the other sleeve, and keep that hand inside the cuff (see Fig. 10–3J,K).

8. Request another person to tie the neck and waist ties snugly without touching the outside of the gown or the person's body. DO NOT ALLOW YOUR HANDS TO EXTEND THROUGH THE GOWN CUFFS when the gown is being tied (see Fig. 10–3L,M).

9. When a disposable gown is applied, with assistance from another person, care must be used to avoid contamination of the waist tie. Figure 10–3N,O shows proper handling of the tag of the tie so the tie and gown remain sterile; the upper portion of the tag is sterile, and the bottom portion is not.

10. Carefully open the inner packet containing your gloves, and pick up one glove with your hand, which is still inside the gown cuff. Place the glove palm down on its proper hand, so that the thumb of the glove rests on the thumb of your hand and the fingers of the glove are directed toward your elbow (see Fig. 10–3P–R).

Procedure text continued on page 287

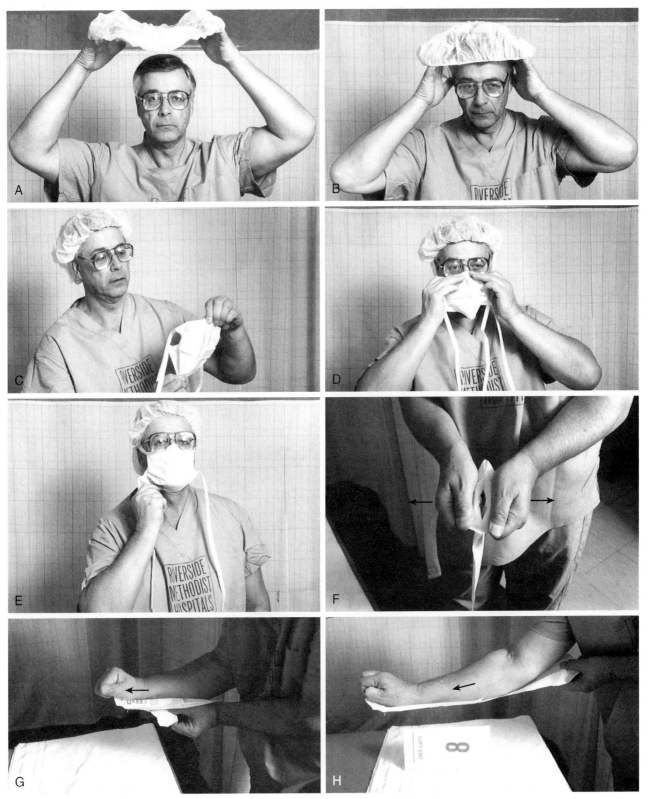

■ **FIGURE 10–3**
Application of protective garments.

continued

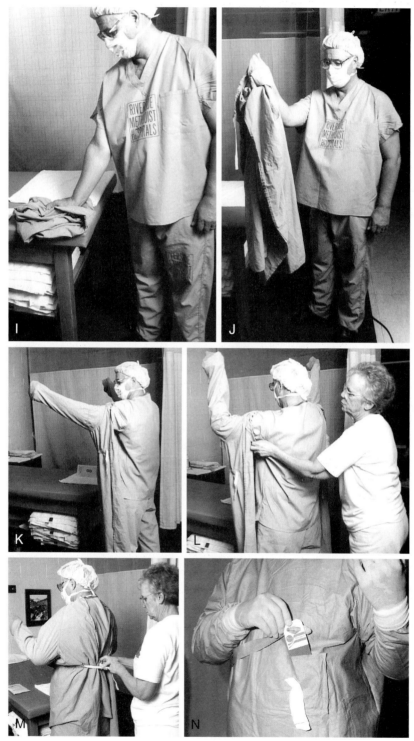

■ **FIGURE 10–3** *Continued*

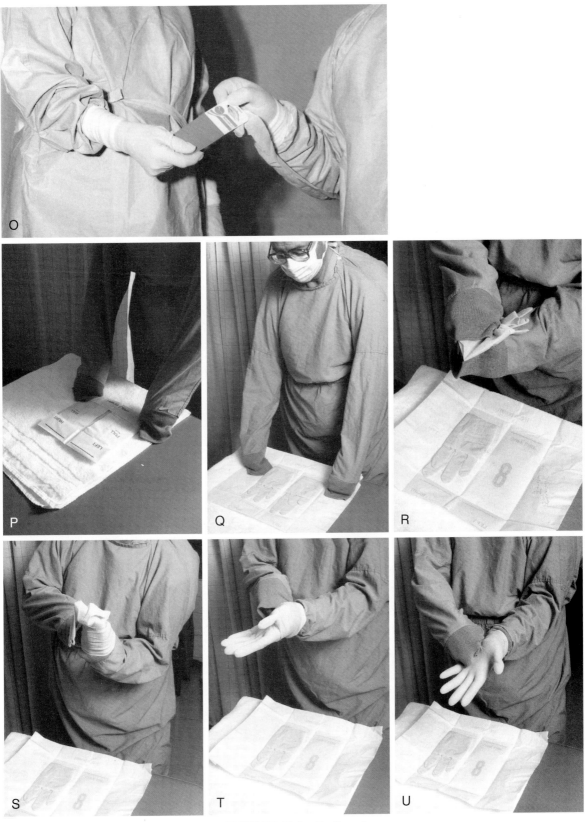

■ **FIGURE 10–3** *Continued*

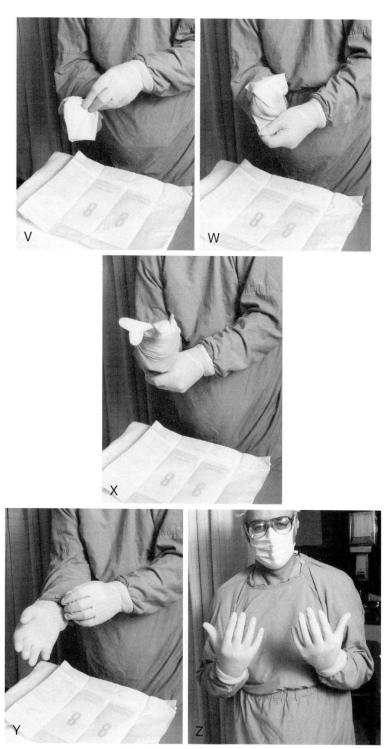

■ **FIGURE 10–3** *Continued*

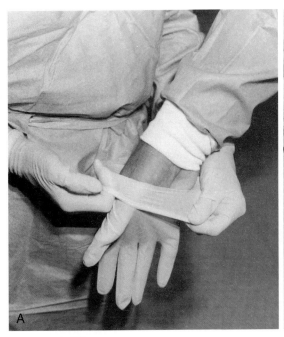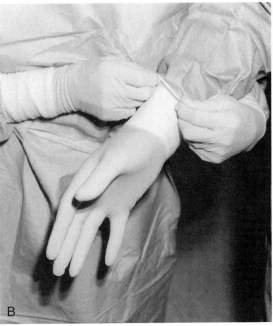

■ **FIGURE 10-4**
A, Two-person method to apply sterile gloves; all garments and gloves are sterile at this time. *B,* Glove is applied over the gown cuff.

PROCEDURE 10-3 *continued*

11. Grasp the cuff of the glove through the cuff of the gown and peel the cuff over your hand to seal or enclose your hand within the glove cuff; then gently maneuver your fingers and hand into the glove. Your other hand remains within the gown sleeve; do not extend it beyond the cuff (see Fig. 10-3*S–U*).

12. Repeat steps 10 and 11 to apply the other glove. Once both gloves have been applied completely, hold them above waist level, and avoid touching your gown or other objects to maintain sterility. A sterile towel can be wrapped over your gloved hands to protect them until it is time to treat the patient (see Figs. 10-3*V–Z* and 10-4*A,B*).

PROCEDURE 10-4
Clothing Removal for Isolation Precautions

1. Untie the waist tie of the gown, and have another person carefully untie the neck tie. He/she should avoid touching your neck, cap, or the outer side of gown when he/she unties the gown (Fig. 10-5*A,B*).

2. Grasp the outer front shoulders of the gown by crossing the arms (i.e., your left hand grasps the right front shoulder, and your right hand grasps the left front shoulder). Gently remove the gown by pulling it over your arms with your arms extended in front of your body. Avoid touching the outer side of the gown with your bare arms or clothing. Gently roll the gown into a ball so that it will be turned inside out, and dispose of it. Avoid touching your skin or clothing with the gown or with your gloves (see Fig. 10-5*C–G*).

continued

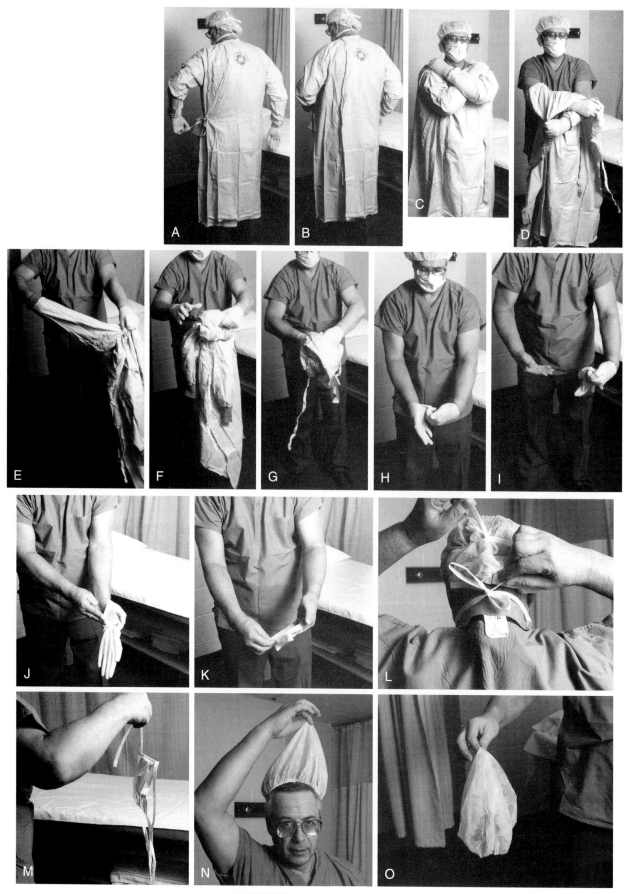

■ **FIGURE 10–5**
Removal of protective clothing.

PROCEDURE 10–4, *continued*

3. The glove cuffs will have been turned down as the gown sleeves are removed from your arms. To remove the right glove, grasp the *outside* of it with your left hand and gently remove the glove so that it is inside out; dispose of it. Use your ungloved right hand to grasp the *inside* of the left glove and gently remove that glove so that it is inside out. Avoid touching the outside of the left glove with your ungloved hand or the ungloved skin with the left glove after the right glove has been removed (see Fig. 10–5*H–K*).

4. Wash your hands as described for medical asepsis.

5. Remove your mask by carefully untying each set of ties and handling it by the ties. Avoid touching the center of the mask with your hands; dispose of it (see Fig. 10–5*L,M*).

6. Remove the cap by handling it by its ties or by gently grasping the center at the top and gently lift it from your head; dispose of it (see Fig. 10–5*N,O*).

7. Wash your hands as described for medical asepsis.

OPEN-GLOVE TECHNIQUE FOR ASEPSIS

There are situations in which the closed-glove technique is impractical or undesirable. The open-glove technique can be used in these situations, but it has a greater potential for glove contamination than the closed-glove technique unless you use extreme caution when you apply the gloves (Procedure 10–5).

REMOVAL OF CONTAMINATED PROTECTIVE GARMENTS

There may be situations in which another person is not available to assist in the removal of the protective clothing after a patient who is infected has been treated (Procedure 10–6). In such a situation, you must be careful when using this method to avoid contaminating yourself.

There are several precautions you should use after you treat a patient who is in strict or respiratory isolation. You must not touch your skin, eyes, hair, or ears with your gloves. Your gloves will be the most contaminated pieces of your clothing; the sleeves and front of the gown are the other items that are apt to be extensively contaminated. Remove your protective clothing carefully, and follow the recommendations for removal that have been provided. Consider the furniture, sinks, linen, and other objects in the room to be contaminated, and therefore avoid touching them with any unprotected surfaces of your body. Re-

member to perform proper hand-washing techniques as you apply and remove your protective clothing. Finally, do not wear protective clothing outside the patient's room or remove equipment from the room for use with patients in another area of the facility.

The following are some of the precautions you should follow when you treat a patient who is in protective isolation:

1. Apply your protective clothing carefully, and follow the recommendations for application that have been provided.

2. Avoid causing excessive air currents in the patient's room by moving slowly and by arranging linen or equipment carefully.

3. Do not enter the patient's room with protective clothing or equipment that has been worn to treat patients in another area of the hospital because you may bring undesired microorganisms into the patient's environment.

4. Remember to perform proper hand washing before applying and after removing your protective clothing.

Adherence to these precautions will help to protect both you and the patient from becoming infected.

THE STERILE FIELD

As the term indicates, a *sterile* field is designed to maintain the sterility of objects contained within the field, such as dressings or bandages, and to prevent

PROCEDURE 10–5
Open-Glove Technique for Asepsis

1. Perform preparatory activities of hand washing and applying the cap, mask, and gown as described in Procedure 10–3, items 1, 2, and 3.

2. Open the package containing the sterile gloves, and place the gloves in the sterile field. Open the inner packet carefully and arrange the gloves so that the cuffs are nearest you by touching only the *inside* of the folded cuffs with your hands. Avoid touching the outer surface of the gloves with your hands as you prepare to apply the first glove (Fig. 10–6A).

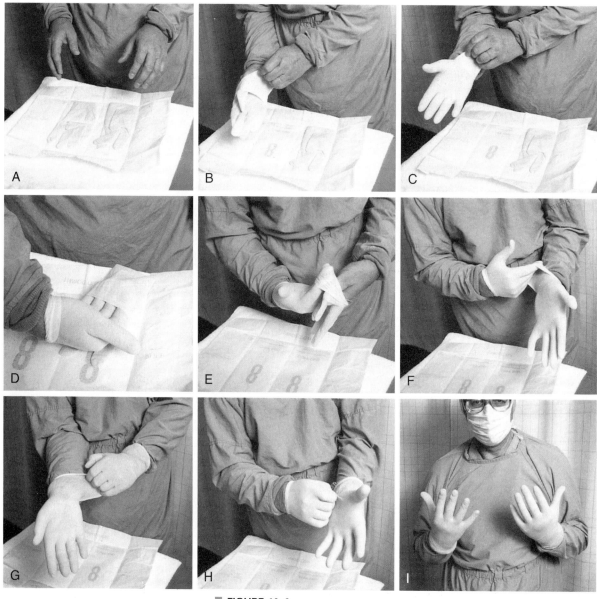

■ **FIGURE 10–6**
Open glove application technique.

PROCEDURE 10–5, *continued*

3. To apply the first glove, grasp the inner side or surface of the folded cuff of the glove. *Caution:* Do not touch the outside of either glove with an ungloved hand. Insert your hand and fingers into the glove, and apply the glove as if you were applying a dress glove, but allow the cuff to remain folded; do not attempt to adjust the cuff or the fit of the glove at this time (see Fig. 10–6*B,C*).

4. Using your gloved hand, lift the other glove by sliding your gloved fingers between the underside of the cuff and the outer side of the palm of the other glove. *Caution:* Do not touch the inside surface of the second glove or your ungloved hand with your gloved hand; to do so will contaminate them. Insert your hand and fingers into the glove but do not allow the thumb of the hand you are using to apply the second glove to touch the inside of the cuff of that glove (see Fig. 10–6*D–F*).

5. Pull the cuff of the second glove over the cuff of the gown by holding the outer surface of the cuff; avoid touching the skin of your hand or the sleeve of the gown with the outside of the first glove that was applied.

6. Once the cuff of the second glove is in place, slide your fingers under the cuff of the first glove, and pull the cuff of that glove over the cuff of the gown (see Fig. 10–6*G*).

7. Adjust the fingers of the gloves as necessary, but avoid touching any nonsterile objects. Keep your hands above waist level and slightly away from your body until you begin the patient care activity (see Fig. 10–6*H,I*).

contamination of the objects, which in turn could contaminate the patient. The sterile field is a form of surgical asepsis designed to keep the area free from pathogens. Usually a nonabsorbent, sterile towel or the outer cover or wrapping of a package that contains sterile supplies is used as the base for the sterile field. Once the field has been established, additional sterile objects can be added to the field cautiously.

It is important to know and to apply the four rules of *asepsis* when you establish the field and when you use items that are part of the field.

1. Know which items are sterile.
2. Know which items are not sterile.
3. Separate sterile items from nonsterile items.
4. If a sterile item becomes contaminated, the situation must be remedied immediately. Contamination occurs any time a sterile item physically contacts a nonsterile item. Often the remedy is to dispose of the contaminated item, and it may also be necessary to reestablish the sterile field.

Only items that have been specifically sterilized or packaged and identified as sterile until the package is opened can be considered to be sterile. If an item has been autoclaved, be certain that black lines appear on the tape used to seal the package. These black lines indicate that the item has been sterilized or can be considered sterile. The outer packages of prepackaged sterile items should be checked to be certain that the

items in the package were labeled to be sterile when packaged and that they are still sterile (i.e., the outer package is completely sealed and dry) (Fig. 10–7).

Once the field has been established (i.e., set up), care must be taken to maintain sterile conditions in

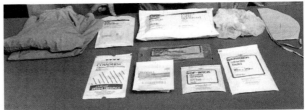
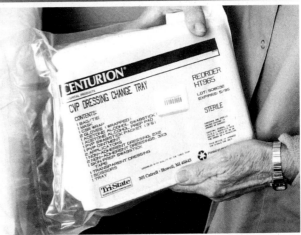

■ **FIGURE 10–7**
Sterile packaging.

PROCEDURE 10-6
Independent Removal of Contaminated Protective Garments

1. Untie the waist tie and then carefully remove one glove by turning it inside out with the opposite hand. *Caution:* Do not touch the bare skin of your hand with the glove of your other hand as the glove is being removed. Dispose of the glove.

2. Untie the neck tie with your ungloved hand but avoid touching the back of the gown, your neck, or your cap. Remove the gown, using your gloved hand to grasp the opposite outer anterior shoulder of the gown and your ungloved hand to grasp the opposite inner anterior shoulder of the gown. Gently turn the gown inside out and remove it from your arms. Avoid touching the outside of the sleeve or cuff with your ungloved hand; dispose of the gown. The remaining glove should roll down to expose the inside of the glove at your wrist.

3. Remove the remaining glove by grasping the inner surface of the glove at the cuff or by inserting one or two fingers at the base of your palm; peel the glove off by turning it inside out. Avoid touching your ungloved hand to the outside of the glove. Dispose of it.

4. Wash your hands as described previously.

5. Remove the mask and cap as described previously.

6. Wash your hands as described previously.

An alternate method is as follows:

1. Untie the waist tie and remove your cap, if it was applied after the mask, by grasping the top of it and lifting it from your head. Avoid touching your hair with your gloved hand. Dispose of the cap.

2. Grasp the outside of one glove at the cuff and fold it down to form a wide cuff; do the same to the opposite glove. Remove one glove by turning it inside out. Avoid touching your exposed hand with the outside of the other glove.

3. Remove the opposite glove by grasping the inside of the cuff of the glove and turning it inside out. Avoid touching the outside of the glove or the sleeve of the gown with your exposed hand. Dispose of the glove. Wash your hands, but avoid getting the cuffs of the gown wet.

4. Untie the mask or grasp the inside of the mask with one hand and the elastic strap with the other hand and remove the mask carefully. Avoid touching the exposed skin of your hands or face with the outer side of the mask. Dispose of the mask.

5. Untie the neck tie of the gown and shrug the gown forward off your shoulders, or grasp the *inside* of the gown at the shoulders and pull it inside out over your extended arms. Roll the gown into a small ball by handling the inside of the gown. Avoid touching your clothing or exposed skin with the outside of the gown. Dispose of the gown.

6. Wash your hands as described previously.

BOX 10–4

Guidelines for Maintaining a Sterile Field

1. Do not talk, sneeze, cough, or reach across a sterile field. The air currents or moisture droplets from your nose or mouth can convey pathogens onto the field.

2. Do not turn your back to the field because contamination of the objects in the field can occur when you are not able to observe the field.

3. Do not allow a nonsterile object to come in contact with a sterile object, and do not allow a sterile object to come in contact with an unsterile object.

4. Do not leave the field unattended, even if it is covered with a sterile towel or other sterile item. In your absence the field can become contaminated.

5. A 1-inch border at the edges of the field is considered to be unsterile. Avoid placing any sterile item within 1 inch of the outer edge of the field, and do not touch this area with sterile gloves or other sterile objects.

6. When you wear sterile protective clothing, the portions that are considered sterile, until they come into contact with an unsterile object or environment, are the gloves, the front of the gown above waist level, and both sleeves of the gown. The remainder of the gown is considered to be unsterile.

7. Remember: Any liquid is affected by gravity. Thus, when forceps or other items that have been stored in a liquid disinfectant are used, they should be handled so the tip or end that has been in the disinfectant is held downward. If the tip or end of the object is held upward, the fluid will flow to a nonsterile area on the object. Then, when the tip or end is held downward again, the fluid will flow from the nonsterile area back to the sterile area, thereby contaminating the object.

8. The base and the area surrounding the field should be void of moisture because moisture is apt to contain microorganisms and can penetrate the field by direct contact, absorption, or the wicking property of any of the materials on the field. Moisture is considered to be a source of contamination, so the field must remain dry. If the base of the field or any of the sterile materials on the field become wet, they should be considered contaminated.

9. To reduce or avoid movement over the field, position the items on the field in the order they will be used so the items that are to be used first are nearest you.

10. The area below the surface of the sterile field, which will usually be tabletop height or waist height, is considered unsterile. Any item that falls to or is located below waist or tabletop level should be considered contaminated.

11. General cleanliness of the treatment area, including the furniture, floor, walls, and lavatories, should be maintained to reduce the proliferation or deposition of microorganisms. Hand-washing techniques and practices described previously should be used when a sterile field is required.

the area and avoid contamination of the field. There are some simple guidelines that when followed, will assist you in maintaining the sterile field (Box 10–4). In general, if you remember and follow the four rules of asepsis, contamination of the field will be avoided. If you have any question as to whether an item is sterile, consider it contaminated and do not use it. If the object has come in contact with other objects that were considered sterile, all of the items should be disposed of and only new items known to be sterile should be used.

It is imperative to maintain the sterile field once it has been established. The healing process, and possibly the patient's life, may be affected by the level of care provided by the caregiver when a sterile technique is required to provide patient care. Procedures designed to protect the patient and the caregiver and to prevent wound contamination must be followed diligently and carefully.

WOUND CARE

Dressings and bandages are important items associated with the care and management of wounds,

Basic Goals of Wound Care

1. Protect the wound and surrounding tissue from additional trauma.
2. Reduce strain on the tissues near the wound.
3. Protect the tissue in the area of the wound from mechanical stress or movement.
4. Reduce the number of pathogenic microorganisms in and around the wound.
5. Expedite the healing process.
6. Decrease or reduce the formation of scar tissue.

and the concept of the prevention of wound infection must be applied by the caregiver. The basic goals of wound care are listed in Box 10–5. Three phases of wound healing are described in the literature: the inflammatory, proliferative, and remodeling, or maturation, phases.

The inflammatory process initiates wound healing. Its function is to limit tissue damage, remove injured or damaged cells, and repair the injured tissue. It is the body's initial local defense response to injury or trauma and it begins immediately after injury or trauma.

The inflammatory process consists of at least three stages: the vascular, exudate, and reparative stages. During the acute phase of healing, the vascular stage is characterized by hyperemia because of a change in cellular filtration pressures and an increase in the permeability of cells. These factors usually produce local edema, warmth, redness, and discomfort, which are the cardinal signs and symptoms of inflammation.

The exudate stage can have any of several appearances: serous (blister), purulent (pus), fibrinous (clotting), or hemorrhagic (bleeding). In this stage, a fluid passes through the walls of vessels into adjacent tissues or spaces to help deposit fibrins and leukocytes, which are necessary to initiate wound healing.

During the reparative stage, damaged cells are replaced, and true wound healing begins. Damaged cells are removed through phagocytosis, which is accomplished by polymorphonuclear cells and monocytes.

The proliferative phase overlaps the inflammatory phase, and granulation, epithelialization, and contraction of the wound site occur. The fibroblastic cells proliferate, and collagen tissue develops to initiate scar formation. According to one theory of healing, the fibroblasts and capillary buds develop at the edges of the wound and gradually advance toward the center of the wound. A bed of granulation tissue forms gradually over the surface of the wound, and the epithelial margins begin to migrate toward the center of the wound on top of this granulation bed. This process leads to contraction of the wound and eventually to formation of a scar.

The remodeling phase overlaps the proliferative phase and is characterized by the organization of the collagen tissue into a more definitive and finite pattern. Another factor associated with this phase is the increase in tensile strength of the tissue that covers the wound (i.e., scar tissue). Because the wound heals from the edges toward the center of the wound, it is important to use care when removing a dressing from the wound. The dressing should be removed gently and from the edges first to avoid disrupting the healing process, particularly if there is an exudate associated with the wound that adheres to the dressing.

Wounds heal by first (primary) or second (secondary) intention. First-intention healing occurs in wounds whose edges are closely related or whose edges have been approximated by sutures, staples, or other similar means. These wounds tend to heal with less likelihood of infection, in a shorter period of time, and with less scar formation. Thus, this is the preferred and most effective method of healing.

Second-intention healing occurs in wounds with large surface areas, with distracted edges, or in which a large amount of tissue has been lost. These wounds may become infected rather easily, usually require an extended healing time, and are apt to exhibit excessive scar formation. When possible, these wounds are transformed into wounds that are better able to heal by the use of skin grafts, skin flaps, or other similar surgical techniques.

Several factors can affect wound healing either favorably or unfavorably. Infection or the presence of high numbers of pathogens in the wound or its surrounding tissue will delay or complicate the healing process. The size, extent, location, and type of wound can all affect healing. A large, deep, irregularly shaped wound usually requires additional time to heal, as does a wound that is located where there is limited or impaired circulation.

The nutritional status of the person is also an important factor. A person with poor nutritional status will experience more difficulty and require a longer healing time. A wound in an elderly patient may not heal as rapidly as a similar wound in a younger adult because of differences in circulation and metabolic responses to the wound. Some medications may aid or enhance wound healing, whereas other medications may delay the healing process. Finally, the patient who has a chronic illness or who is generally debilitated probably will exhibit a delay in the healing of the wound.

WOUND CLASSIFICATION

A wound can be classified as an abrasion, a puncture, a laceration, a burn, an incision, or an ulceration. An abrasion is a wound caused by rubbing or scraping the skin or mucous membrane. A skinned elbow or knee and a floor or carpet burn are examples of an abrasion. A puncture is a wound caused by a pointed object or instrument. Wounds from nails, pin points, or bullets are examples of a puncture wound. A laceration is a wound produced by the tearing of body tissue. A blow from a blunt object or an injury caused by a machine is likely to be a laceration.

A burn is caused when the skin contacts dry heat (fire), moist heat (steam), chemicals, electricity, or radiation. Burns are classified according to their depth and size. A burn may be described as superficial, partial thickness, deep partial thickness, or full thickness. When the upper layer of the epidermis is affected, the wound is superficial; when the lower layers of the epidermis are involved, the wound is a partial-thickness wound; and when the dermis is affected, the wound becomes a full-thickness wound.

An incision is a cut or wound made by a sharp instrument such as a scalpel. An ulceration is the result of an ulcer in which an excavation of the surface of an organ or tissue is produced by the sloughing (i.e., falling away) of necrotic inflammatory tissue. Skin ulcers are often located on the distal lower extremities, especially in the area of the malleoli.

This preceding information is quite limited in its scope and comprehensiveness but is included to provide a basic understanding of the process of wound healing and its relationship to wound management. The reader will have to refer to other sources for additional information about the wound-healing process.

PRESSURE ULCERS

A pressure ulcer, incorrectly referred to as a decubitus ulcer, pressure sore, or bedsore, is one type of wound that can complicate the care of many patients. Although a pressure ulcer may be able to be prevented through an aggressive treatment plan of on-going skin care, frequent changes in the patient's position, proper and adequate nutrition, and the relief of or reduction in pressure to the soft tissue that overlies bony prominences, there is no ensurance these activities will prevent the development of one or more pressure ulcers. The patient's age, body condition and composition, and disease state; the presence of circulation or metabolic disorders; and the mobility capability of the patient are factors that contribute to the risk of pressure ulcers. Therefore, each caregiver who treats the patient must be involved with the prevention of pressure ulcers to maximize the potential of avoiding them (see Box 10–5).

Causes A pressure ulcer is a wound that develops due to two primary factors: pressure to soft tissue that exceeds the normal capillary pressure of the local circulation, and shear force to superficial skin. The soft tissue located over a bony prominence, especially the greater trochanter, sacrum, calcaneus, and ischial tuberosity, is the site at which a pressure ulcer is most likely to occur. In those areas, the capillaries that transport oxygen and nutrients to and remove waste products from the tissue become compressed between the underlying bone and the external pressure source. (*Note:* Table 3–1, in Chapter 3, presents the locations at which pressure ulcers are most likely to develop depending on the patient's position.) When the capillaries are compressed for a period of time, they become occluded, ischemia occurs, and the potential for tissue necrosis exists. If necrosis does occur, tissue is destroyed, and a partial- or full-thickness wound will be evident.

A contributing factor in the development of a pressure ulcer is shear force applied to the patient's skin, which may occur during position changes, transfers, or exercise activities. The shear force may produce friction to the skin, which causes increased surface heat and erosion of the epidermis. The combination of prolonged pressure and episodes of shear force applied to the same area of the body causes trauma to the capillaries, skin, and underlying soft tissue, and a pressure ulcer will develop (see Box 10–7).

Patient Assessment Each patient who is admitted to a health care facility or is being treated at home should be assessed to determine his/her potential or risk to develop a pressure ulcer. In addition, his/her functional abilities such as bed mobility, activity level, wheelchair or ambulatory mobility, feeding, chewing and swallowing capability, and transfer performance should be determined. Information about his/her previous and current medical history, level of mental competence, nutritional status, skin condition, general physical condition, and psychosocial factors are other components of the initial assessment. Identification of specific risk factors should be one of the major outcomes of the initial assessment.

Risk Factors Some of the risk factors related to the development of a pressure ulcer are presented in Box 10–6. A risk assessment at the time of admission of a patient to any health care facility or when he/she is being treated at home by a health care practitioner is a standard of care recommended by several agencies or regulatory bodies, including the Agency for Health Care Policy and Research (AHCPR), National Pres-

BOX 10–6

Primary Risk Factors Associated With Pressure Ulcers

1. Pressure to tissue overlying bony prominences, especially the sacrum, heels, greater trochanters, and ischial tuberosities.
2. Shear and friction forces applied to the skin.
3. Inadequate or improper nutrition, including appropriate and adequate fluid intake.
4. Insensitive body areas, especially those insensitive to pressure.
5. Persistent incontinence, which leads to skin irritation, maceration, or breakdown.
6. Metabolic or systemic disorder or diseases, especially diabetes.
7. Persistent use of tobacco products.

sure Ulcer Advisory Panel (NPUAP), Omnibus Budget Reconciliation Act (OBRA), Association for the Advancement of Wound Care (AAWC), and the Wound, Ostomy, Continence Nurses Society (WOCN). It is important that the patient who is at risk to develop pressure ulcers be identified at admission, his/her risk factors be documented, and a prevention program be initiated promptly. Every person who has contact with the patient, such as housekeeping personnel, family members, aides, and technicians, in addition to primary caregivers, should be considered members of the prevention team. These individuals are apt to observe the patient several times during the day; therefore, observations, comments, or suggestions from nonprimary caregivers can be helpful to the primary caregivers. Prevention should be a responsibility shared by multiple individuals.

Preventive Interventions   Relief of pressure to the soft tissue that overlies a bony prominence is the primary method of pressure ulcer prevention. Relief of the pressure can be accomplished by elevating the area from the pressure source (i.e., use of a pillow beneath the calf to elevate the heel slightly from the mattress when the person is supine), by changing the patient's position frequently so an area is not in prolonged contact with a source of pressure (i.e., use of a turning or positioning schedule to relieve weight bearing on a specific bony prominence), or by positioning him/her so an area is not in contact with a source of pressure (i.e., position him/her in a partial side-lying position with the use of pillows or foam wedges so he/she does not rest directly on his/her lowermost greater trochanter and to separate bony prominences). If the patient is able to independently

alter his/her position, he/she should be instructed on how and when to do so (i.e., perform pushups or lean to one side and then to the other while seated in a wheelchair; lift his/her pelvis from the mattress using his/her lower extremities when he/she is supine; use a trapeze to elevate his/her upper body from the mattress when supine; he/she should perform these activities several times per hour).

Pressure reduction is another preventive method by which the amount of pressure to an area is decreased but not fully relieved. The use of air-fluidized, low–air-loss, or oscillating beds; air or water mattresses; seat cushions (*caution:* do not use the ring, "donut" type of cushion because the rim of the cushion will create pressure, which is apt to occlude capillaries and deprive the local tissue of a proper blood supply and flow); bony joint protectors (i.e., heel or elbow guards); and wound protection dressings are examples of pressure reduction aids or approaches. Shear force can be reduced if a "draw sheet" is used to position or transfer a patient, double socks are used to protect the heels, the head of the bed is elevated to the lowest level of comfort and function for the patient (i.e., at approximately 30 degrees of elevation, the patient will tend to slide down over the bed linen, creating shear to the sacrum and scapulae), the patient is instructed to avoid rubbing his/her heels or elbows on the bed linen when lying supine, and the patient is not

BOX 10–7

Factors That Affect Wound Healing

1. Extrinsic factors
   a. Pressure applied to soft tissue that overlies a bony prominence
   b. Shear force applied to the skin, especially to the heels and sacrum
   c. Maceration of the skin due to body waste, perspiration, or skin-to-skin contact (i.e., skin folds)
   d. Infection
   e. Reduced activity leading to prolonged immobility
2. Instrinsic factors
   a. General health of the patient
   b. Condition of the skin
   c. Body build and composition
   d. Nutritional status
   e. Hydration status

Depending on the presence or absence of these factors, each may have a positive or negative effect or influence on the healing of the wound.

Adapted from Morey S: Pressure ulcer/wound care. Presented at Ohio Physical Therapy Association Annual Conference, April 17, 1997, Columbus, OH.

BOX 10–8

Guidelines for Pressure Ulcer Intervention and Management

1. Provide pressure relief or reduction to the body areas susceptible to ulcer development.

2. Develop and follow a schedule to alter the positions the patient is placed as one method to accomplish the previous guideline.

3. Determine the nutritional and fluid intake needs of the patient; establish an appropriate diet and feeding schedule to meet the needs.

4. Initiate mobility activities for the patient that are possible, safe, and appropriate; include bed, wheelchair, and ambulation activities. Shear forces must be avoided.

5. Perform debridement of necrotic tissue, as necessary, to promote healing.

6. Perform wound and skin cleansing as necessary; avoid the use of toxic agents, including many types of soaps, hydrogen peroxide, and povidone-iodine (Betadine).

7. Perform consistent and thorough perineal care, especially when the patient is incontinent.

8. Rinse the ulcer with a sterile saline solution with an appropriate pressure at the time of dressing changes.

9. Develop and follow a schedule to observe, evaluate, remove, and apply dressings that is appropriate for the patient and personnel involved.

10. Provide education to all caregivers involved with the patient's care, including his/her family members; include information on prevention, care, and management.

11. Develop and follow a program designed to prevent the development of pressure ulcers, especially for persons who demonstrate a high risk of developing pressure ulcers.

dragged across the bed linen when turning, positioning, or transferring him/her (Box 10–8).

Skin Care Frequent inspection of and attention to care of a patient's skin, particularly for the patient who is incontinent, are important preventive activities. Prompt cleansing of the skin; maintenance of dry, clean skin of the perineum, buttocks, and upper thighs; and the use of topical agents to provide a mois-

ture barrier or moisturize dry skin may be necessary for many patients. In addition, the use of lubricants, protective dressings (i.e., films, hydrocolloids, hydrogels), and paddings should assist to minimize shear and friction. *Caution:* Massage of the tissue that overlies a bony prominence should be avoided because it may traumatize the local capillaries, which are apt to be fragile and susceptible to injury.

Caregivers whose treatment requires handling of the extremities, especially the upper extremities, should be aware of the possibility of causing a skin tear when treating elderly patients because their skin tends to be fragile and can be torn quite easily. Skin tears should be assessed and measured before treatment. The area should be cleaned gently with normal saline solution, and the wound edges should be dried by patting the area with gauze. Small pieces of detached epithelium that appear to be traumatized can be debrided by a qualified caregiver, and skin that appears to be viable and nontraumatized should be repositioned gently over the wound. A nonadherent dressing should be applied and covered with a protective bandage.

All caregivers should use care to avoid activities or procedures that intensify the established risk factors for a given patient. Prolonged, excessive pressure over time to areas of bony prominences and shear and friction forces must be avoided during exercise, transfers, mobility activities, and turning or positioning of the patient. Straps used to attach splints or orthoses must not be applied too tightly, and footwear must fit properly to avoid friction or blister development. The caregiver must be aware of the potential for injury or damage to the patient's skin and must adjust the treatment program to avoid trauma to the skin.

Wound Classification and Staging A pressure ulcer should be assessed and classified according to its stage or level of tissue destruction (Table 10–1). The stage designation also provides a diagnosis of the amount or type of tissue insult and injury that has occurred. If the epidermis and a portion of the dermis are involved, the wound is considered to be a partial-thickness wound, and the ulcer is considered to be superficial. When the entire dermis and underlying fascia, muscle tendon, or bone are involved, the wound is considered to be a full-thickness wound, and the ulcer is considered to be deep. Box 10–9 lists and describes the four stages associated with a pressure ulcer. These stages can be described as being progressive: stage 1 becomes stage II and stage II becomes stage III; however, the stages cannot be described regressively. That is, as a stage III ulcer heals, it does not revert to stage II. Instead, as a stage IV wound heals, it continues to be classified as stage IV, but the percentage of the wound that has healed is reported or a measurement and description of the open area of the wound are

	Table 10–1 GOALS OF WOUND MANAGEMENT DEPENDENT ON WOUND STAGE AND APPEARANCE	
Stage	**Appearance**	**Goals**
I	Erythema that does not blanch when pressure is intact.	Remove, relieve pressure, keep area clean; avoid friction and shear forces.
II, III	Granulation/nondraining	Maintain moist wound bed; protect surrounding tissue; observe for infection.
II, III	Granulation/draining	Maintain moist wound bed; protect surrounding tissue; observe for infection; absorb exudate.
IV	Necrotic/nondraining	Maintain moist wound bed; protect surrounding tissue; observe for infection; soften and remove eschar, necrotic tissue.
IV	Necrotic/draining	Maintain moist wound bed; protect surrounding tissue; observe for infection; absorb exudate.
II, III, IV	Infected wound	Protect the surrounding tissue; absorb exudate, and contain infection.

Adapted with permission from Kendall K, Porter C, Carroll C, Lamare RNC, Tilley JG: Evolution of Sacred Heart Hospital's wound assessment sheet. In *Acute Care Perspectives,* Newsletter of the Acute Care/Hospital Clinical Practice Section, Alexandria, VA: American Physical Therapy Association, Summer 1995, p. 8.

used to indicate the improvement or healing of the wound. A wound cannot be staged if its depth cannot be measured or visualized; therefore, a wound covered with eschar or necrotic tissue cannot be staged until the wound surface is exposed through debridement of the eschar.

Wound Assessment Several methods or parameters can be used to assess many characteristics of the wound; examples are provided in Box 10–10. The size is determined by measuring the longest and widest portions of the wound. The measurements are stated in centimeters, and a disposable, plastic overlay can be used to measure the wound. The overlay should be positioned on the wound so its top is directed toward the patient's head and the measurements are made based on the configuration of the face of a clock. Length measurements are made along a line from 12 o'clock (head) to 6 o'clock (foot), and width measurements are made from 9 o'clock (left) to 3 o'clock (right).

The depth is measured by inserting a sterile cotton-tipped swab vertically into the wound until it contacts the bottom or floor of the wound. The caregiver uses his/her finger or thumbnail to indicate where the upper portion of the shaft of the swab exits the wound; the distance from the end of the swab to the mark on the shaft indicates the depth. The swab and plastic overlay must be disposed immediately after each is used for a patient. A swab also can be used to determine the amount of undermining of the edge of the wound or tunneling of the wound into surrounding soft tissue. A technique similar to the one described for measuring the depth can be used to measure undermining and tunneling by inserting the swab horizontally. Probing of these areas should be performed gently and cautiously because it will not be possible to observe the tissue that the swab contacts. It is recommended the caregiver wear nonsterile gloves when he/she performs these measurements.

BOX 10–9

Staging a Pressure Ulcer

Stage I—Erythema is present; the skin is intact, and the erythema does not blanch when pressure is applied.

Stage II—Skin loss occurs, which may affect only the epidermis or may penetrate into the dermis, but not through it; the wound bed is free of necrotic tissue and usually appears moist and pink. Classified as a partial-thickness wound.

Stage III—Tissue loss that includes the epidermal and dermal skin layers with penetration into the subcutaneous tissue; some necrotic tissue may be present; tunneling or undermining may occur; an exudate may be observed; and the wound may be infected. Classified as a full-thickness wound.

Stage IV—Destruction of deep tissue such as fascia, joint tissue, and bone may be affected; necrotic tissue is likely to be present; tunneling or undermining may occur; an exudate may be observed; and the wound may be infected.

Partial thickness indicates the epidermis and upper portion of the dermis are involved, but the wound does not reach the subcutaneous tissue; the wound is considered to be superficial. Full thickness indicates the epidermis and entire dermis and subcutaneous tissues are involved; fascia, joint tissue, and bone may be affected; the wound is considered to be deep.

Adapted with permission from Kennedy KL: *Wound Caring.* Copyright 1997 Professional Education Systems, Inc. (800-647-8079). No further reproduction may be made without consent from the publisher.

Adapted from Morey S: Pressure ulcer/wound caring. Presented at the Annual Conference of the Ohio Physical Therapy Association, April 17, 1997, Columbus, OH.

Pressure Ulcer Assessment Factors

1. Identify the wound stage.
2. Measure the wound size.
3. Measure the wound depth.
4. Observe and describe the tissue at the wound edges.
5. Examine the wound for areas of tunneling or undermining; measure the length or depth.
6. Observe and describe the characteristics of any exudate (viscosity, amount, color).
7. Observe and describe the characteristics of any necrotic tissue (color, adherence, texture, consistency, amount).
8. Describe any wound odor.
9. Observe and describe the characteristics of the surrounding skin (dry, macerated, color, texture, blistered, edematous, firm, soft).
10. Observe and describe characteristics of wound healing
    a. Granulation
    b. Epithelialization
    c. Budding
    d. Wound contraction

Another assessment component is to observe and describe the color patterns or necrotic tissue of the wound and to estimate their percentage of content in the wound. Red color is indicative of the process of granulation, yellow or grayish-brown is the color of slough, and eschar will appear black. Epithelial tissue will appear to be pink and shiny and indicates that coverage of the wound by new skin is occurring. Photographs taken periodically using a Polaroid camera can be used to document the condition of the wound and the surrounding tissue (skin).

Wound Care Usually, nursing personnel will be the primary caregivers responsible for the care of a pressure ulcer; however, other caregivers are involved with various aspects of wound management and care. The basic elements of wound care include debridement of necrotic tissue, wound cleaning, wound dressing, and the possible use of adjunctive therapies or interventions.

Debridement The removal of necrotic tissue from the wound allows the wound to heal more effectively. Debridement can be performed with sharp instruments (i.e., scalpel, scissors), mechanically, chemically, or with autolysis. Sharp debridement is the most rapid method, and a scalpel or scissors are used to remove thick adherent eschar and other devitalized tissue. Depending on state statutes, practice acts, and the policies and procedures of the facility, a variety of persons who have the appropriate training may legally perform sharp debridement. Mechanical debridement can be performed through pressure irrigation, the removal of dressings, hydrotherapy, electrical stimulation, a combination of hydrotherapy and ultrasonography, and the use of dextronomers. The use of enzymes to debride is another method in which enzymes are applied to the wound or the patient's self-produced enzymes are the active agent; this is known as *autolysis* or *autolytic debridement.* Enzymatic debridement tends to be more effective for small areas of necrosis or when the patient is unable to tolerate other methods. Nutritional support may be necessary to promote improvement in skin condition to increase the development of subcutaneous tissue and improve or maintain the patient's metabolism. Some patients may require supplemental enteral or parenteral feedings to ensure sufficient nutrient levels are attained (see Box 10–6).

Dressings Care of the wound usually requires the selection and application of one or more types of dressings. The purposes of the dressing are to protect the wound, assist the healing process, reduce infection or contamination of the wound, and remove exudates and toxic waste when the dressing is removed. Tables 10–2 and 10–3 present information about the selection and effects of several types of dressings. Dressings that prohibit observation of the wound may need to be removed more frequently than dressings that permit observation. Some dressings cause maceration of the surrounding skin, and a moisture barrier may need to be applied when those dressings are used. Finally, dressings should be removed carefully to avoid trauma to the wound surface or surrounding tissue. The wound and its surrounding skin should be observed and assessed each time a dressing is removed, and documentation should be made of noticeable changes from previous observations.

Summary Pressure ulcers are caused by pressure to the soft tissue that overlies a bony prominence. When the tissue is trapped between the bony prominence and a source of external pressure, the capillaries in the tissue are occluded, leading to local ischemia and tissue necrosis. A contributing factor is shear force applied to the skin. There are many risk factors that predispose the patient to the development of a pres-

Table 10–2
DRESSING CHOICES AND PREFERRED USES

Stage or Condition	Type of Dressing						
	TF	HC	HyG	AL	WD	WW	PS
I	X	X					
II	X	X	X			X	
III		X	X	X		X	X
IV				X		X	X
Necrotic/draining				X	X	X	
Necrotic/nondraining			X		X	X	
Noninfected	X	X	X	X	X	X	
Infected				X	X	X	

TF = transparent film, HC = hydrocolloid, HyG = hydrogel, AL = alginate, WD = wet to dry, WW = wet to wet, and PS = packing strip.
Adapted with permission from Kendall K, Porter C, Carroll C, Lamar RNC, Tilley JT: Evolution of Sacred Heart Hospital's wound assessment sheet. In *Acute Care Perspectives,* Newsletter of the Acute Care/Hospital Clinical Practice Section, Alexandria, VA: American Physical Therapy Association, Summer 1995, p. 8.

sure ulcer; therefore, every patient, on admission to a health care facility or who is treated at home, should be assessed for these risk factors. If one or more risk factors are identified, a specific, aggressive prevention program should be initiated. Integral components of such a program are proper skin care, pressure relief or reduction, proper positioning, and frequent position changes.

If a pressure ulcer occurs, it should be classified and described accurately and objectively so appropriate documentation can be made (Box 10–11). Wound care such as debridement, the use of dressings, and proper nutrition are important aspects of treatment. An interdisciplinary care team should be established to maximize the care and management of the patient and the wound.

PERIPHERAL VASCULAR CONDITIONS

Wounds caused by venous or arterial insufficiency or diabetes should be differentiated from a pressure ulcer. In some instances, the location and appearance of the wound will be sufficient to determine the type of wound and its cause. For example, a wound located directly over a bony prominence suggests a pressure ulcer; a wound located in the area of the medial malleolus accompanied with edema and dark, dusky skin

Table 10–3
PRODUCT SELECTION BASED ON WOUND SEVERITY

Dressing	Value/Effects
Transparent film (Bioclusive, Tegaderm, OpSite)	Dressing of choice for stages I and II wounds with blister formation over bony prominences; resists shear; may be applied to heels prophylactically; self-adherent and allows wound to be observed; may be used for autolytic debridement. Do not use on draining or infected wounds.
Hydrocolloid (Duoderm, Restore [paste or granules])	Dressing of choice for stages II and III wounds with minimal drainage; provides moist wound bed; absorbs small amount of drainage; self-adherent and provides cushioning over bony prominence. Do not use on infected wounds; medications cannot be used under the dressing.
Hydrogel (Vigilon, ClearSite, NuGel)	Recommended for stages II and III wounds with dressing covering the gel; moist wound bed is maintained; recommended for use on skin tear, cover with rolled absorbent material (Kling); may cause maceration of surrounding healthy tissue; does not protect wound from external soiling.
Wet to wet	Safe choice for unstaged wounds; use on stage II partial-thickness wounds and stages II and IV wounds; dressing will need to be changed every 8 hours to maintain moist wound base; should moisten dressing with saline solution before removal if dressing is dry to prevent bleeding and disruption of granulation bed; moisture barrier must be used on surrounding tissue to prevent maceration.
Wet to dry	Use on stages II and IV wounds for debridement; slough and necrotic tissue adhere to dressing and are removed with dressing.
Calcium alginates (CaAl) (Kaltostate, Algosteril)	Use to absorb heavy drainage but will require a secondary dressing to cover the CaAl; may be used on infected wounds.

Adapted with permission from Kendall K et al: Evolution of Sacred Heart Hospital's wound assessment sheet. In *Acute Care Perspectives,* Newsletter of the Acute Care/Hospital Clinical Practice Section, Alexandria, VA: American Physical Therapy Association, Summer 1995, p. 8.

Pressure Ulcer Documentation Guidelines

1. Describe the site or location of the ulcer.
2. Identify the stage of the ulcer based on the classification system of the National Pressure Ulcer Advisory Panel (NPUAP).
3. Measure and report the size of the total surface area of the ulcer.
4. Measure and report the depth of the ulcer.
5. Determine the evidence or extent of ulcer tunnels or undermined areas; report tissue destruction underlying intact skin along the margins of the ulcer; measure the width and length.
6. Estimate and describe the percentage of color (black, red, yellow) and the percentage of the ulcer covered with new skin; describe the composition of the ulcer (i.e., granulation and epithelialized tissue).
7. Estimate and describe the type and amount of exudate (i.e., viscosity, color, consistency).
8. Describe the odor associated with the ulcer after it has been rinsed with sterile saline solution.
9. Observe for and report whether edema or induration exists in the tissue surrounding the periphery of the ulcer.
10. Observe for and report whether signs of inflammation are present in the tissue surrounding the ulcer; measure and report the area in which signs appear.
11. Observe and describe the condition of the skin surrounding the ulcer (i.e., dry, moist, loose, taut, warm, discolored).

discoloration suggests a venous insufficiency wound; and a small wound located below the ankle accompanied by localized edema suggests an arterial insufficiency wound or a wound due to diabetes.

Several assessment methods or tests are available to evaluate the status of venous and arterial circulation in the lower extremity. Peripheral venous circulation dysfunction can be caused by defective or deficient valves, occlusion of the veins, or limited function of the "calf-pumping" mechanism. Peripheral arterial circulation dysfunction usually is due to some form of occlusion of arteries, which is associated with atherosclerosis. Both circulatory systems may exhibit acute or chronic conditions. Some tests that can be performed to determine the function of the venous and arterial peripheral circulation are presented in Boxes 10–12 and 10–13. Other evaluative procedures are examination of the patient's skin, measurement of the skin temperature, palpation of the pulse at various sites, evaluation of sensation, auscultation of an artery, and measurement of blood pressure. Doppler ultrasonography and air plethysmography may be performed but they require specific training and special equipment.

Treatment procedures or activities for these types of wounds are beyond the scope of this text. However, the caregiver should be aware of his/her responsibility to notify the patient's physician when one of these conditions is identified. For most patients, prompt medical care and management of any condition that affects the peripheral venous or arterial circulation will be necessary to prevent a serious complication.

GRADUATED COMPRESSION GARMENTS

Uses of graduated compression garments include control of edema in an extremity, assist in the return of venous circulation in a lower extremity, and decrease in the formation of extensive scar tissue resulting from a burn. The garments are fabricated for an individual patient from a fabric that because of its elastic properties, produces an external, graduated compression force to the tissues. The compression decreases from the distal portion to the proximal portion at approximately every 1½ inches. In addition to their use on the extremities, the garments can be fabricated for a patient's head or trunk. These applications would be beneficial to decrease the development of scar tissue for the person who has been burned.

Disadvantages of these garments are that they tend to contain body heat and restrict heat loss; they may be difficult to apply, especially when they are applied initially to an edematous extremity; and their elastic properties are reduced over time and with use, so frequent replacements may be needed.

Measurements for a pressure gradient garment for the upper or lower extremity can be performed easily by using the paper measuring tapes supplied by the manufacturer. The tapes allow circumferential measurements of the extremity to be made approximately every 1½ inches from the distal to the proximal aspect of the extremity. Specific landmarks on each extremity are used to properly position the tape before the application of the individual strips that are wrapped around the extremity. Complete instructions and directions, including diagrams, are provided with each

BOX 10–12

Peripheral Venous and Arterial Circulation Tests

I. Venous sufficiency tests
  A. Percussion test—Used to assess the function of the values of the saphenous vein
    1. With the patient standing, the caregiver palpates a proximal segment of the saphenous vein with the fingers of one hand; he/she uses the fingers of the other hand to tap (percuss) a distal segment of the vein.
    2. A fluid movement will be sensed by the fingers on the proximal segment during percussion if the valves are not functioning properly.
    3. Both lower extremities can be tested, and the results compared.
  B. Deep vein thrombophlebitis test—Used to assess the possible presence of a thrombus
    1. The caregiver grasps and squeezes the patient's calf while passively forcing the foot into dorsiflexion. If the patient complains of pain in the calf, a positive response is reported; this is known as a positive *Homan's sign.*
    2. Another method is to apply a blood pressure cuff around the patient's calf and to inflate it gradually; a patient with an acute condition would not tolerate an inflation pressure higher than 40 mm Hg; once the pain threshold has been reached, do not further inflate the cuff; test the noninvolved lower extremity first if only one extremity is suspected of having a deep vein thrombosis (DVT).
II. Arterial sufficiency tests
  A. Rubor of dependency test—Used to evaluate the arterial circulation by observing skin color changes that occur with the lower extremity elevated and level.
    1. When the patient is supine, observe and record the color of the plantar surface of the foot (normal = pinkish); elevate the lower extremity. approximately 45 to 60 degrees for 1 minute (abnormal = rapid loss of color).
    2. Return the extremity to level; observe and record the color of the plantar surface (normal = rapid pink flush; abnormal = 30 seconds or longer for color to appear, color will be bright red).
  B. Venous filling time test—Used to determine the length of time required for superficial veins to refill, after they have been emptied, due to arterial flow through the capillaries into the veins. *Note:* Patient must have a normal venous system.
    1. The patient is supine and his/her lower extremities are elevated to 45 to 60 degrees for 1 minute; then he/she dangles the legs over the edge of the bed or table; refilling of the veins is observed and timed (normal = 10 to 15 seconds for refilling).
  C. Claudication—Used to measure the length of time a patient can walk before he/she experiences claudication.
    1. The patient walks on a level grade treadmill at 1 mile per hour until claudication occurs; the time elapsed is recorded when calf pain prevents him/her from continuing to walk.
    2. The test can be repeated at specified intervals, and the time elapsed values can be compared.

Adapted from Morey S: Pressure ulcer/wound care. Presented at the Ohio Physical Associated Annual Conference, April 17, 1997, Columbus, OH; and O'Sullivan SB, Schmitz TJ: *Physical Rehabilitation Assessment and Treatment.* 3rd edition. Philadelphia: F.A. Davis, 1994.

BOX 10–13

General Assessment Activities for Peripheral Vascular Conditions

I. Objective activities
   A. Skin examination
      1. Observe color and compare with that of opposite extremity.
      2. Observe the condition of the skin (dry, scaly, flexible, firm, loose, adherent, moist, presence of exudate).
      3. Palpate to sense temperature, edema, and general condition.
      4. Observe for absence of hair.
      5. Evaluate superficial sensation; use objects with different textures; apply light pressure; use a monofilament "feeler."
   B. Measure skin temperature
      1. Use a thermistor with a probe; measure temperature at various sites or locations along the extremity.
      2. Compare values with those obtained from similar sites or locations on the opposite extremity.
   C. Palpate pulses
      1. Evaluate all major arterial pulses; refer to techniques and procedures in Chapter 4.
      2. Evaluate the quality and rate.
      3. Compare findings of involved extremity with those of noninvolved extremity.
   D. Auscultation
      1. Use a stethoscope to listen for blood flow in the major arteries of the neck, abdomen, groin, and extremities.
      2. Listen for a swish-like sound, which indicates fluid turbulence known as bruit; a narrow vessel lumen will produce turbulence.
   E. Blood pressure
      1. Perform measurement on both upper extremities; use a proper size cuff.
      2. Follow the techniques and procedures presented in Chapter 4.
   F. Edema
      1. Observe for and measure edema using palpation, girth, or volumetric measurements.
      2. Compare values obtained from involved extremity with values of noninvolved extremity.
      3. Remeasure periodically to determine whether edema is regressing, progressing, or static.
II. Subjective information
   A. Obtain past history of the current condition from the patient or a family member.
   B. Obtain specific information about the current condition or a previous similar or different condition and the effects or result of previous treatments.
   C. Determine personal habits that may affect the condition (i.e., eating, use of tobacco, reaction to heat or cold, sensory changes).

Adapted from O'Sullivan SB, Schmitz TJ: *Physical Rehabilitation Assessment and Treatment.* 3rd edition. Philadelphia: F.A. Davis, 1994.

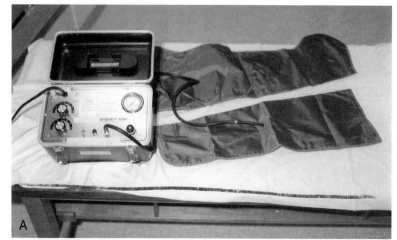

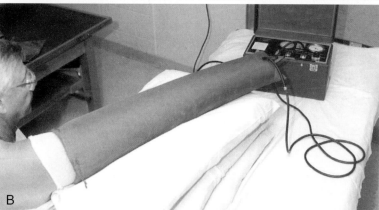

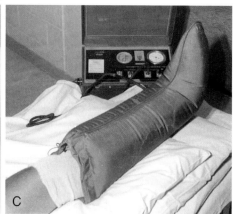

■ **FIGURE 10–8**

A, Equipment used for intermittent compression to the extremities; controls on the left side of the unit allow the time of inflation and deflation to be designated, and the dial in the upper right indicates the amount of pressure in the sleeve during inflation. *B,* Upper extremity compression with elevation of the extremity and use of stockinet. *C,* Lower extremity compression.

measuring tape (Procedure 10–7). It is recommended two garments be ordered simultaneously so one garment will be available for use while the other garment is being washed. Use of the two garments alternately will extend the life of each garment. Furthermore, replacement garments should be ordered so they will be available before the time the current garment has no therapeutic value. Instructions about the application, removal, and care of the garment are provided by the manufacturer.

Intermittent compression through the use of a mechanical pump and sleeve is a method of treatment for chronic or acute edema or swelling and venous insufficiency. Sleeves are available for the upper and lower extremity, and they are inflated and deflated with the pump (Procedure 10–8). The inflation cycle provides an external compression force to the extremity that assists to expel the edema or assists the return of venous blood from the extremity. (*Caution:* Before using compression to the lower extremity for a venous condition, arterial insufficiency and thrombophlebitis must be ruled out. If arterial insufficiency is present, the inflation phase of the intermittent compression cycle may cause additional occlusion of the arterial circulation and possibly tissue ischemia. If thrombophlebitis is present, the potential exists of causing an embolus to enter the venous system.) The patient is

positioned supine or sitting, the sleeve is applied, and the extremity is elevated above the level of the heart. (*Note:* Tubular stockinet can be applied to the person's extremity before application of the sleeve to help to maintain cleanliness of the inside of the sleeve.) The amount of pressure in the sleeve and the parameters of the cycle should be established for each patient. Generally, the maximum compression force should not exceed pressure that is slightly below the patient's diastolic blood pressure to avoid possible cardiovascular complications. Treatments may be scheduled for up to 1 hour and may be repeated several times per day. A program of mechanical intermittent compression will be advantageous to reduce the edema in an extremity before measurement for a graded compression garment. When this approach is used, the garment can be measured more accurately and will be more likely to control the residual edema. The application of low stretch compression wraps or tubular elastic gauze to the extremity after each pumping session will help to minimize redevelopment of the edema and should be performed until a permanent graded compression garment is available (see Fig. 10–8*A–C*).

In addition to the mechanical compression, the patient can be instructed to perform active pumping exercises and to elevate the extremity two or three

P R O C E D U R E   1 0 – 7
Measurement of a Pressure Gradient Garment

1. Upper extremity
   a. Seat the person and provide a support for his/her upper extremity to elevate it; expose the entire upper extremity from the top of the shoulder to the ends of the fingers.
   b. Apply the spine of the measuring tape along the length of the extremity; apply the paper strips at the specified landmarks (elbow, base of the thumb/wrist).
   c. Wrap each individual strip around the extremity; keeping it flat, in close contact with the skin, perpendicular to the spine, and parallel to the strip above and below; do not pull the strip so tight that it causes an indentation in the soft tissue; attach the strip to the spine, and follow the manufacturer's instructions for pleating the spine to ensure the garment's length will be appropriate.
   d. After all the strips are in place, use bandage scissors to cut each strip along the side of the spine that is scalloped (the side that has round indentations); it may be helpful to use cellophane tape to reinforce the attachment of each strip to the spine.
   e. Label the tape with the patient's name; indicate whether it is the left or right extremity; list any specific information or instructions regarding the fabrication; fold the tape and place it in the mailing envelope.

2. Lower extremity
   a. Position the patient supine and provide support for his/her lower extremity to elevate it from the mattress or mat; expose the lower extremity from the groin to the end of the toes. *Note:* If a leotard ("panty hose")-type garment is to be fabricated, it will be necessary to provide waist and hip measurements.
   b. Apply the spine of the measuring tape along the length of the extremity; apply the paper strips at the specified landmarks (heel/ankle).
   c. Wrap each individual strip around the extremity; follow the same procedure outlined in item C for upper extremity measurements.

continued

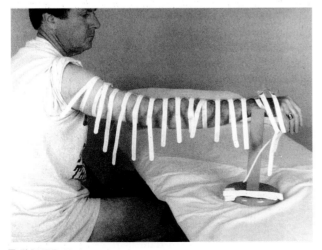

■ **FIGURE 10–9**
Application of measurement tapes for graduated compression (pressure gradient) garment; upper extremity.

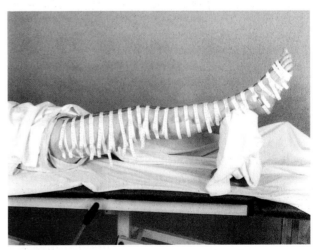

■ **FIGURE 10–10**
Application of measurement tapes for graduated compression (pressure gradient) garment; lower extremity.

continued

PROCEDURE 10–7, *continued*
> d. Follow items d and e for upper extremity measurement procedures. *Note:* Extension strips may be added to strips that are not long enough to encircle the extremity; pleats (folds) can be made on the measuring tape to adjust the length of the garment; when edema control is the goal, the extremity should be measured when the least amount of edema is present (i.e., measure early in the morning); many options and modifications are available for the garments (Figs. 10–9 and 10–10).

times per hour to assist with edema control. Isometric muscle pumping exercises for the upper extremity and active ankle pumping (i.e., repetitive dorsi/plantar flexion) for the lower extremity, with the extremity elevated and supported, are two activities that are used frequently.

It is important to observe and converse with the person periodically during each treatment session. Complaints of numbness, tingling, or other forms of paresthesia by the patient may indicate the treatment should be terminated. To conclude a treatment session, the sleeve should be in the deflated mode so the sleeve can be removed. If the treatment is terminated with the sleeve inflated, disconnect the hose attached to the control unit from the sleeve. Pressure to the outside of the sleeve will cause it to deflate; when the sleeve has been removed, remove and discard the stockinet. Observe and palpate the extremity and measure the circumference (girth) periodically if lymphedema was the condition being treated. Be observant for skin or circulatory changes that may have occurred due to the treatment; document your activities, observations, and measurements as necessary.

These pump units may be rented by or loaned to a person to use at home, and he/she should be provided with written instructions and directions about use of the unit. Precautions that he/she should follow and a method of communication between the patient and caregiver should be established. In addition, periodic reevaluation of the person's response to or effect of the home treatments should be performed by the caregiver. Contraindications to the use of the pump are severe arterial insufficiency, cutaneous infection, acute dermatitis, wet dermatosis, and a recent thrombosis. These symptoms may also contraindicate the use of support stockings for vascular conditions.

PROCEDURE 10–8
Intermittent Compression Pump

1. Explain the procedure to the patient and obtain consent; measure the blood pressure; examine the extremity; measure the circumference (girth) of the extremity if treating edema.

2. Position and drape the patient according to his/her diagnosis or condition and extremity involved; apply tubular stockinet and then apply the sleeve to the extremity.

3. Adjust the controls of the unit as necessary (i.e., pressure, inflation-to-deflation ratio); turn on the unit.

4. Periodically monitor the patient during the treatment session.

5. To conclude the treatment, turn off the unit when the sleeve is deflated. *Note:* If the unit is turned off when it is inflated, it can be deflated by detaching the inflation hose of the unit from the sleeve. Remove the sleeve and stockinet; discard the stockinet.

6. Examine the extremity; measure the circumference (girth), if treating edema; document your activities and findings.

DRESSINGS AND BANDAGES

The composition of a dressing and its bandage varies, but in many instances several layers are involved. As an example, a topical medication may be applied directly to the wound, with a nonabsorbent material (e.g., a Telfa pad) placed over the medication along with a second layer consisting of a cotton gauze pad; for large wounds or wounds that exhibit excessive drainage, a third layer of an absorbent material may be used. These three layers comprise the dressing.

A fourth layer of a material such as roller gauze and a fifth layer of a material such as an elastic wrap may be used as a bandage. Depending on the purpose of or need for the dressing, the type of wound, and the purpose of or need for the bandage, various layers may be omitted or added. However, you should be able to differentiate the purposes or functions of a dressing and a bandage.

The functions of a dressing are to prevent additional wound contamination, keep microorganisms in the wound from infecting other sites, prevent further injury to the wound, apply pressure to control hemorrhage, absorb wound drainage, and assist in wound healing.

The functions of a bandage are to keep the dressing in place, maintain a barrier between the dressing and the environment, provide external pressure to control swelling, provide support or stability to an area, hold splints in place, and assist the dressing in accomplishing its functions.

Removal of a Dressing The caregiver should presume that the wound and dressing are contaminated and therefore should apply nonsterile gloves before removing the dressing for self-protection. Once the gloved hand has touched the dressing or the wound, it must not touch any other object, especially the patient's or caregiver's skin, the clean (sterile) dressing, or any other object in the area. Once the dressing has been removed, it and the gloves should be disposed of in a closed container or nonporous bag. The caregiver should remove the gloves without touching the outside of either glove with his/her exposed skin as described previously. Immediately after the removal and disposal of the gloves, the caregiver must wash his/her hands to further reduce the possibility of cross-contamination.

To remove a nonadherent dressing, the bandage may be removed independently of the dressing or with the dressing. If you are unfamiliar with the site and shape of the wound, request information about it from the patient or other personnel who are familiar with it. The patient may be able to indicate the size and location of the wound on his/her corresponding

extremity or on the caregiver's extremity. Bandage scissors are used to cut through the various layers of the bandage. The blunt tip of the scissors is placed under the edge of the material so the tip is next to the patient's skin. The initial cut should be made a safe distance from any edge or from the center of the wound. If you are uncertain where or how to cut the dressing, attempt to unwrap or remove the bandage without using scissors to expose the dressing; then carefully remove the dressing layers. As you remove the bandage and dressing materials, mentally note how many layers there are, the materials used, and the sequence of application of the materials. By doing this, you will be prepared to reapply the dressing properly.

The deepest layer of the dressing should be removed by carefully loosening and freeing the dressing from the wound edges and gently pulling it toward the center of the wound; this method least disrupts the healing process. After the dressing has been removed, all dressing materials and your gloves should be disposed of into a closed container as described previously, and you should wash your hands before you perform any other activity (Fig. 10–11).

When the wound has been exposed, its condition should be evaluated carefully (Box 10–14). The caregiver should gently and carefully palpate the tissue in the area of the wound to determine the following:

1. Temperature of the wound tissue in comparison with the temperature of tissue away from the wound on the same or another extremity.

2. Tone of the tissue.

3. Integrity of the wound edges or the area of healing.

4. Condition of the skin (e.g., dry, moist, pliable, or taut).

5. Sensory response or capacity of the tissue.

Your observations and findings should be reported and documented using specific and objective terms. A nurse or physician should be notified if you observe adverse changes or a regression in the healing process or condition of the wound since your previous observation of the wound.

To remove a dressing that adheres to the wound, it may be necessary to soak the bandage and dressing first to reduce disruption of the healing surface of the wound when the dressing is removed. This can be accomplished by soaking the area in a basin, whirlpool, tub, or other similar container. An alternative method is to pour water or a saline solution over the bandage and dressing repeatedly until the hardened exudate has softened. The actual removal of the dressing should be performed as described previously. If a whirlpool is used, the turbine should not be activated until the dressing has been removed from the water. Removal of the dressing material before the turbine is

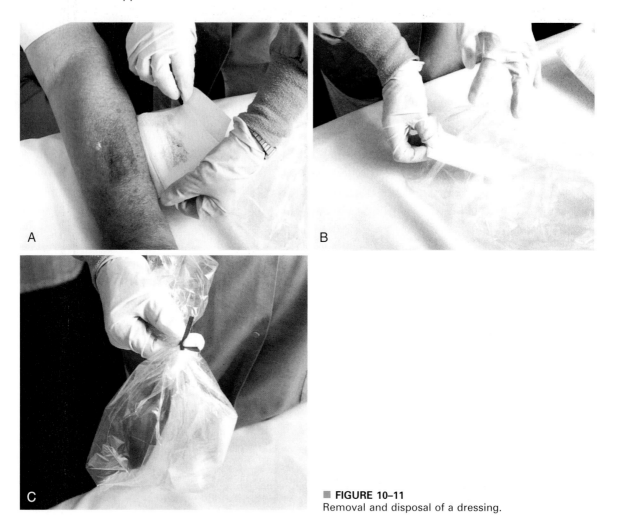

■ **FIGURE 10–11**
Removal and disposal of a dressing.

turned on will prevent it from being drawn into the turbine or occluding the drain when the water is released. If edema is associated with the wound, the use of a whirlpool may increase production and decrease removal of excess interstitial fluid (edema) because of the warmth of the water and the dependent position of the extremity when it is immersed.

Application of a Sterile Dressing After the removal of the bandage and dressing, the wound may require care to enhance its healing. Before a new dressing can be applied, necrotic tissue may have to be removed from the surface of the wound through the process of debridement. Debridement may be accomplished by using a gauze pad to gently rub the surface of the wound, running water over the surface of the wound, or using a scalpel or scissors to excise the necrotic tissue. A description of the specific methods and techniques used to debride a wound is beyond the scope of this text. Debridement may or may not require the approval of a physician before it can be performed by a caregiver other than a physician. In some situations, only the physician will be permitted to perform wound debridement.

A sterile field, along with the appropriate wound care materials, should be established, and the caregiver should wear sterile, protective clothing appropriate for the patient's condition. If it is necessary to dry the patient's skin before the dressing is applied, a sterile towel should be used. The patient should be positioned so that he/she is comfortable and the wound is accessible (Fig. 10–12*A–C*).

Medications can be applied directly to the wound or to the dressing material and then onto the wound. Medication in a tube or jar should be applied to a cotton swab, gauze pad, or other acceptable applicator and then applied to the wound. The sterile applicator must not contact the unsterile exterior of the tube or jar, and care must be used to avoid contaminating the contents of the tube or jar with the applicator once it has contacted the patient (see Fig. 10–12*D,E*). Therefore, a new swab or gauze pad should be used each time the medication is obtained from the tube or jar.

Select the appropriate dressing material and apply it directly to the medication base over the wound. Be certain you maintain its sterility as it is applied by handling it with sterile gloves or sterile forceps (see Fig. 10–12*F*). Once the initial layer has been applied

Wound Evaluation

1. Observe and palpate the condition of the skin surrounding the wound; record your findings.
2. Observe and record the color of the tissue surrounding the wound.
3. Observe and record the color and appearance of the wound.
4. If an exudate is present, note the type and amount.
5. Determine whether there is an odor; if so, indicate what the odor is and how pervasive it is.
6. Determine whether there are signs of inflammation or infection.
7. Determine whether there are signs of pressure or irritation.
8. Determine whether there is edema or swelling; if so, observe where it is located and in what amount.
9. State the location and measure the size and depth of the wound.
10. Determine the type of wound or lesion (e.g., abrasion, puncture, laceration, burn, incision, ulceration).

over the wound, the upper layers of the dressing and the bandage do not need to be applied using sterile technique. Cover the dressing with the appropriate bandage, and evaluate the tension, location, and coverage of the bandage. The bandage should have sufficient tension to secure the dressing and control edema, if edema is present or anticipated, but it must not occlude or impede the local circulation. You may have to question the patient about the tension, or you can slide a finger under the outer edges of the bandage to determine the tension force.

Some suggestions for the proper application and evaluation of a bandage are listed in Box 10–15. Some indicators of an improperly applied or functioning bandage are the following:

1. If the color of the segment distal to the bandage becomes excessively red, blue, or pale, the bandage is usually too tight and is constricting the local circulation.
2. If the patient complains of pain, numbness, tingling, or a burning sensation in the segment distal to the bandage, the bandage is usually too tight and is affecting local neural receptors.
3. If the exposed distal segment feels cold to the touch when compared with the similar, opposite segment,

the bandage is usually too tight proximally and is constricting the flow of arterial blood to the area.
4. If edema develops in the segment distal to the bandage, the bandage is usually too tight and is constricting the local lymphatic and venous circulation.
5. If the bandage changes position, it is usually too loose.

When any of these conditions occur, the bandage should be removed and reapplied. The patient should be informed of these problems and should become responsible for monitoring the bandage when he/she is not being treated or under the direct care of another person. After the bandage has been applied, the caregiver should evaluate the bandage to determine how well it has been applied. The proximally and distally exposed areas of tissue should be observed and palpated; the patient should be questioned about the sensations he/she perceives in the extremity; and the tension of the bandage should be tested. This last activity can be accomplished by simultaneously inserting a finger beneath the deepest layer of the bandage at the proximal and distal edges of the bandage. The pressure should be essentially equal at both sites or slightly greater distally than proximally.

The patient or a family member should be instructed to evaluate the bandage periodically and to remove and reapply it when any of the signs or symptoms of improper application are evident. The length of time the bandage should remain in place; when it should be routinely removed, such as for bathing, for exercise, or if it becomes wet; and how long it can remain removed before it is reapplied should be explained to the patient. You should instruct him/her how to remove and apply the bandage. By observing his/her performance, you can be more certain he/she understands and can perform the procedure. Written instructions may be useful for him/her and the family.

Bandages may be applied and used for purposes other than to cover and protect a dressing. Additional applications and uses, as well as types of bandage materials, are presented in Chapter 9.

CONTROL OF DISEASE IN THE HEALTH CARE ENVIRONMENT

There are many resources available to obtain information about the prevention of disease transmission and the spread of pathogenic microorganisms. Much of the information is not new, but in recent years a greater emphasis has been placed on the concept that each patient should be treated as if he/she had a transmissible or infectious disease. The spread

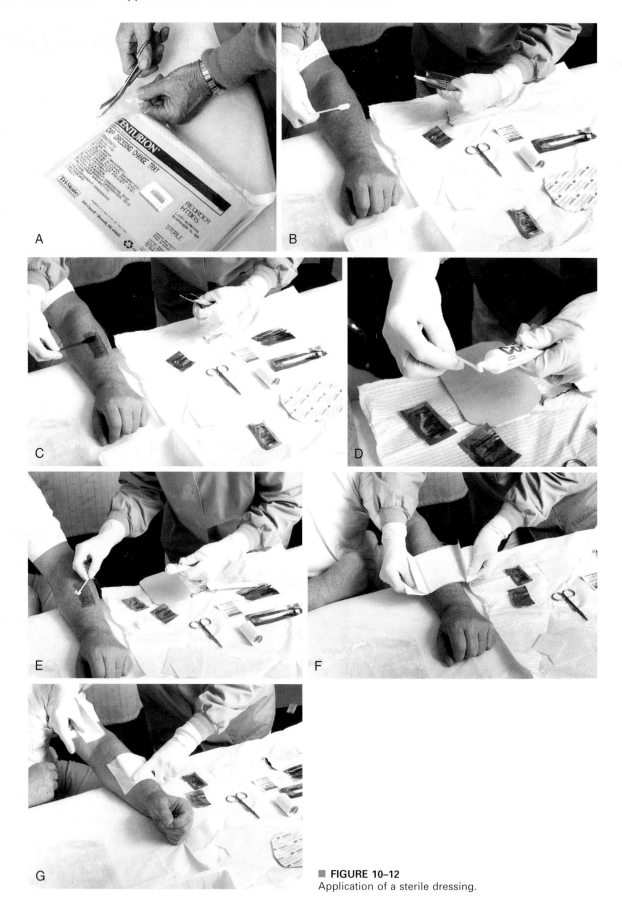

■ **FIGURE 10–12**
Application of a sterile dressing.

BOX 10–15

Guidelines for Applying Bandages

1. The tension at each turn of the bandage should be equal unless edema is to be controlled. To control edema, the general guideline is to have greater pressure distally than proximally so the edema is passively moved toward the proximal areas of the extremity. This can be accomplished with a low stretch compression bandage providing gradually decreasing pressure from distal to proximal.

2. Spiral turns are preferred over circular turns because they are less likely to occlude the local circulation.

3. Each turn should overlap approximately one half of the previous turn to produce pressure and protect the wound.

4. Avoid wrinkles in the deep layers of the bandage to reduce unnecessary local pressure to the skin caused by the wrinkles.

5. Bony prominences should be wrapped with caution to avoid excessive pressure; it may be helpful to pad around, but not over, the prominence to reduce pressure to it.

6. The patient's fingers or toes should not be included in the bandage unless the wound is located on them. They should be visible so they can be observed for signs of excessive pressure such as edema, cyanosis, or temperature change. The patient should be instructed to inform the caregiver if numbness, tingling, or paresthesia develops in his/her fingers or toes.

7. Avoid bandaging techniques that cause or create direct contact between two skin surfaces. Use a small gauze or cotton pad between the fingers and toes to separate them. Failure to separate a skin-to-skin contact may lead to skin breakdown as a result of the effects of the accumulation of moisture and heat.

8. Do not secure the bandage directly over the wound, over a bony prominence, or where the patient's body weight is apt to rest on the item securing the bandage. If tape is used to secure the bandage, it should not completely encircle the extremity or the segment where the wound is located, and it should not be applied to the patient's skin if the bandage will be removed frequently. Safety pins and metal clips must be applied carefully to avoid injury to the patient during and after application. When a safety pin is used, the caregiver should insert a finger under the bandage to elevate it off the patient's skin and avoid puncturing the skin with the pin.

9. The bandage used to cover a dressing should extend approximately 1 inch above and below the dressing.

10. The bandage should be removed and reapplied if it turns, slides down or up, becomes wet, or becomes soiled with drainage or if the patient complains of discomfort. Whenever the bandage is removed and the dressing is changed, you should observe the wound and the surrounding tissue.

of and serious consequences associated with AIDS, which is caused by HIV, and hepatitis, especially the type caused by the hepatitis B virus (HBV), have created the need for health care workers and others who may have close, personal contact with a person with one of these two diseases to use caution during contact. Both diseases are life threatening. Hepatitis B is more easily contracted but can be prevented with a vaccine. Currently there is no vaccine to prevent AIDS, nor is there any satisfactory treatment for AIDS. Because these two life-threatening diseases have be-

come more prevalant and are spread through contact with various body fluids, the emphasis on cleanliness and sterile techniques has increased.

Some excellent and basic sources of information about infection control are the Centers for Disease Control and Prevention (CDC); Occupational Safety and Health Administration (OSHA); Environmental Protection Agency (EPA); city, county, and state health departments; and the infection control department, or a similar department, of a local hospital. Furthermore, seminars and other types of continuing education programs, including hospital-based programs for employees regarding AIDS and hepatitis, are available to health care personnel. Many brochures, textbooks, pamphlets, newspapers, magazines, and visual aids contain information about these and other diseases; some of these sources are listed in the Bibliography.

Individual institutions and agencies have enacted policies and procedures to control the spread or transmission of infection and disease. The caregiver and all other persons who treat patients, handle soiled patient linen, remove wound dressings, or collect disposed items (i.e., needles and other sharps) used to treat patients must become familiar with and adhere to established policies and procedures and develop proper personal habits for maximal protection.

Patients must be protected from nosocomial infections that can be spread from patient to patient or to a given patient by a caregiver who is careless or does not follow accepted infection control measures. Basic measures of prevention include frequent hand washings (before and after treatment of each patient), the use of proper hand-washing technique, and the wearing of appropriate protective clothing such as gloves, gown, cap, and mask. A caregiver may try to avoid one or more of these measures because of a perceived lack of time, poor access to the items, or poor location of the sink; a lack of proper-sized apparel; dermatitis as a result of frequent washing or a reaction to the available soap or detergent; a lack of understanding of the importance of using infection control methods for each patient; or poor motivation to comply with the policies and procedures for other reasons. Therefore, it may be necessary for the employer or department supervisor to reduce as many of these factors as possible, whether they are real or perceived, to make it more convenient for the caregiver to comply with the policies and procedures.

In 1985, the CDC developed the strategy of "universal blood and body fluid precautions" (or "universal precautions") to address concerns regarding the transmission of HIV in the health care setting. The concept stresses that *all patients should be assumed to be infectious for HIV and other blood-borne pathogens.* In a health care setting, universal precautions should be followed when any worker is exposed to blood, selected other body fluids (peritoneal fluid, pleural fluid, synovial fluid, cerebrospinal fluid, semen, and vaginal secretions), or any body fluid visibly contaminated with blood. HIV transmission has not been documented after exposure to body fluids such as feces, nasal secretions, sputum, sweat, tears, urine, or vomitus, but HBV can be transmitted by many of these fluids or body waste products; therefore, the caregiver may need to protect himself/herself when handling these fluids to reduce the transmission of other pathogenic microorganisms, and the use of universal precautions is recommended when contact with

these items is likely to occur. Exposure, as defined by the CDC, means contact with blood or other body fluids through percutaneous inoculation or contact with an open wound, nonintact skin, or a mucous membrane (Box 10–16).*

DISINFECTION, DECONTAMINATION, AND DISPOSAL

Careful handling is necessary to prevent injuries from needles, scalpel blades, and other sharp instruments or equipment during their use, disposal, cleaning, or handling during or after patient care. Needles should not be uncapped until they are used and should not be manipulated by hand when uncapped. They should be placed in a puncture-proof container after use, along with scalpel blades and other sharp items.

Hands and other skin surfaces should be washed immediately and thoroughly after they have been contaminated by blood, wound drainage, or other body fluids to which universal precautions apply, even if gloves have been worn. The gloves should be removed by being careful not to contact your skin with the external surface of the gloves when the gloves are removed. The soiled gloves should be disposed of in a nonporous container; the same pair of gloves must not be worn to treat more than one patient.

Soiled linen should be handled as little as possible and with minimal movement to prevent contamination of the air and the persons who handle the linen. It should be disposed of and transported in bags that are leak proof and clearly designated as containing potentially contaminated linen. The risk of disease transmission from soiled linen contaminated with pathogenic microorganisms is negligible, but reasonable care should be taken when such linen is handled.

Protective clothing contaminated with blood or other body fluids subject to universal precautions should be disposed of and transported in bags or other containers that are nonporous and leak proof. Any person who is involved with the bagging, transporting, or laundering of contaminated clothing should wear gloves.

Infective waste products such as feces, urine, bulk blood, or suctioned fluid can be disposed of by carefully pouring them into a drain or toilet connected to a sanitary sewer, if this is permitted by institutional or local public health policies and procedures. In some instances, the waste product may have to be placed in a plastic bag that can be sealed so it can be transported. Individual bedpans and urinals, if not made of

---

*This information was obtained from *Morbidity and Mortality Weekly Report,* Volume 38, Number S–5–S–6, 1989.

BOX 10–16

Universal Precautions

Universal precautions represent a system of infection control in which it is assumed that every direct contact with a patient's body fluids is potentially infectious.

1. Barriers
   a. Gloves
   b. Protective clothing
   c. Eye protection
   d. Face shield
   e. Mask
   f. Mouthpiece, intubation device, resuscitation bag during CPR

2. Hand care
   a. Avoid wearing artificial fingernails; they may separate from the real nail, producing a pocket for pathogen growth.
   b. Always wear gloves when treating a patient who places you at risk to contact a body fluid, especially blood; avoid contact with the outer surface of the gloves when they are removed.
   c. Thoroughly wash your hands before and after patient care, especially if your hands were in contact with a body fluid.

3. Sharps (needles, scalpel blades)
   a. Dispose of all sharps in a puncture-proof container immediately after their use.
   b. Do not uncap or expose needles until they are needed.
   c. Use caution when you handle and dispose of the item to avoid wounding yourself.

4. Miscellaneous
   a. Avoid eating, drinking, smoking, applying cosmetics or lip balm, and handling contact lenses in a patient care area.
   b. Avoid hand contact with mucous membranes of your eyes, nose, mouth, or ears.
   c. Handle all linen carefully, especially linen soiled by a patient's body fluid or waste; dispose of and transport it in the proper bag, hamper, or container.
   d. Avoid unnecessary contact with a patient who places you at risk to contact a body fluid or waste product, especially his/her blood.
   e. Report incidents of contact with a patient's body fluid or waste product on an unprotected area of your body; seek immediate assistance if a direct blood-to-blood contact occurs between you and a patient.

a disposable material, must be cleaned thoroughly and sterilized before use by another patient. Persons who are involved with the handling of these waste products should wear gloves, and a gown may be necessary if soiling of the handler's clothing is anticipated.

Protective clothing and apparel should be available to all caregivers and other personnel who treat, transport, or handle items used for the patient whose condition requires the use of universal precautions. Items that should be available are gloves, either disposable or reusable; gowns; masks; and protective eyewear, such as eye shields or safety glasses. The necessary items should be applied before treatment of the patient or before items associated with the patient are handled. Disposable gloves usually do not provide as much protection as individually sized, reusable gloves.

Disposable gloves are usually one-size-fits-all gloves and will not conform closely to the wearer's hands and wrists. Furthermore, these gloves can slip easily and can be removed inadvertently during patient care. However, they can form an effective barrier between the caregiver's hands and the patient when applied and used properly. *Remember:* Regardless of the type of gloves you use, be careful when removing them so you avoid any contact between the outside of the glove and your skin. Gloves should be worn routinely in situations in which it is necessary to control bleeding, perform a venipuncture, perform oral or nasal suctioning, perform endotrachael intubation, change a contaminated dressing, and handle or clean contaminated instruments or equipment. Usually it is not necessary to wear gloves to measure blood pressure or temperature. However, if there are other reasons to wear gloves when performing these two procedures, they should be worn.

A gown, mask, and protective eyewear should be worn when there is spurting blood and in any other situation in which splashing of blood is anticipated or expected. Again, these examples are related to the patient for whom universal precautions are in effect. There can be several other reasons or patient conditions that could necessitate the wearing of protective clothing. Remember to follow specific institutional or agency policies and procedures regarding the use of protective clothing.

Spills of body fluids should be cleaned as soon as possible, and the surface where the spill occurred should be cleansed with a solution of one part 5.25% sodium hypochlorite (bleach) diluted in 10 parts water or with an EPA-approved hospital disinfectant. Towels or linen used to clean up the spill must be disposed of properly, and the person involved in cleaning the spill should wear gloves and may have to consider whether a gown should be worn. Generally, it is better to be overprotected than underprotected when dealing with body fluids.

OSHA has established regulations for health care facilities designed to protect the employees of these facilities. The facility has the responsibility to provide its employees with information and instruction in techniques to protect themselves from infectious diseases, especially blood-borne diseases. Specifically, each health care facility must do the following:

1. Educate its employees on the methods of transmission and the prevention of HBV and HIV.

2. Provide safe and adequate protective equipment, and teach the employees where it is located and how to use it.

3. Teach the employees about work practices used to prevent occupational transmission of disease, including, but not limited to, universal precautions, proper handling of patient specimens and linens, proper cleaning of body fluid spills, and proper waste disposal.

4. Provide proper containers for the disposal of waste and sharp items, and teach the employees the color coding system used to distinguish infectious waste.

5. Offer the HBV vaccine to employees who are at substantial risk of occupational exposure to HBV.

6. Provide education and follow-up care to employees who are exposed to communicable disease.

OSHA also has outlined the responsibilities of health care employees. These include the following:

1. Use protective equipment and clothing provided by the facility whenever the employee contacts, or anticipates contact, with body fluids.

2. Dispose of waste in proper containers, using knowledge and understanding of the handling of infectious waste and color-coded bags or containers.

3. Dispose of sharp instruments and needles into proper containers without attempting to recap, bend, break, or otherwise manipulate them before disposal.

4. Keep the work and patient care area clean.

5. Wash his/her hands immediately after removing gloves and at all other times required by hospital or agency policy.

6. Immediately report any exposures such as needle sticks or blood splashes or any personal illnesses to his/her supervisor and receive instruction about any further follow-up action.

Decontamination There are several methods that can be used to clean or decontaminate equipment or a surface area. By definition, *decontamination* means "to remove, inactivate, or destroy blood-borne pathogens on a surface or item to the point where they are no longer capable of transmitting infectious particles and the surface or item is rendered safe for handling, use, or disposal."*

Sterilization *Sterilization* is used to destroy all forms of microbial life, including high numbers of bacterial spores. An item can be sterilized by being subjected to steam under pressure, or autoclaved; by being subjected to ethylene oxide, a gas; by being subjected to a dry heat source; or by being immersed in an EPA-approved chemical sterilant for 6 to 10 hours or according to the manufacturer's instructions. This last method should be used only for instruments or equipment that are impossible to sterilize with heat, usually instruments or items that penetrate skin, such as needles or scalpel blades, or that contact areas of the body that are not contaminated.

Disinfection High-level *disinfection* destroys all forms of microbial life except high numbers of bacterial spores. Hot water pasteurization, at 80°C to 100°C for 30 minutes, or exposure to an EPA-approved sterilant chemical as mentioned previously for 10 to 45 minutes or as directed by the manufacturer are the common methods used for this type of disinfection. This method can be used for reusable instruments or items that come into contact with mucous membranes (e.g., endotracheal tubes).

Intermediate-level disinfection destroys most viruses, most fungi, vegetative bacteria, and the tuberculosis bacterium, but it does not kill bacterial spores. EPA-approved hospital disinfectant chemical germicides labeled for tuberculocidal activity and commer-

---

*Rules and Regulations. Federal Register. December 6, 1991; 56:64175.

cially available hard-surface germicides or solutions that contain at least 500 ppm of free available chlorine are the solutions most commonly used to accomplish this type of disinfection. Common household bleach in a solution of approximately ¼ cup per gallon of water will produce an appropriate solution.

Low-level disinfection destroys most bacteria, some viruses, and some fungi but it does not kill the tuberculosis bacterium or bacterial spores. EPA-approved hospital disinfectants without a label claim for tuberculocidal activity are used for this type of disinfection. These types of agents are excellent cleaners and can be used for routine housekeeping or to remove soiling in the absence of visible blood contamination.

Environmental disinfection is used to clean and disinfect surfaces that have become soiled and is done by using any cleaner or disinfectant that is intended for environmental use. Environmental surfaces include floors, woodwork, mat or treatment table pads, countertops, sliding or transfer boards, and sinks.

When liquids are used as cleaning agents, the person who uses them should protect his/her skin from repeated or prolonged contact with the agent by wearing gloves and other protective clothing as necessary.

Any item that is to be disinfected or sterilized should be cleaned thoroughly first to remove residual organic matter such as blood, excrement, or tissue. Different microorganisms will require different methods and levels of disinfection. The CDC, the local health department, or a hospital infection control department can be contacted for current information regarding the best method to use and the level necessary to destroy or control various microorganisms.

The patient's room and the treatment area should be cleaned routinely by housekeeping personnel using EPA-approved cleansing products according to institutional policies and procedures. It is unlikely that the pathogenic microorganisms that are usually present on the walls, floors, carpet, furniture, and other objects in the area will be transmitted to persons or patients. Simple actions such as disposing of linen that drops onto the floor; avoiding shaking or rapidly moving linen, which could create air currents and lift microorganisms from the floor onto clothing; avoiding placing contaminated linen or protective clothing against your clothing to reduce the transfer of microorganisms; and promptly discarding dressings and soiled linen according to institutional or agency policies and procedures will assist in reducing the transmission of microorganisms.

Protective Clothing As described previously, protective clothing is recommended to safeguard the caregiver and the patient when it is necessary to reduce the transmission of pathogens from the caregiver to the patient, or vice versa. Gloves offer protection to the caregiver's hands to reduce the likelihood that he/she will become infected with microorganisms from an infected patient. They also reduce the likelihood that the patient will receive microorganisms from the caregiver and reduce the possibility that a colony of microorganisms will develop on the caregiver's hands that could be transmitted to patients or to other personnel. Suggestions on the application, use, and removal of gloves have been presented elsewhere in this chapter.

The mask is designed to reduce the spread of microorganisms that are transmitted through the air. It protects the wearer from the inhalation of particles or droplets that may contain pathogens. It also acts as a filter to reduce the transmission of pathogens from the wearer to the patient. The proper techniques for application, positioning, and removal of the mask have been presented elsewhere in this chapter.

A gown is used to protect the wearer's clothing from becoming contaminated or soiled by contact with a contaminant. It also provides a barrier to decrease the transmission of microorganisms from the caregiver's clothing to the patient or to his/her environment. Techniques for the proper application and removal of the gown have been presented elsewhere in this chapter.

Protective eyewear, such as goggles, facial shield, or eyewear with side shields, should be worn to prevent fluids from entering the eyes. It is especially important that protective eyewear be worn when blood splashes or spurts are likely to occur and when other body fluids are likely to be sprayed or splashed onto the face.

Disposal Instruments and equipment used to treat a patient should be cleaned or disposed of according to institutional or agency policies and procedures. Contaminated reusable equipment should be placed carefully in a container, labeled, and returned to the appropriate department for sterilization. Contaminated disposable items should be placed carefully in a container, labeled, and disposed of according to institutional or agency policies and procedures.

Anyone who handles any of these instruments or equipment should wear gloves and should wash his/her hands before and after the gloves have been applied and removed. Needles, scalpels, and other sharp instruments should be placed in puncture-proof containers. No attempt should be made to recap, bend, or break the needle before it is disposed. The ear tips of a "community" or departmental stethoscope should be wiped with alcohol before and after each use. In some instances, it may be necessary to clean the diaphragm with alcohol. If the cuff of the sphygmomanometer becomes contaminated, it should be disinfected in a manner similar to that used for clothing items. Each patient in isolation should have his/her own individual thermometer. If this is not possible, the thermometer must be sterilized or receive high-level disinfection before it is used for another patient.

Contaminated or soiled linen should be disposed of with minimal handling, sorting, and movement. It can be bagged in an appropriate bag and labeled before transport to the laundry, or the bag can be color coded to indicate the type or condition of linen it contains.

Contaminated dressings, bandages, materials, paper items, and other disposable items should be properly placed in a nonporous container or bag, labeled, and disposed of according to institutional or agency policies and procedures.

Other contaminated items such as toys, magazines, personal hygiene articles, dishes, and eating utensils should be disposed of or disinfected and should not be used by others until they have been disinfected.

These precautions require greater emphasis when caring for patients whose susceptibility to infection is greatest. Patients with extensive burns, with a disease that compromises the immune system, or who are receiving chemotherapy or body irradiation are examples of patients who are more susceptible to transmitted pathogens. Protection of patients from pathogens is important for all patients but is particularly important for patients who have a reduced capacity to resist or overcome infection.

SUMMARY

The caregiver may be required or find it necessary to treat a patient who has a transmissible pathogen or who needs to be protected from pathogens that may be in the environment. Therefore, the caregiver must be aware of methods he/she can use to protect both the patient and himself/herself. The most effective method for the caregiver to use to reduce the transmission of pathogens is to routinely wash his/her hands. Other methods include maintaining a barrier between the caregiver and the patient and to dispose of dressings, sharps, and contaminated items properly. Most hospitals require all employees to adhere to the procedures established in the CDC's universal precautions for blood-borne pathogens.

The caregiver should be able to apply and remove a dressing to protect the patient and himself/herself from contamination. The method of selecting the appropriate dressing and its application should be

known by the caregiver so proper wound care will be provided.

Each institution has the responsibility to protect its employees from occupational exposure and transmission of pathogens. The institution's employees have the responsibility to follow the institution's policies and procedures regarding infection control. The desired outcome is to protect patients, visitors, and employees from contracting or transmitting pathogens. Information about the use of aseptic techniques and protective clothing, the proper handling of dressings and bandages, and methods to control the spread of disease in the hospital or a similar health care setting has been provided.

■ SELF-STUDY/DISCUSSION ACTIVITIES

1. Explain the difference between medical and surgical asepsis.

2. Describe at least five signs or symptoms of an improperly applied bandage, and state a corrective action for each.

3. Describe at least four instructions or precautions you should give a patient to whom you have applied a bandage.

4. List the four rules of asepsis, and indicate the importance or significance of each rule.

5. Describe and demonstrate how you would evaluate a bandage's tension.

6. Describe how you would evaluate a wound at the time a dressing is changed.

7. Explain your duties or obligations when you treat a patient in isolation and when you treat a patient in protective isolation.

8. Describe the principles you would use to establish a sterile field.

9. Demonstrate the sequence you would use to apply and remove protective clothing when treating a patient in isolation and when treating a patient in protective isolation.

10. Explain the concept and principles associated with universal precautions, and describe the actions you would perform to comply with those principles when you provide patient care or treatment.

11. Demonstrate how to measure a person for a graded compression garment for the upper and lower extremity.

Chapter 11

■ Incidents and
■ Emergencies

OBJECTIVES

After studying this chapter, the reader will be able to:

1 Explain basic, immediate actions to take after selected types of patient injury or acute illnesses.

2 Describe precautions to apply to improve safety and reduce patient and employee injury in the treatment setting.

3 Differentiate between heat exhaustion and heat stroke through the observation of signs and symptoms and the application of appropriate treatment.

4 Differentiate between an insulin reaction and acidosis through the observation of signs and symptoms and the application of appropriate treatment.

5 Differentiate between autonomic hyperreflexia and postural (orthostatic) hypotension through the observation and measurement of various signs and symptoms and the application of appropriate treatment.

6 Identify the signs and symptoms of choking and apply the Heimlich maneuver.

7 Analyze patient care activities and determine the need to modify, reduce, or discontinue treatment.

8 Describe at least five ways or means to maintain personal and patient safety.

9 Identify factors to consider to maintain a safe treatment environment.

Acidosis: A pathologic condition resulting from the accumulation of acid or depletion of the alkaline reserve in the blood and body tissues; characterized by an increase in hydrogen ion concentration.

Autonomic hyperreflexia (dysreflexia): An uninhibited and exaggerated reflex of the autonomic nervous system as a result of a stimulus.

Cardiac arrest: The sudden and often unexpected stoppage of effective heart action.

Cardiopulmonary resuscitation (CPR): The reestablishment of heart and lung action as indicated for cardiac arrest.

Convulsion: A series of involuntary contractions of the voluntary muscles.

Emergency medical technician (EMT): A person trained to manage the emergency care of sick or injured persons during transport to a hospital or at the scene of injury.

Fracture: A break in the continuity of a bone.

Insulin: A double-chain protein hormone formed from proinsulin in the beta cells of the pancreatic islets of Langerhans.

Laceration: A wound produced by the tearing of body tissue, as distinguished from a cut or an incision.

Orthostatic/postural hypotension: A fall in blood pressure associated with dizziness, syncope, and blurred vision that occurs on standing or when standing motionless in a fixed position.

Patent: Open, unobstructed, or not closed.

Seizure: A convulsion or attack, as in epilepsy.

Shock: Acute peripheral circulatory failure caused by derangement of circulatory control or loss of circulating fluid.

Sternum: A plate of bone forming the middle of the anterior wall of the thorax; the breast bone.

Vasoconstriction: A decrease in the caliber of blood vessels.

Vasodilation: An increase in the caliber of blood vessels.

Xiphoid: The distal portion of the sternum.

INTRODUCTION

All employees of the patient care area have the responsibility to provide and maintain a safe environment for patient care. In free-standing service units, or the provision of services in a patient's home, the caregivers and employees should be qualified to provide immediate emergency care. Hospital caregivers and employees should be aware of and follow departmental or institutional policies and procedures regarding emergency situations. In either situation employees should know how to contact and request assistance (e.g., the use of 911 or local fire, emergency medical, or police telephone numbers and special emergency terms such as "code blue," "code red," and "Captain Thermo").

All caregivers should be informed of their required legal responsibilities and limitations in providing emergency aid, especially as they relate to the "Good Samaritan" statutes of the state in which they work. In some states the employee may be more liable for his/her actions when emergency care is provided by the employee in a hospital or other similar setting where medical equipment or support personnel are available. In most states there is some legal protection for the person who causes additional injury or trauma when he/she provides emergency care, particularly if the aid was a lifesaving or life-sustaining measure. A review of specific professional practice acts and other state statutes may be necessary to determine one's emergency care responsibility in that state.

It should be recognized that the potential for patient and employee injuries becomes greater under certain conditions. Some examples are when there are too few personnel available to manage the patients in the area, too few qualified personnel, excessively busy personnel, personnel who are inattentive to patient needs, poorly maintained or defective pieces of equipment, inadequately trained personnel, and personnel who display careless behavior. The supervisor and all employees should be especially alert when changes in personnel occur. Examples of such personnel changes include shift changes; times when some personnel are on vacation or ill, and no replacement personnel are provided; during a holiday or weekend, when fewer personnel are apt to be used; and when several acutely ill patients are being treated simultaneously.

Some general types of patients that may necessitate closer attention and care by the service unit personnel include elderly patients; debilitated patients; patients with decreased mental competence or cognitive deterioration; patients whose physiologic status has been compromised as a result of extensive burns, a spinal cord injury, a chronic respiratory condition, an acute or chronic cardiac condition, or acute or chronic diabetes; psychologically or emotionally disturbed patients; very young patients; febrile patients; and patients who have been injured or involved in an unusual incident during a previous hospitalization or treatment program.

Caregivers should be aware of and prepared to respond properly to an improper referral or prescription by refusing to treat the patient. Precautions or contraindications associated with various treatments should be recognized and applied judiciously to reduce the incidence of injury or trauma to the patient or caregiver. In addition, the caregiver should understand and be aware of the potential problems that may develop in a patient secondary to the primary diagnosis, and more care should be used when treating the person with a serious illness or extensive trauma. Supportive personnel should be supervised and guided so that they are not requested or expected to perform any treatment activities beyond their education, training, skill, and competence.

Treatment programs or sessions may need to be modified, reduced, or terminated in response to the observed or reported changes in a patient's condition. The patient who convulses without a known cause, experiences incontinence of bowel or bladder without a known cause, loses consciousness without a known cause, or exhibits new or different symptoms from those observed previously should be evaluated carefully before his/her treatment is continued.

The patient who exhibits signs or symptoms of an acute illness or who appears to be experiencing an adverse response to treatment (e.g., unusual vital signs, vertigo, syncope, nausea, or vomiting) should have his/her treatment terminated temporarily, and he/she should be reevaluated by a physician before being treated again. Nursing and other medical personnel should be apprised of changes in the patient's condition, and appropriate documentation must reflect the change.

A mentally competent patient should be informed by the caregiver about the intent, anticipated outcome, and potential risks associated with the planned treatment. The patient should have the opportunity to ask questions or seek additional information about the treatment. If he/she refuses the treatment, his/her decision should be accepted and nursing and other medical personnel notified. All patients should have the opportunity to participate in the process of informed consent before receiving treatment, and his/her autonomy regarding deciding whether to receive treatment should be respected. The caregiver may find it helpful or necessary to confer with a physician, nurse, or other practitioner involved with caring for the patient to assist with the resolution of a dilemma related to a patient's nonconsent. The incident should be documented in the patient's medical record by the caregiver.

Injuries or trauma that may occur to a patient who receives treatment includes burns, lacerations, muscle strains, ligamentous sprains, heat stress, hematomas, fractures, respiratory distress, and cardiovascular distress.

The physical environment in which the patient is treated and the equipment used to treat patients should be maintained to meet the standards established by various agencies. These agencies include the

Occupational Safety and Health Administration (OSHA), Joint Commission on the Accreditation of Healthcare Organizations (JCAHO), Commission on the Accreditation of Rehabilitation Facilities (CARF), and National Institute on Occupational Safety and Health (NIOSH); the policies and procedures established by the hospital or treatment facility must also be followed.

PRINCIPLES AND CONCEPTS

Many health care providers overlook the need to maintain a safe environment for treatment. The service unit supervisor or department manager is responsible for developing a safety education and awareness program for all of the employees in the department. Staff meetings and orientation programs regarding environmental, employee, and patient safety should be developed, implemented, and repeated periodically. General guidelines to reduce and avoid patient or employee injury should be included in the unit's policy/procedure or safety manual. Employees should be required to read this material periodically, and their comprehension of this material should be evaluated. Failure to provide information and training sessions on safety could create increased organizational or personnel liability and reduce the level of the quality of care.

Written policies and procedures should identify and explain the following:

1. Patient scheduling patterns, the least acceptable ratio of personnel to patients, and what is to be done when unacceptable ratios occur.
2. The maintenance and monitoring of records such as referrals, patient status documentation, treatment protocols, and incident reports.
3. Plans for the evacuation and care of patients and the expected function of all personnel at the time of an emergency, such as a fire or disaster.
4. First aid or immediate emergency care plans.
5. Restriction or access of visitors to the treatment areas.
6. Security measures for patient and employee valuables and procedures for items that are lost or found.
7. The establishment of equipment inspection, repair, and maintenance records.
8. The process and procedures for general infection control and handling of toxic materials.
9. The application and use of protective clothing, handling of body fluids, management of patients

who are placed in isolation, and changing the dressings of infected wounds.

10. Employee job duties, descriptions, and responsibilities.

11. Supervisory relationships, lines of communication, a table of organization, the span of control, and the chain of command of the facility and the service area.

The physical environment and equipment should be prepared, inspected, and maintained so that

1. Proper levels of ventilation, temperature, humidity, light, and noise are provided.

2. Routine janitorial and housekeeping services are available and provided.

3. Equipment functions according to the manufacturer's standards.

4. Structural hazards are minimized or eliminated.

5. Equipment is properly attached or fixed to structurally sound and strong areas (i.e., it should be attached to wall studs, bolted to the floor, or attached to ceiling joists or rafters).

6. Equipment and supplies not in use are stored, line cords and electrical outlets are protected by a built-in ground, and wheels on movable equipment have locks.

7. Emergency exits and evacuation routes are clearly marked and displayed for patients, visitors, and employees.

8. Emergency equipment, such as fire extinguishers or hoses, first aid kits, and intubation airways, is available, accessible, and ready for use.

9. A metabolic cart is available with its components clearly marked and ready to use.

10. Floor surfaces are clean and dry, and loose or torn carpeting and other similar hazards are eliminated.

Safety related to patient care both affects and is the responsibility of the service unit personnel. It is imperative that all personnel understand and comply with safe personal and patient care practices. Regardless of the goal of treatment, the primary responsibility of any practitioner is to "do no harm" to the patient. Employee injuries are frequently associated with activities that require lifting, carrying, pushing, pulling, and reaching. The development, use, and application of proper body mechanics was presented in Chapter 2. It may be helpful to review it for suggestions to prevent injury to yourself and to the patient. You should always be alert to the possibility that patient injury can occur, and you should anticipate or "expect the unexpected" to happen.

BOX 11–1

Responsibilities of Supervisors

1. Be certain each employee is qualified and competent for his or her assigned duties and responsibilities. This will require the supervisor to observe and evaluate each employee's performance not less often than once a year.

2. Be certain each employee understands his/her duties and responsibilities and what he/she is expected to do. This can be accomplished during the orientation of a new employee and during performance evaluation sessions.

3. Develop and implement an ongoing safety training and awareness program for unit personnel.

4. Instruct and teach personnel how to establish appropriate professional interpersonal relations with each patient. Each patient must receive individualized care and should be considered as an entire person rather than as a patient with a specific disability or condition.

5. Instruct and teach personnel how to obtain informed consent from each patient before initiating or extensively altering his/her treatment.

6. Instruct personnel to explain all treatment procedures to each patient and to monitor, guide, instruct, or direct the patient during his/her treatment.

7. Instruct personnel to refer the patient to another caregiver when he/she is not skilled or competent to treat the patient.

8. Instruct personnel to clarify a referral or prescription that is considered to be inaccurate or incomplete, or to contain a contraindicated procedure before treating the patient by contacting the referring person.

9. Instruct personnel to clarify any referral or prescription if he/she is unsure of its intent or expected outcome before initiating treatment. A verbal referral or prescription should be transferred to written form within 24 to 48 hours of its receipt and the written form signed by the person who originally provided it.

10. Be certain personnel report malfunctioning equipment or other forms of breaches of safety and that they correct such situations when appropriate.

PROCEDURE 11 – 1
Treatment of Patient Injuries

1. Immediately provide or obtain emergency care for the patient according to established organizational policies and procedures and the competence of the caregiver. Do not leave the patient unattended, but do attempt to prevent any further injury and act to stabilize the patient's physiologic status. When it is apparent that assistance from trained personnel (e.g., emergency medical technicians, trauma team, cardiopulmonary resuscitation team) is needed, they should be contacted before on-the-scene emergency care is initiated to reduce response time. If two or more persons are at the scene, one person should contact the support team while the other begins emergency care.

2. After the emergency phase is concluded, document the incident with objective and factual information. Indicate the type of emergency care that was given and by whom. List the persons who witnessed or observed the incident, who was notified about the incident, the time the incident occurred, and any events leading up to the incident. Do not confer with the patient or his/her relatives about the incident, and do not express information to anyone that would indicate you were negligent or at fault.

3. Notify your immediate superior or the department supervisor or risk manager of the incident.

4. File the incident report with the appropriate person within the organization.

5. Notify the insurance carrier of the incident. In a large facility, this may be done by the risk manager.

The supervisor or department manager has several specific responsibilities, as listed in Box 11–1.

Prevention is an important aspect of patient and employee safety. You should be particularly careful during a patient-assisted transfer, lifting activities, and ambulation activities and when equipment is used. Certain patient conditions, such as wound management, require special attention to avoid infection of the wound and cross-contamination of other persons. Personal cleanliness in the form of proper hand washing before and after each patient's treatment is essential for successful infection control. Your personal safety can be maintained best through the use of proper body mechanics, proper personal hygiene, familiarity with the operation of equipment, and familiarity with the methods of infection control and by performing those safety techniques or procedures for which you have been educated or trained.

An injury to a patient can occur even though safety measures are applied with diligence and consistency. However, it is less likely to occur when safe practices are used. The person who is most directly involved with providing care to the patient to whom an injury occurs should follow the steps given in Procedure 11–1.

These procedures may vary slightly from facility to facility, but they are necessary to protect the employee, facility, and patient.

Each employee must be aware of the need for the consistent application of preventive measures to maintain a safe environment and the safe care of each patient. The employee's thoughts and behavior should be directed to promote safety for himself/herself, the patient, visitors, and other employees. Each employee should be prepared to react to emergency situations quickly, decisively, and calmly. Any emergency or first aid treatment provided by departmental personnel should be performed according to institutional policies and procedures and the training of the employee. Institutional and community agency emergency telephone numbers should be posted by each telephone, and employees must use these numbers when assistance is required or desired.

EMERGENCY CARE

Although the role of the caregiver may be to provide immediate first aid, the caregiver should make an effort to obtain immediate assistance from the most qualified individual available, such as a physician, a nurse, an *emergency medical technician,* or other medical personnel. In the hospital this may be relatively easy, and trained personnel who will react quickly when called are likely to be readily available. However, in the patient's home, an outpatient clinic, a school, an athletic facility, or even an extended care facility, assistance may be difficult to obtain and may require a period of time. Sources of assistance within and external to the setting should be known by the caregiver, and the most appropriate source should be contacted promptly. It will require judgment by the caregiver to determine whether he/she should attempt to obtain assistance before or after initiating emergency care or first aid. *Note:* In most situations, it will be best if assistance is requested before initiating emergency care unless the delay of immediate aid is life threatening to the patient. Whatever care has been provided before assistance arrives will have to be explained to the person who provides additional care. Any objective information about the patient's condition should be provided to the person as well.

EMERGENCY CARE FOR SPECIFIC CONDITIONS

When an injury or change in the patient's condition requires first aid or emergency care, you should be aware of some of the emergency aid that could be provided. The best way to be prepared to provide emergency care is to participate in an educational program or course provided by a qualified instructor or agency.

Bandages This section presents information on the application and use of bandages when an emergency situation occurs and first aid is necessary. In general, the bandage is used to support or stabilize a segment; restrict motion of a joint; or to control edema, swelling, or joint effusion and a dressing would not be required. The most common injury that would require the use of a bandage for any of these purposes is a sprain or strain.

Types of Bandage Materials Materials that are used frequently for a bandage are muslin, which is unbleached cotton; woven, elastic, porous cotton; rolled gauze; a stockinet, which is loosely knit cotton formed into a tube; and adhesive tape (Fig.

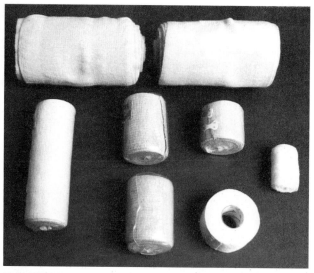

■ **FIGURE 11–1**
Types of bandages. *Left* to *right* and *top* to *bottom,* 6-inch elastic extra long, 6-inch, 4-inch, 3-inch, and 2-inch bandages; adhesive tape; and roller gauze.

11–1). Some of these items will have to be laundered, whereas other items should be disposed of after they have been used once. The woven elastic bandage can be used multiple times, but care must be taken when it is washed and dried to preserve its shape and elasticity. It should be washed by hand in lukewarm water, similar to the way a wool sweater would be washed. Excess water should be gently squeezed from the bandage, and the bandage should be laid flat on an absorbent towel to dry. Do not hang the bandage from a clothesline because it will stretch as a result of the weight of the water that remains in its fibers. After it is completely dried, it should be rolled up so it will be ready for application. The patient should be given or should purchase several of these bandages so he/she will have a clean one to apply while a previously used one is being laundered and dried. The patient or a family member should be instructed in the proper care of this type of bandage.

Bandages may be named according to their shape, appearance, purpose, design, or material used. Several types of bandages are discussed in the sections that follow. However, a description of the application and use of a bandage, wrap, or strapping with adhesive tape to an area after injury or to prevent an acute injury is beyond the scope of this text.

Triangular The triangular bandage is a large piece of cloth cut or formed into a triangle. (For example, a square piece of cloth folded diagonally becomes a triangle.) It is most often used as a temporary sling to support the weight of a patient's upper extremity as a first aid approach. When it is used for this purpose, you must be certain the cloth triangle is large enough to contain the patient's forearm and hand. To apply the sling, use the following procedure:

1. Flex the elbow of the injured extremity to slightly more than 90 degrees with the palm facing the patient's chest.
2. Place the apex of the sling at the elbow, and bring the outer end of the sling over the forearm and shoulder of the injured upper extremity (Fig. 11–2A).
3. Bring the other end of the sling under the forearm and over the shoulder of the uninjured upper extremity (see Fig. 11–2B).
4. The patient may have to elevate the shoulder of the injured extremity until the sling ends are tied.
5. Secure the sling by tying the ends in a square knot positioned to one side of the spinous processes of the patient's neck.
6. Have the patient relax his/her shoulder, and be certain the sling trough supports the forearm.
7. Pull the free apex end of the sling over the elbow and pin or tape it to the front of the sling.
8. Position the patient's hand within the sling, and

evaluate the height of the hand and forearm, which should be horizontal or elevated slightly above a horizontal position (see Fig. 11–2C and Fig. 11–3).

Cravat A cravat can also be used as a sling but will not support the patient's upper extremity as well as the triangular sling; it is used as a first aid approach.

1. To form the cravat, fold a square or rectangular cloth into a series of overlapping layers to the width desired. A belt, necktie, or scarf can be used to form a cravat.
2. Loop the cravat over the forearm of the injured upper extremity.
3. Tie the two free ends behind the patient's neck using a square knot or, if a belt is used, the belt buckle.

Roller Bandage A roller bandage is an elastic or nonelastic material formed in a cylindrical roll and fabricated in various widths and lengths. It is used to maintain and protect a dressing, to provide pressure, to maintain a splint, to provide support to a joint, or to restrict motion.

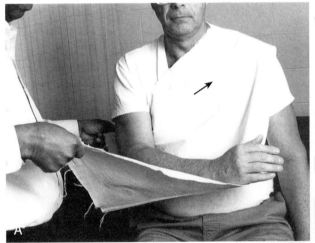
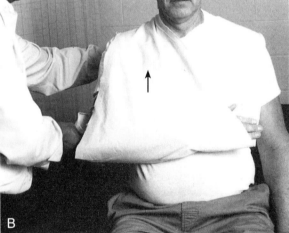
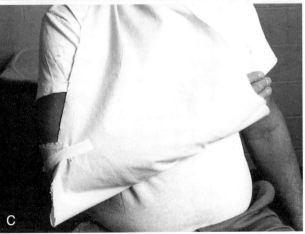

■ **FIGURE 11–2**
Application of a triangular bandage.

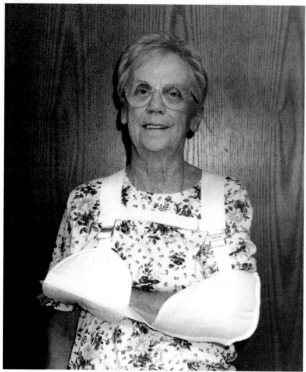

■ **FIGURE 11–3**
Adjustable sling designed to eliminate pressure to the neck.

1. Patterns of application
   A. *Circular.* The bandage is applied in a series of overlapping circular turns around a part to initially or terminally anchor the bandage. It must be applied carefully to avoid occlusion of the local circulation, which could result in decreased blood flow and development of swelling distal to the bandage (Fig. 11–4*A*).
   B. *Spiral.* The bandage is applied in a series of overlapping diagonal turns around a part; these turns may be applied upward or downward. A spiral bandage is less apt to occlude the circulation and will cover a larger area than the circular bandage with the same amount of material (see Fig. 11–4*B*).
   C. *Open spiral or oblique.* The open spiral is a series of diagonal turns that do not overlap and that have an open space between each turn. The bandage begins and terminates with circular anchors and will cover a larger area than the spiral bandage with the same amount of bandage (see Fig. 11–4*C*).
   D. *Spiral reverse.* The spiral reverse is a series of spiral turns, each of which is folded or reversed on itself midway through each turn. The bandage begins and terminates with circular anchors and is used when the part or segment being bandaged varies excessively in its shape and circumference (e.g., forearm or lower leg). The reverse component allows a nonelastic bandage to conform to the change in circumference, so this pattern is usually used with a nonelastic gauze roller bandage (see Fig. 11–4*D,E*).
   E. *Recurrent.* The recurrent pattern is a series of lengthwise layers applied to the anterior-posterior or dorsal-volar surfaces of an extremity or digit. It is used to cover the most distal aspect of a residual limb or the digits. The bandage is anchored with circular turns and may be completed with spiral or figure-of-eight turns (see Fig. 11–4*F,G*).
   F. *Figure-of-eight.* The figure-of-eight is a series of spiral turns applied in alternate directions. The first turn progresses in an inferior-to-superior direction and level, and the second turn progresses in a superior-to-inferior direction and level. Additional turns follow in the same alternating pattern. This type of bandage can be applied to the foot and ankle, knee, shoulder, hand and wrist, and elbow.
      (1) *Foot and ankle.* Anchor the bandage at the base of the toes, and then cross it diagonally over the dorsum of the foot and around the foot (see Fig. 11–4*H*). Bring the bandage diagonally across the anterior ankle, return it to the foot, and repeat the diagonal turns (see Fig. 11–4*I*). Repeat this pattern until the bandage is applied completely. Terminate the bandage with a circular anchor on the lower leg below the belly of the gastrocnemius muscle (see Fig. 11–4*J*). Use a 4-inch bandage for most adults and a smaller width for children.
      (2) *Hand and wrist.* Anchor the bandage at the distal palm, proximal to the metacarpophalangeal (MCP) joints (see Fig. 11–4*K*). Then cross it diagonally through the palm, over the wrist, and diagonally over the dorsum of the hand (see Fig. 11–4*L*). Continue with the figure-of-eight pattern over the hand and wrist. The thumb and fingers are not incorporated in the bandage. Terminate the bandage on the lower forearm with a circular anchor (see Fig. 11–4*M*). Use a 1- or 2-inch bandage for most adults and a 1-inch bandage for children.
      (3) *Knee.* Anchor the bandage slightly below the knee, cross diagonally to the medial or lateral aspect of knee, and make a circular anchor above the knee (Fig. 11–4*N*). Return to the lower leg with a diagonal turn and continue with the figure-of-eight pattern until the area is covered (Fig. 11–4*O*). Terminate the bandage on the thigh with a firm circular anchor (Fig. 11–4*P*). Use a 4-inch bandage for most adults and a 3-inch bandage for most children.

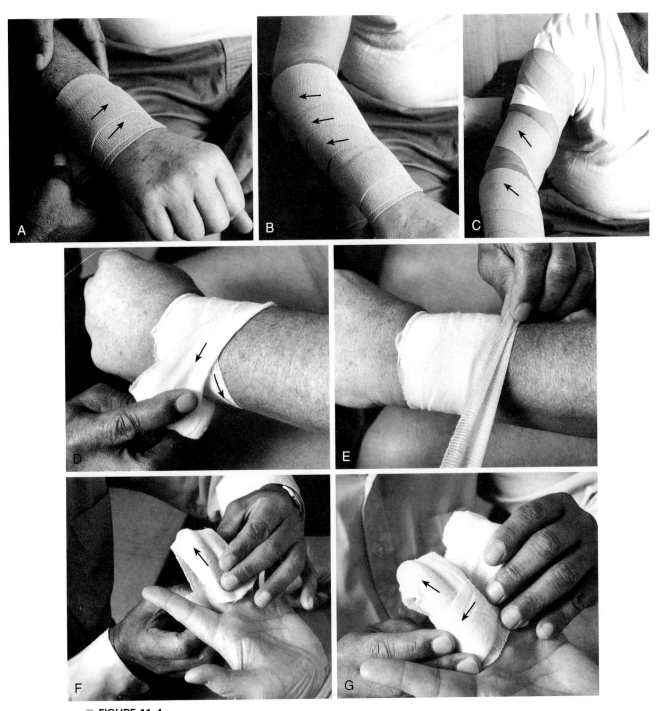

■ **FIGURE 11–4**
Patterns of application of elastic roller bandage. *A,* Circular. *B,* Spiral. *C,* Open spiral. *D* and *E,* Spiral reverse. *F* and *G,* Recurrent for fingers.

continued

(4) *Elbow.* Follow the same pattern as described for the knee, substituting the upper arm and forearm for the thigh and lower leg. Use a 3- or 4-inch bandage for most adults and a 2- or 3-inch bandage for most children.

G. *Spica.* A spica bandage incorporates the figure-of-eight pattern, but a large anchor or spica is applied around the upper trunk or pelvis to prevent the distal portion of the bandage from sliding down the extremity to which it is applied.

(1) *Shoulder.* Anchor the bandage on the injured upper arm slightly below the level of the injury (see Fig. 11–4Q). Bring the bandage across the back of the patient's upper trunk, through the opposite axilla, and diagonally across the chest (see Fig. 11–4R). Bring the

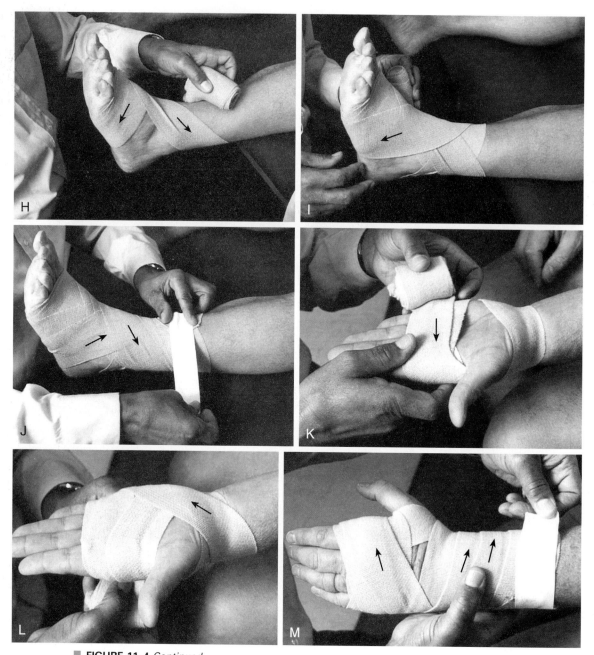

■ **FIGURE 11–4** *Continued*
H through *J*, Figure 8 for the foot and ankle. *K* through *M*, Figure 8 for the hand and wrist.

bandage over the injured shoulder and through the axilla on injured side and apply several spiral or figure-of-eight turns on the upper arm (see Fig. 11–4*S*). Wrap the bandage around the upper trunk periodically as described, and terminate the bandage on the trunk spica or the upper arm portion of the wrap. Use a 3- or 4-inch bandage for most adults and a 2- or 3-inch bandage for most children.

(2) *Hip.* Anchor the bandage around the patient's thigh, below the level of the injury (see Fig. 11–4*T*). Wrap the bandage diagonally around the thigh several times using a figure-of-eight or spiral pattern (see Fig. 11–4*U*). Bring the bandage completely around the pelvis, between the iliac crests and the greater trochanters several times, and then return the bandage to the thigh (see Fig. 11–4*V*). Complete the bandage with a figure-of-eight or spiral pattern and anchor the bandage on the pelvic spica or on the thigh portion of the bandage. Use a 6-inch bandage for most adults and a 4-inch bandage for most children or small adults. Usually several bandages sewn together or an extremely long bandage are required to accomplish this pattern.

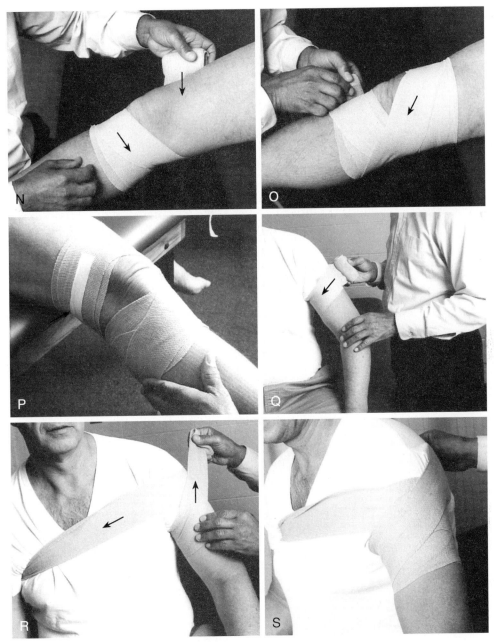

■ **FIGURE 11–4** *Continued*
N through *P*, Figure 8 for the knee; *Q* through *S*, Spica for the shoulder.

Remember: It is important to select the proper-width bandage for the size of the area being wrapped. For most adults the following bandage widths are recommended: a 3- or 4-inch bandage for the foot and ankle; a 1- or 2-inch bandage for the hand or wrist; a 2-, 3-, or 4-inch bandage for the elbow; a 3- or 4-inch bandage for the knee; a 6-inch bandage for the thigh; and a 3- or 4-inch bandage for the upper arm. If the bandage is too wide for the area, wrinkles will develop or the bandage will not conform properly to the area. If the bandage is too narrow, it will be insufficient to cover the area or may cause undesired pressure. An elastic bandage is the best type to use for most of these patterns.

Lacerations The objectives are to prevent contamination of the wound and control the bleeding. Treatment is described in Procedure 11–2.

Shock The objectives are to identify and reduce or remove the cause when possible and to prevent or reduce the extent of the physiologic state of shock.

Signs and symptoms of *shock* include pale, moist, cool skin; shallow and irregular breathing; dilated pupils; a weak, rapid pulse; diaphoresis; dizziness or nausea; and syncope. Treatment is described in Procedure 11–3.

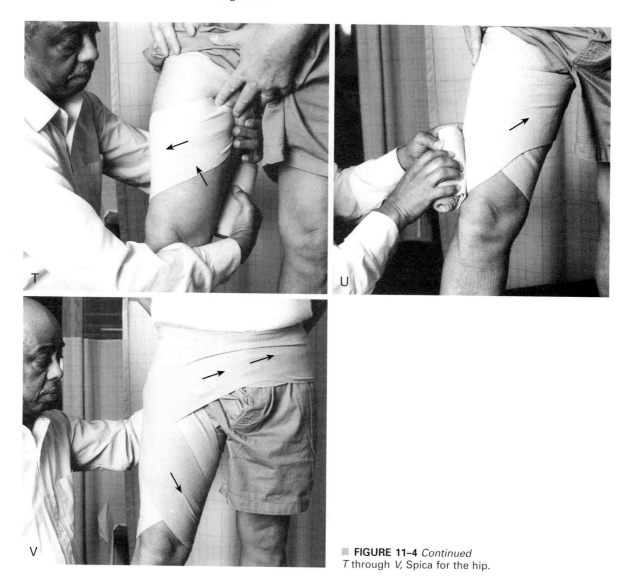

■ **FIGURE 11–4** *Continued*
T through *V,* Spica for the hip.

Orthostatic or Postural Hypotension Some patients may experience *orthostatic* or *postural hypotension*. This condition usually is accompanied by signs and symptoms similar to those described for shock. This condition occurs most frequently when the person attempts to stand rapidly from a stooped, kneeling, recumbent, or sitting position. The elderly person, the person who uses antihypertension medication, the person who has a decreased ability to return venous blood from the periphery to the heart (e.g., the spinal cord–injured person), and the person who has been immobilized in a recumbent position for an extended period of time are those who are most apt to demonstrate orthostatic hypotension. The reduced venous return from the lower extremities results in decreased filling of the left ventricle, which leads to decreased cardiac output and, eventually, decreased cerebral perfusion. As a result, the person experiences dizziness and possibly syncope when he/she stands up.

The first aid measures used to resolve this condition are the same as those listed in Procedure 11–3.

Some measures that can be taken to prevent this condition are to wrap the patient's lower extremities, from the feet to the groin, with elastic bandages; apply an abdominal binder or corset; apply elastic hose (half or full length); instruct the patient to perform active ankle dorsiflexion–plantar flexion exercises ("ankle pumps") and alternate knee-to-chest exercises frequently while he/she is supine or sitting; allow the person to accommodate to the upright position gradually by slowly elevating the head of the bed to various levels; or use a tilt table to stand the patient by increments.

In a severe case, it may be necessary to apply a full-body pressurized garment (a G suit) to stabilize the venous circulation. The abdominal binder, elastic lower extremity wraps, elastic hose, and G suit provide external pressure to the veins of the extremities and trunk, which assists to return venous blood to the heart and reduces the pooling or collection of venous blood in the lower extremities and abdomen. The active use of the lower extremity muscles will assist in

PROCEDURE 11-2
Treatment of Lacerations

1. Wash your hands and apply protective gloves; apply a clean or sterile, nonabsorbing towel or similar object to the wound. Continue to wear protective gloves during the treatment of the wound. Obtain additional assistance and contact emergency service personnel as necessary.

2. Elevate the wound above the level of the heart to reduce blood flow to the area if blood flow is excessive.

3. In some instances, the wound can be cleansed with an antiseptic or by rinsing it with water.

4. Place a clean towel or sterile dressing over the wound and apply direct pressure to the wound.

5. Encourage the patient to remain quiet and avoid using the extremity.

6. If there is arterial bleeding (demonstrated by spurting blood), it may be necessary to apply intermittent, direct pressure to the artery above the level of the wound. This is done most frequently to the brachial and femoral arteries to restrict blood flow to the distal wound site. However, prolonged pressure by the use of a tourniquet should be avoided. The person should be transported to a site where appropriate medical care can be provided unless assistance can be brought to the patient.

PROCEDURE 11-3
Treatment of Shock

1. Determine the cause of shock (e.g., excessive bleeding, inability to adjust to moving from a supine to a sitting or standing position, response to excessive heat) and remedy it if possible. Monitor the patient's blood pressure and pulse rate. Obtain additional assistance and contact emergency support personnel as necessary.

2. Place the person in a supine position with his/her head slightly lower than the lower extremities. If there are head and chest injuries or if respiration is impaired, it may be necessary to position the person in a supine position, level, or with the head and chest elevated slightly. If bleeding is the apparent cause and the wound is visible, attempt to control bleeding as described for a laceration.

3. A cool compress applied to the person's forehead may be of comfort, and a light blanket may be used to prevent loss of body heat.

4. Have the patient remain quiet and avoid exertion.

5. After the symptoms have been relieved, gradually return the person to an upright position, and monitor him/her to ensure regression of his/her condition.

6. Request transportation so the patient can be taken to a facility where he/she can receive proper care and treatment.

PROCEDURE 11–4
Treatment of Fractures

1. Obtain information about the injury from the conscious patient (i.e., its cause, its location, the extent of discomfort, and any restriction of motion). Obtain additional assistance and contact emergency service personnel as necessary.

2. Observe the site of injury or the position of the extremity, and evaluate the patient's general appearance and condition. Monitor his/her blood pressure and pulse rate.

3. Gently palpate the area and surrounding tissue to evaluate swelling or edema and tenderness. Deformity and soft tissue bruising are indications of an underlying fracture.

4. Avoid movement or activity that has the potential to cause additional damage.

5. Apply support to the site to stabilize it, but do not attempt to align the bone ends. Use a firm object to stabilize the fracture prior to transporting the patient. A pillow folded around the site, canes or crutches applied on either side of a lower extremity fracture, or a flat piece of wood applied to either side of the fracture site can be used; on small extremities a large magazine can be wrapped around the site.

6. Cover an open fracture site with a sterile towel or dressing, but do not attempt to reinsert the bone ends beneath the skin.

7. If a spinal fracture is suspected, use extreme caution when handling the patient. Place him/her on a firm, flat board, and maintain the head and neck in a neutral position. To insert the spinal board, logroll the patient, avoiding forward, backward, or side bending of the spine. At least three persons will be required to roll or lift the patient. Evaluate the level of neurologic sensation and function by asking the patient to move an extremity or report his/her response to a stimulus applied to the skin. Evaluate the patient for signs of shock, bleeding, and additional injuries. Obtain qualified medical assistance rather than attempting to transport the patient with minimal assistance or without sufficient immobilization. This is a serious injury, and the patient must be handled carefully.

8. Request transportation so the patient can be taken to a facility where he/she can receive proper care and treatment.

"pumping" or moving the venous blood toward the heart and reduce the pooling of venous blood in the lower extremities. The gradual elevation of the patient from a recumbent to a sitting or standing position will assist the vascular system to accommodate physiologically to the changes in position.

Fractures The objectives are to protect the fracture site and avoid further injury to it, prevent shock, reduce pain, and prevent wound contamination if the bone ends have penetrated the skin. Emergency care *should not* include any attempt to align the fracture segments or "set" the fracture. Treatment is described in Procedure 11–4.

Burns The objectives are to prevent wound contamination, to relieve or reduce pain, and to prevent shock. Treatment is described in Procedure 11–5.

Convulsions/Seizures The objectives are to protect the person from injury should he/she fall or experience excessive involuntary movements of the extremities and to protect the patient's modesty or privacy. Treatment is described in Procedure 11–6.

PROCEDURE 11-5
Treatment of Burns

1. Remove or eliminate the agent causing the burn, or remove the patient from the agent; contact skilled personnel when the burn wounds are extensive or involve the face, hands, perineum, or feet. Obtain additional assistance and contact emergency service personnel as necessary.

2. Cut away or remove clothing near the site of the burn, but do not attempt to remove clothing that lies over or is part of the wound. Remove jewelry from the patient if edema has not developed and the jewelry can be removed without causing additional trauma.

3. A clean or sterile dressing or towel can be loosely laid over the wound. In some instances a moist dressing will be more comfortable for the patient. Do not apply any cream, salve, ointment, or similar substance (e.g., butter or lard) to the wound, because this will mask the appearance of the wound and may lead to infection or a delay in healing.

4. If the wound has been caused by a toxic chemical, use a copious amount of water over the wound site to dilute the substance. However, avoid washing the chemical onto an unaffected portion of the skin to prevent causing a burn to that area.

5. Observe the patient for shock, respiratory distress, and other injuries. Prepare the patient for transportation or transport him/her to a facility that is prepared to manage this type of injury.

PROCEDURE 11-6
Treatment of Seizures

1. Place the person in a safe location and position; do not attempt to restrain or restrict his/her body convulsions. Obtain additional assistance and contact emergency service personnel as necessary.

2. Monitor the rate and quality of respiration. There may be a period of tonic contraction of all body muscles, which will cause respiration to cease for up to 50 to 70 seconds. After this has ended, respirations may be slower and deeper than normal for a brief period.

3. Assist in keeping the patient's airway patent, but do not attempt to open the mouth by placing any object between the teeth. Never place your finger or a wooden or metal object in the patient's mouth, and do not attempt to grasp or position the tongue.

4. When the convulsions subside, turn the person's head to one side in case he/she vomits.

5. Allow the patient to rest after the convulsions cease, and protect his/her modesty and privacy. It may be helpful to cover the person with a blanket or screen him/her from view. Some patients' sphincter control may be lost during or at the conclusion of the seizure, resulting in the involuntary discharge of his/her bladder or bowel contents.

6. The patient should be evaluated by a physician to determine the cause of the seizure if the cause is not known.

PROCEDURE 11–7
Treatment for Choking

1. When assisting a *conscious* adult or a child who is more than 1 year old:
   a. Ask the person if he/she is choking. If he/she can speak, cough, or breathe, do not attempt to assist him/her.
   b. If the person is unable to speak, cough, or breathe, check his/her mouth and remove any visible foreign object.
   c. If the person cannot speak, cough, or breathe, position yourself behind him/her. Clasp your hands over the person's abdomen slightly above the umbilicus but below the diaphragm.
   d. Use the closed fist of one hand, covered by your other hand, to give three or four abrupt thrusts against the person's abdomen by compressing the abdomen in and up forcefully (Heimlich maneuver; Fig. 11–5). Continue to apply the thrusts until the obstruction becomes dislodged or is relieved or the person becomes unconscious.
   e. Obtain advanced medical assistance.

2. When assisting an *unconscious* adult or child who is more than 1 year old:
   a. Place the person in a supine position, and request help from others in contacting advanced medical assistance.
   b. Open the person's mouth, and use your finger to attempt to locate and remove the foreign object (finger sweep).

continued

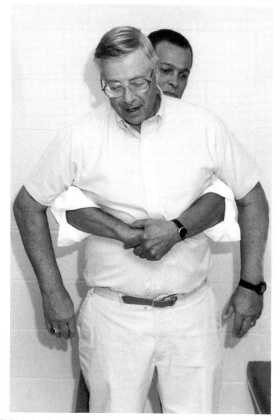

■ **FIGURE 11–5**
Application of the Heimlich maneuver; hands are positioned above the umbilicus and below the diaphragm; and pressure is exerted in and up.

PROCEDURE 11–7, *continued*

  c. Open the airway by tilting the head back and lifting the chin forward, and attempt to ventilate using the mouth-to-mouth technique.
  d. If this approach is unsuccessful in initiating respiration, give 6 to 10 subdiaphragmatic abdominal thrusts using the heel of one hand reinforced by the other hand (Heimlich maneuver; see 1d).
  e. If this approach is unsuccessful in initiating respiration, repeat the finger sweep, open the airway, attempt to ventilate, and perform the abdominal thrusts. Be persistent and continue these procedures until the object is removed or advanced medical assistance arrives. (*Note:* Avoid performing a blind finger sweep in children who are younger than 8 years old. Instead, lift the chin to expose the oral cavity, and remove a foreign body if you see it.)
  f. It may be necessary to initiate cardiopulmonary resuscitation (CPR) techniques after the object has been removed to stabilize the person's cardiopulmonary functions.

3. When assisting a *conscious* infant (younger than 1 year old):
  a. Support his/her head and neck with one hand, and place him/her in a prone position over your forearm, with the head lower than the trunk and your forearm supported on your thigh.
  b. Perform four forceful interscapular blows with the heel of your free hand.
  c. Immediately after applying the blows to the upper back, turn the infant supine with the head lower than the trunk, and perform four thrusts to the lower sternum with two fingers.
  d. Repeat the back blows and sternal thrusts until the object is expelled.

4. When assisting an *unconscious* infant:
  a. Place the infant supine, and request help from others in contacting advanced medical assistance.
  b. Perform a tongue-jaw lift, and remove any foreign object if it is visible.
  c. Open the airway using the head tilt–chin lift technique described previously and attempt to ventilate the infant.
  d. Perform four back blows and four sternal thrusts if respiration has not been started.
  e. If the foreign body has not been removed, repeat the sequence until the foreign object is extracted.
  f. If the foreign body has been removed and the infant is not breathing, initiate basic CPR techniques (i.e., open the airway, use mouth-to-mouth and nose ventilation and perform chest compressions to initiate a heart rate).

(**Note:** *All persons who have experienced a choking incident should be examined by a physician as soon as possible. This information is based on the recommendations of the American Heart Association. A pamphlet containing diagrams and this information can be obtained from most affiliate offices of the American Heart Association.*)

Choking   The objectives are to restore and maintain a *patent* airway and normal breathing. Treatment is described in Procedure 11–7.

Heat-Related Illnesses   The objectives are to remove or reduce the cause of the illness and to return the individual to a state of normal homeostasis.

The two primary forms of heat-related illness are heat exhaustion and heat stroke (Table 11–1). Of the two, heat exhaustion poses the least threat to life, whereas heat stroke is considered a medical emergency because it can be life threatening. Both illnesses can result from a hot, humid environment; vigorous physical activity; dehydration; and depleted body elec-

Table 11–1
SIGNS AND SYMPTOMS OF HEAT-RELATED ILLNESSES

	Heat Exhaustion	Heat Stroke
Skin	Profuse diaphoresis	Dry; no diaphoresis
Nausea	Present	Present
Headache	Present	Present
Breathing	Shallow, rapid	Labored
Pulse	Weak, rapid	Strong, rapid
Color	Pale	Flushed or changes to gray
Temperature	Normal or slightly elevated	Very elevated (106°F to 110°F)
Behavior	Exhaustion, collapse	Exhaustion, collapse, convulsions
Consciousness	Unconscious	Unconscious
Eyes	Pupils normal	Pupils contract, then dilate

trolytes. Persons who are treated with hydrotherapy and persons who participate in vigorous aerobic exercise in a warm, humid environment should be observed periodically for signs or symptoms of heat exhaustion or heat stroke. Heat stroke may follow heat exhaustion if the person is not treated properly when the signs of heat exhaustion appear. Muscle cramps in the legs and abdomen may be the initial indicators of a heat-related illness. Rest, increased fluid intake, and gentle stretching and massage to the affected areas are methods used to relieve these symptoms.

Heat Exhaustion When the signs and symptoms of this condition are observed, it is important to cool the person and counteract the effects of dehydration. Emergency first aid treatment procedures are pre-

sented in Procedure 11–8. You may need to treat the person for shock, and you should monitor him/her for signs or symptoms of heat stroke. The person should not be given salt tablets by mouth as part of the treatment. The ingestion of excess salt may interfere with the person's ability to readjust his/her electrolyte balance to a normal state.

Heat Stroke This condition is life threatening, and its signs and symptoms must be recognized quickly so emergency, first aid treatment can be initiated promptly. Emergency, first aid treatment procedures are presented in Procedure 11–9. The individual with heat stroke will require care and treatment by qualified medical personnel, and he/she must be transported to a medical facility as soon as possible.

Insulin-Related Illnesses The objectives are to restore the person to his/her normal *insulin*–glucose state and to remove, correct, or compensate for the cause of the condition.

It is important to differentiate between the conditions of hypoglycemia (hyperinsulinemia, or an insulin reaction) and hyperglycemia (*acidosis*), as outlined in Table 11–2. An insulin reaction can be caused by too much systemic insulin, too little food intake, or excessive exercise in relation to the metabolic state of the person. Acidosis can be caused by too little systemic insulin, the intake of too much food or improper food (i.e., excessive sugar), or insufficient physical activity in relation to the metabolic state of the person.

Insulin Reaction If the person is conscious, provide him/her with some form of sugar (e.g., candy or orange juice). If the person is unconscious, glucose

PROCEDURE 11–8
Treatment for Heat Exhaustion

1. Place the person in a comfortable position in a shady or covered area or room that is well ventilated. Loosen or remove the person's outer clothing, and monitor his/her vital signs. Obtain additional assistance and contact emergency service personnel as necessary.

2. Sponge the person's forehead and neck with a cold compress or ice bag. Cool wet towels or sheets can be used to cool the person, and water may be given by mouth if he/she is conscious.

3. Observe the person for shock or other changes in his/her condition, and treat his/her symptoms as appropriate. Vomiting, refusal of fluids, or loss of consciousness indicates his/her condition is becoming worse.

4. Request transportation so the person can be taken to a facility where he/she can receive proper care and treatment if he/she does not exhibit relief of his/her signs and symptoms within a short time or if the previously listed signs or symptoms occur.

PROCEDURE 11–9
Treatment for Heat Stroke

1. Place the person in a semireclining position in a shady or well-ventilated covered area or room. Remove his/her outer clothing, and monitor his/her pulse and respiration rates. Obtain additional assistance and contact emergency service personnel immediately.

2. Cool the person quickly with large amounts of cool or cold water or apply cold, wet compresses, towels, or sheets to his/her body. Ice bags can be applied to his/her wrists, ankles, each groin area, each axilla, and lateral neck areas to cool the large blood vessels.

3. This is a life-threatening condition, and prompt emergency care must be provided; the person should be transported to a medical facility as rapidly as possible.

may have to be provided intravenously. The person should rest, and all physical activity should be stopped. This condition is not as serious as acidosis, but the person should be given the opportunity to return to a balanced metabolic state as soon as possible. It may be necessary to counsel the person on how he/she can balance his/her food intake and exercise or monitor his/her blood glucose levels and insulin dosage more carefully.

Acidosis Acidosis can lead to a diabetic coma, and death can occur if this state is allowed to persist. It should be considered a medical emergency that requires prompt action, including assistance from qualified personnel. The patient should not be given any form of sugar. Usually an injection of insulin is needed, and a nurse or physician should provide care as quickly as possible.

Autonomic Hyperreflexia (Dysreflexia) The objectives are to determine and remove the noxious stimu-lus causing the condition and to return the person to his/her level of normal homeostasis.

Autonomic hyperreflexia occurs in individuals with a relatively recent complete injury to the cervical and upper thoracic portions of the spinal cord down to the T6 cord level. Signs and symptoms include severe hypertension, bradycardia, profuse diaphoresis above the level of the cord lesion, a pounding headache, a general feeling of discomfort, red skin blotches, and piloerection ("goose bumps"). The person may convulse, respiration may become difficult, and the person may become unconscious.

Various noxious stimuli below the level of the spinal cord lesion (e.g., bladder distention caused by urine retention, fecal impaction, open pressure ulcers, tight straps from an orthosis or urine retention bag, localized pressure, or exercise) may cause a massive sympathetic system response that can't be controlled or counteracted by higher centers in the brain because of the location of the spinal cord injury. The result is uncontrolled, widespread peripheral arterial *vasoconstriction*, which causes severe hypertension. This condition should be considered a medical emergency, and a physician should be contacted for immediate assistance. Treatment is described in Procedure 11–10.

Cardiac Arrest The objective is to maintain the cardiopulmonary system at a level sufficient to sustain life until the person can be transported to a medical facility.

All health care practitioners should be trained and certified to perform *cardiopulmonary resuscitation* (CPR). The information presented in this section is a summary of the CPR techniques developed by the American Heart Association. This group advocates the use of the acronym "ABC" to identify the three impor-

Table 11–2
WARNING SIGNS AND SYMPTOMS OF INSULIN-RELATED ILLNESSES

	Insulin Reaction	Acidosis
Onset	Sudden	Gradual
Skin	Pale, moist	Flushed, dry
Behavior	Excited, agitated	Drowsy
Breath odor	Normal	Fruity odor
Breathing	Normal to shallow	Deep, labored
Vomiting	Absent	Present
Tongue	Moist	Dry
Hunger	Present	Absent
Thirst	Absent	Present
Glucose in urine	Absent or slight	Large amounts

PROCEDURE 11–10
Treatment of Autonomic Hyperreflexia

1. Initially place the person in a sitting or semirecumbent position because this will tend to reduce the hypertension. Do not place the person in a supine position.

2. If the noxious stimulus can be identified, it should be removed or relieved if possible. A common stimulus is an occluded catheter or a completely filled urine retention bag, which prevents drainage of urine from the bladder.

3. Monitor the person's vital signs frequently. Provide reassurance to the patient, and obtain qualified medical assistance.

4. Be aware that this condition could occur at any time, and be prepared to assist the patient.

PROCEDURE 11–11
Cardiopulmonary Resuscitation (CPR)

1. Determine the condition of the patient by gently shaking him/her and asking "Are you all right?" or "How do you feel?"

2. If the patient does not respond, place him/her in a supine position on a firm surface. Open his/her airway by lifting up on the chin and pushing down on the forehead to tilt the head back.

3. Check for respiration by observing the chest or abdomen for movement, listen for sounds of breathing, and feel for his/her breath by placing your cheek close to his/her mouth. If none of these signs are present, the patient is not breathing, and you should proceed to initiating breathing techniques.

4. Pinch the patient's nose closed, and maintain the head tilt to open the airway. Place your mouth over the patient's open mouth and form a seal with your lips; perform two full breaths, and then proceed to evaluating the circulation. Some persons prefer to place a clean cloth over the patient's lips before initiating mouth-to-mouth respirations. If available, a plastic intubation device can be used to decrease the contact between the caregiver's mouth and the patient's mouth and any saliva or vomitus.

5. Palpate the carotid artery for a pulse. If there is no pulse, you must begin external chest compressions.

6. To initiate chest compressions, kneel next to the patient, place the heel of one hand on the inferior portion of the *sternum* just proximal to the *xiphoid* process, and place your other hand on top of the first hand. Position your shoulders directly over the patient's sternum, keep your elbows extended, and press down firmly, depressing the sternum approximately 1½ to 2 inches with each compression. Relax after each compression, but do not remove your hands from the sternum. The relaxation and

PROCEDURE 11–7, *continued*

compression phases should be equal in duration. This can be accomplished by mentally counting "1001," "1002," "1003," etc., for each phase.

7. If you perform all CPR procedures without assistance, you should perform 15 chest compressions and then perform 2 breaths. You must compress at the rate of 80 to 100 times per minute. Continue these procedures until qualified assistance arrives or the patient is able to sustain independent respiration and circulation. If you are alone, attempt to gain assistance from other persons by calling loudly for help. If a second person is present, he/she should contact an advanced medical assistance unit before beginning to assist with CPR. In most instances the patient will require hospitalization and evaluation by a physician.

(**Note:** *Extreme care must be used to open an airway in a patient who may have experienced a cervical spine injury. In such cases, use the chin lift, but avoid the head tilt. If that technique does not open the airway, the head should be tilted slowly and gently until the airway is patent.*)

These procedures are appropriate to use for adults and for children 8 years of age and older. A pamphlet or booklet containing diagrams and instructions for CPR techniques can be obtained from most affiliate offices of the American Heart Association.

tant components of CPR—airway, breathing, and circulation—and the sequence in which they should be managed.

In 1992, new guidelines for CPR recommended that qualified medical assistance be contacted by using the 911 emergency telephone service or by calling a community emergency medical technical support unit (e.g., an emergency medical service or a local fire department, police department, or hospital) *before* the initiation of CPR by an individual. Early contact with a medical assistance team or unit will permit the team to reach the victim as rapidly as possible. If CPR is initiated before contacting more qualified medical assistance personnel, such assistance will be delayed. Therefore, when more than one person is available at the scene, one should perform CPR while another contacts advanced medical assistance immediately. CPR is described in Procedure 11–11.

In 1992, new guidelines for basic life support (BLS) were adopted by the American Heart Association and the American Red Cross based on the proceedings of a conference of physicians published in the *Journal of the American Medical Association (JAMA)*.

These guidelines advocate the application of interposed abdominal compression (IAC) as well as sternal (chest) compression when the two-person approach is used. It has been determined that abdominal compressions assist in moving the blood to the periphery and brain more effectively than sternal compressions alone. Further information about these new guidelines can be obtained from local offices of

the American Heart Association or American Red Cross.

SUMMARY

The guidelines presented elsewhere in the text regarding the environment, general patient safety considerations, and the employment of qualified, competent, and properly trained personnel should be reviewed. The patient must be informed of the intent and expected outcome of treatment and the action that will be performed if an adverse reaction to treatment occurs.

Emergency equipment and supplies should be accessible in the treatment area, and the telephone numbers of qualified advanced medical assistance personnel should be posted (e.g., 911, internal emergency numbers or codes ["Doctor Blue," "Doctor Heart," "Captain Thermo"], and other external numbers). Periodic reviews of emergency procedures should be included in staff education programs and CPR retraining of personnel should be performed annually by qualified instructors.

Special care and attention should be provided to any patient whose condition is more apt to lead to an emergency. For instance, patients who require full-body immersion or who use a therapeutic pool should be provided with fluids before, during, and after treatment to avoid heat exhaustion. The patient injured at or above the T6 cord level should be monitored for noxious stimuli, especially retention of urine to avoid autonomic hyperreflexia. Treatment for patients with diabetes should be scheduled so that patients will not be adversely affected by an insulin injection or food intake prior to receiving treatment. These persons should be counseled to adjust their food or insulin intake according to the type of treatment or amount of physical activity required and in his/her usual amount of exercise and food or insulin intake. The patient with a history of convulsions should be reminded to use his/her anticonvulsive medications consistently and according to the prescriptive instructions.

Each patient's vital signs should be monitored frequently, especially patients whose conditions have the potential to lead to an emergency. The Valsalva maneuver should be avoided by requiring the patient to breathe regularly during exercise. A patient who has been recumbent for extended periods of time or who has a reduced ability to return peripheral venous blood to the heart should be observed and monitored when he/she moves from a recumbent or sitting position to a more upright position. This individual should be given the opportunity to accommodate gradually to an upright position, or preventive measures should be used to relieve symptoms of hypotension. The patient should be protected until it is determined that he/she has accommodated sufficiently to sit or stand safely and without experiencing the symptoms of orthostatic hypotension.

Finally, the caregiver should observe each patient for signs or symptoms of an abnormal physiologic response to treatment and should be prepared to act when an emergency occurs.

■ SELF-STUDY/DISCUSSION ACTIVITIES

1. Describe your responsibilities and obligations to a patient who experiences an injury during or as a result of his/her treatment.

2. Explain how you would treat a person who has experienced heat stroke, heat exhaustion, an insulin reaction, acidosis, or autonomic hyperreflexia.

3. Differentiate the signs and symptoms of heat exhaustion and heat stroke.

4. Differentiate the signs and symptoms of orthostatic hypotension and autonomic hyperreflexia.

5. Outline what you believe should be included in a safety orientation and prevention program for caregivers in an inpatient and an outpatient facility.

6. Describe the activities you would perform to monitor a patient's response to his/her treatment.

7. You find it necessary to apply a bandage for each of the conditions listed. For each condition state the type of bandage you would select, state the rationale for your selection, and apply it on another person: (1) to control joint effusion/swelling after a recent right ankle sprain; (2) to protect the distal aspects (tips) of the center two fingers of the left hand; and (3) to support the proximal, medial tissue of the left thigh after a recent muscle strain.

Chapter 12

Americans With Disabilities Act: A Review

After studying this chapter, the reader will be able to:

1 Explain the purpose of the Americans With Disabilities Act (ADA).

2 Describe the emphasis of the four primary titles of the act.

3 Define the terms associated with the act.

4 Discuss the roles a consultant could perform related to the ADA.

5 Describe actions an employer or business person can perform to respond to the employment and accessibility requirements of the ADA.

INTRODUCTION

Discrimination toward employment and access to workplaces, businesses, and transportation has existed for many years for persons with disabilities. Groups and organizations such as the Equal Employment Commission, President's Committee on Employment of People with Disabilities, National Easter Seal Society, Paralyzed Veterans of America, Multiple Sclerosis Society, Arthritis Foundation, and American Physical Therapy Association have advocated improvement in mobility, access, and employment opportunities for persons with disabilities. Previous federal legislation was designed to protect persons with disabilities from discrimination through the use of certain requirements or incentives. The Fair Housing and Architectural Barriers Act of 1968 and its amendments in 1988, Section 504 of the Rehabilitation Act of 1973, Civil Rights Act of 1964, and Education for all Handicapped Children Act of 1975 are examples of legislation that pertains to persons with disabilities. However, the Americans With Disabilities Act (ADA), which was signed on July 26, 1990, provided enforceable prohibitions and standards that ban discrimination based on disability. The ADA was designed to extend the civil rights for people with disabilities to improve their opportunity for employment by private sector employers; for access to public bus and train service, including AMTRAK; for access to public accommodations and services; and for access to certain types of telecommunications. The ADA is federal anti-discrimination legislation designed to remove employment and access barriers for individuals with disabilities.

The ADA has five titles: Title I, Employment; Title II, Public Service (including public transportation); Title III, Public Accommodations; Title IV, Telecommunications; and Title V, Miscellaneous Provisions. Compliance with most of the regulations and requirements of the ADA was mandated to occur no later than 2 years after the act was signed. At this time, all deadlines for compliance with all regulations have been exceeded, and the legislation is in full effect. It is important to understand the ADA interfaces or is related to other state and federal laws, such as the Family and Medical Leave Act (FMLA), Occupational Safety and Health Act (OSHA), and Worker's Compensation laws in effect in each state. Employers, owners, managers, administrators, and persons who are involved with the employment of workers should become familiar with these acts and laws to understand how they may interact with the ADA. Information and assistance with these relationships can be obtained from state and federal departments of labor and local or federal Equal Employment Opportunity Commission, (EEOC) offices.

It has been estimated there are approximately 49 million persons of all ages with disabilities in the United States. To date, only approximately 25% of these persons are full-time employees.

DEFINITIONS

1. Individual with a disability—Person who has a physical or mental impairment that substantially limits one or more major life activities. Self-care, walking, speaking, breathing, learning, working, and performance of manual skills are major life activities according to the ADA. The ADA protects an individual if he/she has a record of or is regarded as having an impairment.

2. Reasonable accommodation—Making modifications at the job site or workplace that will enable persons with disabilities to easily perform a specific job. Some examples of reasonable accommodations are having a physically accessible workplace, restructuring a job, or adjusting a work schedule or hours of work to meet an individual's needs.

3. Undue burden—An action necessary to provide a reasonable accommodation that would cause the employer or owner significant difficulty or expense. Several factors are considered to determine whether a hardship would occur for the employer or owner; these factors include the size of business, number of its employees, type of operation of the business, nature and cost of the needed accommodation, and whether the accommodation would have an adverse effect or pose a risk to other employees.

4. Qualified individual with a disability—A person who can perform the essential functions of a given job or activity, with or without the benefit of reasonable accommodation. In other words, the person must have the knowledge, skills, and mental and physical capabilities to perform the essential elements of a particular job.

5. Covered entity—Employer, employment agency, labor organization or joint labor management organization, or state and local governments.

Many of the terms in these definitions are not specific and therefore subject to interpretation. The person with a disability, the employer, an attorney, and state or federal agency personnel may differ in their interpretation of the language contained in the ADA. At the time the act became effective, it was anticipated there would be a great amount of litigation related to the meaning and interpretation of ADA language; however, that has not occurred.

GENERAL ASPECTS OF THE ADA

It previously was indicated the ADA contains four primary titles, each of which addresses a specific protected category and has separate compliance requirements. Persons in the private sector who own, manage, or lease a business or are employers and who are involved with any type of business, public service, housing, or workplace regulated by Titles I and III should become familiar with the provisions of those titles. All private sector employees who employ 15 or more employees are required to comply with Title I. In addition, because of the requirements of Title III related to accessibility to public accommodations and most commercial facilities, employers and business owners and their agents are affected even if they employ fewer than 15 persons.

Title I prohibits an employer from discriminating against a qualified individual with a disability on the basis of that disability alone. This prohibition affects job application and hiring procedures, opportunities for advancement, compensation and salary matters, and job training activities. An employer could be considered to have discriminated against a qualified person with a disability if the employer does not make reasonable accommodations for the individual or denies employment based on the need to make reasonable accommodations unless the employer can demonstrate the needed accommodations would cause an undue hardship on the operation of the business.

When a qualified individual with a disability is hired, the employer is required to make accommodations for a known disability that would enable that employee to achieve the same level of performance and to enjoy benefits equal to those of an average, similarly situated person without a disability. However, the accommodation does not have to ensure equal results or provide exactly the same benefits. The employee must request the accommodation, and he/she may suggest an appropriate accommodation. The employer is allowed to review and propose more than one type of accommodation and to select that which is most appropriate or reasonable without leading to undue hardship, providing it effectively allows the person with a disability to perform the job. Accommodations must be determined based on each individual's needs because the nature and extent of a disabling condition and the requirements of a job will vary. Examples of reasonable accommodations, depending on the disabling condition and job requirements, are adjusting the height or changing the cutout area of a desk, adjusting the height and location of shelves, relocating file cabinets, repositioning telephones and other pieces of office equip-

ment, modifying standard office or telecommunications equipment, modifying testing and training activities or procedures, and providing readers or interpreters for persons with a vision or language impairment.

Title III is designed to protect persons with disabilities on the basis of his/her disability from discrimination related to full and equal access to services, facilities, accommodations, goals, privileges, and advantages of any place of public accommodation by the person who owns, leases, or operates a site, place, or facility classified as public accommodation. Virtually every type of private entity or business whose operation affects commerce is considered to be a public accommodation. Examples of public accommodations are a hotel or motel; restaurant or bar; theater or auditorium; convention center or lecture hall; grocery store, shopping center, or sales or retail establishment; laundromat, gas station, or professional office; public transportation building; museum or library; park or zoo, amusement park or places of education; day care center or senior center; and, gymnasium, spa, or bowling alley. For existing facilities and those to be constructed, structural physical barriers must be removed or not included. Removal, modification, or alteration of structural barriers is usually required by Title III when the changes can be made reasonably and accomplished without significant difficulty or expense. The installation of ramps; widening of doorways; use of door hardware that is more functional than a knob that must be turned; provision of an alternative pathway with a firm surface to buildings, parking areas, or areas within a building; installation of support (grab) bars or rails; increase in space in restrooms to accommodate a wheelchair; creation of accessible parking

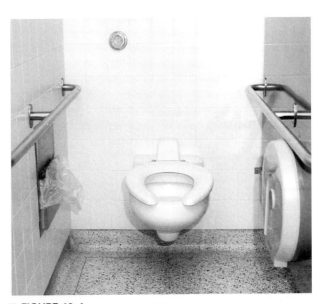

■ **FIGURE 12–1**
Addition of "grab" rails in a public restroom with a slightly elevated commode.

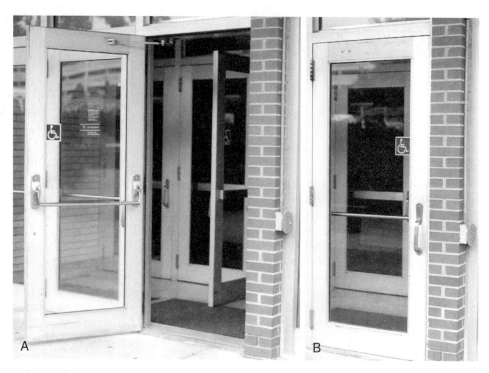

■ **FIGURE 12–2**
A, Pressing the control disk opens the outer and inner doors; the threshold of the outer door may be difficult for some persons in wheelchairs to wheel over. *B,* Electrically operated door on a public building; the control disk is located on the brick column; doors close after a preset time period has elapsed.

spaces; use of telephones and water fountains accessible from a wheelchair; and curb cutouts are typical adjustments that can be made to provide greater access for persons with disabilities (Figs. 12–1 and 12–2*A,B*). In addition, auxiliary services and aids must be provided to individuals with a vision or hearing impairment (Fig. 12–3). Auxiliary services could be as simple as having the server in a restaurant read the menu selections to persons who are visually impaired or having the server prepared to use a pad and pencil to communicate with persons who are hearing impaired. An aid that may be required is a telephone or an outlet for a portable device that will serve the needs of persons with hearing impairments, such as a telecommunication display device (TDD). The provisions of Title III do not apply to exempted entities, including private clubs and establishments that are exempt from Title II of the Civil Rights Act of 1964, religious organizations or entities

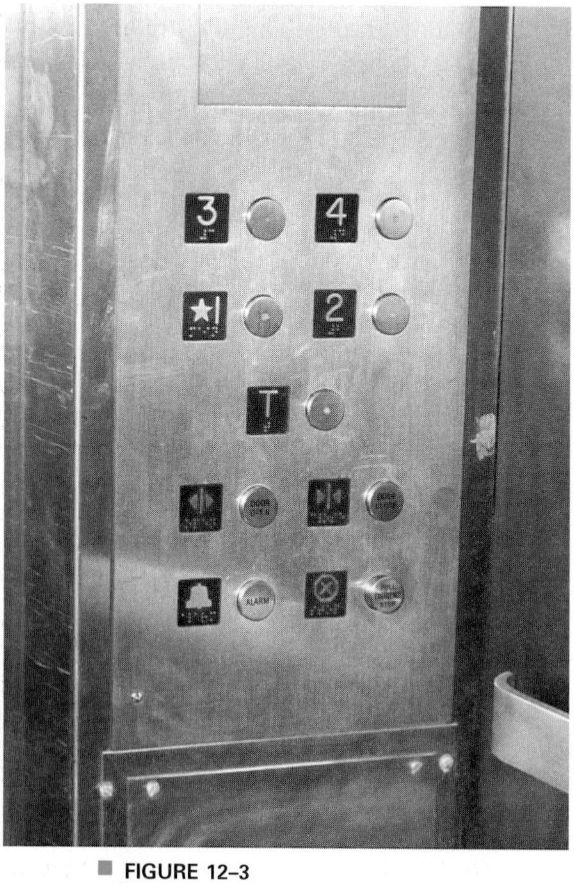

■ **FIGURE 12–3**
Elevator controls with braille symbols.

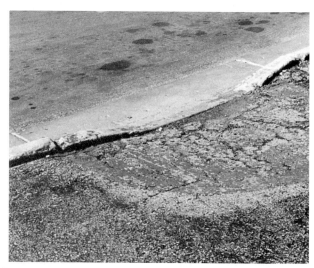

■ **FIGURE 12–4**
Curb cut out showing uneven surfaces, narrow opening, and lack of cross-walk markings. Unfortunately, some cutouts may not be in good repair or functional for wheelchair access.

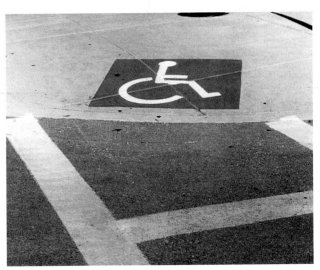

■ FIGURE 12–5
Curb cut out showing smooth, gradual elevation from street level to sidewalk; width of cut out; cross-walk markings; and large turning area on sidewalk in all directions.

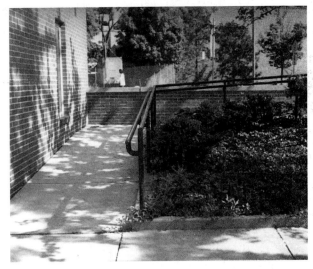

■ FIGURE 12–6
Ramp to public building showing ramp width, even surface, and adequate space to turn wheelchair where direction and slope of ramp change.

controlled by religious organizations, and entities operated by governments that are not covered by Titles I and II (Figs. 12–4 to 12–9).

COMPLIANCE AND IMPLEMENTATION OF REGULATIONS

Employers, managers, administrators, and persons with disabilities should become educated about the employment of persons with disabilities. Consultation with human resource personnel, legal counsel, external qualified consultants, current employees with disabilities, and department supervisors is a recommended initial step. Review of the application form, process, and procedures; selection and hiring procedures; and evaluation, advancement, and training opportunities and activities will help to determine the current and necessary level of compliance with Title I. Time should be spent to determine the essential functions of a job; prepare a comprehensive job description, written in functional terms; observe the workplace layout and environment; and, prepare an on-site job analysis for each job of the business. The physical and mental requirements of the job should be identified as well as any special skills or abilities that are needed. Specific education and training qualifications and any certification or licensure credentials that are required should be listed. The employer and his/her agents involved with the hiring process must be aware of restrictions associated with the limits imposed on preemployment inquiries of applicants. During the preoffer, application phase of the employment process, disability-related questions, medical history information, and medical examinations are prohib-

ited by the ADA unless they are specifically job related. An applicant can be asked whether he/she can perform specific essential job functions such as lift and carry objects, stand for prolonged periods of time, climb a ladder, or use specific pieces of office equipment. When an interview is conducted, the questions asked and the discussion should relate to the information requested on the application and the functional requirements of the job. The interviewer is permitted to ask the applicant about the duties he/she performed in a previous job. Questions about any visible physical characteristics of the applicant, his/her present health status, and his/her psychiatric history or previous addiction to drugs are prohibited.

Medical examinations or evaluations are permitted if they are performed after an offer of employment has been made providing all employees in a specific job category receive the same type of examination. The medical information that is obtained must be placed in a file or separated from his/her personnel file. Preemployment tests for illegal drug use are permitted because such testing is not considered to be part of a medical examination by the ADA. However, employers and their agents should understand that a person who has successfully completed a drug or alcohol abuse rehabilitation program or is enrolled in such a program and is drug free is protected from discrimination by the ADA. When a person with a disability is hired and the disability is made known, the employer should be prepared to address the need for reasonable accommodation to provide a better opportunity for the employee to perform the job. This issue was described previously.

The employer must consider the requirements for accessibility contained in Title II that are different from the reasonable accommodation requirements of Title I. Consultation with a knowledgeable architect,

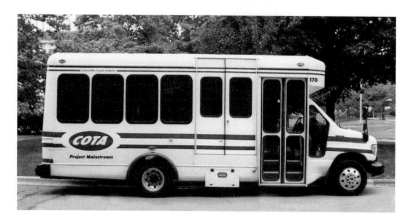

■ **FIGURE 12–7**
Vehicle used to transport persons from home to another location and then back to home. A lift is used to accommodate wheelchair users, and open space with restraints for wheelchairs is available in the vehicle.

qualified design professional or health care professional (i.e., physical therapist, occupational therapist, industrial health specialist), or current employees with disabilities may assist the employer to reach decisions necessary to comply with Title III. Existing facilities classified as public accommodations are required to remove structural architectural barriers where removal is readily achievable. Access into a facility or establishment for persons with disabilities, freedom of movement, and access to goods and services once inside the facility should be given immediate attention. Suggestions and examples of how this can be accomplished have been presented previously. If the re-

moval of existing architectural barriers is not readily achievable, the facility, establishment, or entity must provide its goods, services, facilities, privileges, advantages, or accommodations through alternative methods if such methods are readily achievable. To comply with these requirements, a business may need to provide a "drive-through" window, offer home deliveries, or provide catalog sales. *Note:* "Readily achievable" is defined as being able to be accomplished easily and performed without much difficulty or expense. The categories of the accessibility audit requirements for public accommodations are contained in Box 12–1. Specific requirements, specifications, and guidelines for each of these categories are contained in the *Code of Federal Regulations,* Department of Justice, Civil Rights Division; 28 CFR, Part 36; July 1, 1994 (revised). According to data available from the Presi-

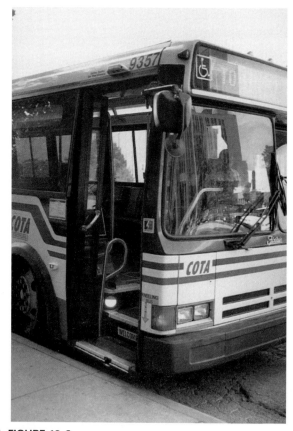

■ **FIGURE 12–8**
Kneeling bus in lowered position (operated by Central Ohio Transit Authority).

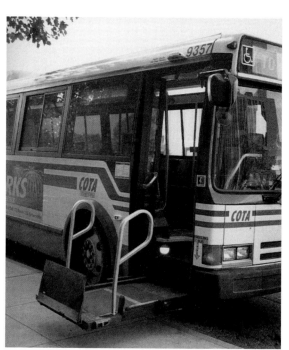

■ **FIGURE 12–9**
Bus with lift being lowered; vertical panel prevents a wheelchair from rolling off the lift, and another panel or bar prevents the chair from rolling toward the bus (not in photograph).

BOX 12–1

Accessibility Audit Requirement Categories

1. Ramps and slopes
2. Doors and hallways
3. Signage
4. Stairs and elevators
5. Flooring
6. Obstacles and protrusions
7. Reach range and clear space
8. Seating
9. Equipment (i.e., telephones, drinking fountains, controls and receptacles, toilet rooms)
10. Accessible path and walkway
11. Parking and loading zone
12. Alarms and warnings
13. Area for emergency refuge

dent's Committee on Employment of People with Disabilities, approximately 80% of the costs to make existing facilities accessible have been less than $1000.00 and 50% of the changes have cost less than $50.00. Extensive remodeling of a facility usually is not required, but creative and innovative ways of thinking

BOX 12–2

Activities for an Americans With Disabilities Act Consultant

1. Educate employers, managers, supervisors, employees, and persons with disabilities about the ADA, particularly Titles I and III.
2. Perform on-site job analysis; identify essential job functions.
3. Perform on-site environmental evaluation.
4. Assist to develop function-based job descriptions.
5. Advise on job-related accommodation needs.
6. Advise on the removal of physical barriers and the improvement of access internally and externally.
7. Perform physical capacity and functional ability testing of current and prospective employees based on essential job functions.
8. Assist to develop policies and procedures related to compliance with the ADA.

BOX 12–3

Suggestions for Employers for Hiring Persons With Disabilities

1. Learn where to locate and how to recruit people with disabilities.
2. Learn how to communicate and interact with people who have disabilities.
3. Be certain company applications and employment forms do not ask for disability-related information and they are formatted so they are accessible to all persons with disabilities.
4. Prepare written job descriptions that clearly and specifically identify the essential functions of a job.
5. Be certain company medical examinations, evaluations, or tests comply with the ADA.
6. Be prepared to provide reasonable accommodations needed by a qualified applicant to compete for the job.
7. Treat the individual with a disability with dignity and respect.
8. Know that persons protected by the ADA include persons with acquired immune deficiency syndrome or cancer or who are mentally retarded, deaf, blind, learning impaired, or brain injured due to trauma.
9. Train supervisors and other employees about making reasonable accommodations.
10. Use procedures to maintain and protect medical records as confidential.
11. Prepare and train all employees to communicate, interact, and work with people with disabilities.

are important elements to use to resolve the majority of accommodation or accessibility problems.

A qualified and knowledgeable health care professional consultant is a valuable resource for an employer. Activities or roles that could be expected of such a consultant are presented in Box 12–2. The employer should review and evaluate the person's credentials, qualifications, and postconsultation experiences to determine his/her level of expertise before contracting for his/her services. The desired and expected outcome or product of the consultation; time frame for the consultation, costs and expenses anticipated, and method of payment for the services should be clearly identified to the satisfaction of the persons involved with the consultation.

The ADA also provides some tax incentives to encourage employers and business owners to comply with the act (Box 12–3). The Internal Revenue

Service allows a deduction of up to $15,000 per year for expenses associated with the removal of qualified architectural and transportation barriers. In addition, small businesses are eligible to receive a tax credit of up to $5000 for certain costs that are incurred to comply with the ADA. When the two incentives are added, a small business owner could accrue $20,000 in tax incentives in 1 year. As in all tax-related matters, consultation with a tax advisor is recommended to review and assist with the preparation and filing of the appropriate documents.

SUMMARY

On July 26, 1990, the ADA was signed, and most requirements contained in it became effective on July 26, 1992. Each of the four primary titles contains regulations, guidelines, and prohibitions specific to that title. The purpose of the ADA is to prohibit discrimination against persons with disabilities, based on the disability, through comprehensive and enforceable prohibitions. The act was designed to extend the civil rights for people with disabilities in the areas of employment (Title I); access to goods, services, and facilities classified as public accommodations (Title III); access to certain types of public transportation, including AMTRAK (Title II); access to government employment, facilities and services (Title II); and access to auxiliary devices and aids such as telecommunications (Title IV) (Box 12–4).

The ADA is complex legislation that requires careful study before an individual can become reasonably familiar with the act. Many terms and concepts are not defined specifically and at times may appear to be ambiguous and subject to interpretation; therefore, assistance or consultation with a variety of persons, including an architect, attorney, or industrial health specialist or a health care professional, may be necessary to gain information and suggestions on compliance with the act. There are many resources available that provide specific information about the many requirements of the ADA; several of them are located in the Bibliography.

Although most of the requirements of the act have been in effect since July 1992, increased education of employers, persons with disabilities, members of many professions, students enrolled in health care education programs, and society about the purpose and extent of the ADA is needed. Many health care professionals profess themselves to be advocates for persons with disabilities, but they have not been active in promoting or providing information about the ADA. Graduates of many professional education programs have limited knowledge of the ADA; this limits their ability to educate others or serve as advocates for

---

BOX 12–4

Summary of Americans With Disabilities Act Titles I Through IV

Title I: Employment
Employers may not discriminate against an individual with a disability in hiring or promoting if the person is otherwise qualified for the job. Employers will need to provide "reasonable accommodations" to individuals with disabilities, including job restructuring and equipment modification, but they need not provide accommodations that impose an "undue hardship" on business operations. Regulated by the Equal Employment Opportunity Commission.

Title II: Public Service
State and local governments may not discriminate against qualified individuals with disabilities. All government facilities, including public transportation and communication, must be accessible. Regulated by the Secretary of Transportation.

Title III: Public Accommodations
Public accommodations operated by private entities such as restaurants, hotels, retail stores, and theaters may not discriminate against individuals with disabilities. Auxiliary aids and services must be provided to individuals with vision or hearing impairments or other individuals with disabilities, unless an undue burden would result. Physical barriers in existing facilities must be removed if removal is readily achievable; if not readily achievable, alternative methods to provide service or access, if they are readily achievable, must be provided. All new construction and alterations to public accommodations must be accessible. Regulated by the Attorney General.

Title IV: Telecommunications
Companies or businesses offering telephone service to the general public must offer telephone relay services to individuals who use telecommunication devices for the deaf (TDDs) or similar devices. Regulated by the Federal Communications Commission.

---

persons with disabilities. Minimal research has been performed and published related to the effect or outcomes of the act for employers, persons with disabilities, or society; therefore, continued investigation of the values, limitations, costs, enforcement, and awareness of the effects of the ADA on society seems warranted.

■ SELF-STUDY/DISCUSSION ACTIVITIES

1. State the purpose of the ADA.

2. List and describe the major theme of Titles I through IV of the ADA.

3. Describe how you could serve as a consultant to an employer to assist him/her to comply with Titles I and III of the ADA.

4. Visit several workplaces or businesses and identify structural architectural barriers; explain how they could be eliminated or modified to comply with Title III of the ADA.

5. Outline activities an employer could perform to become prepared to employ persons with disabilities.

6. Propose three or four topics that would be appropriate for investigation and research.

BIBLIOGRAPHY

The Accessible Housing Design File. Florence, KY: Barrier Free Environments, Inc.

The ADA: An Easy Checklist. Chicago, IL; National Easter Seal Society.

ADA Title 1 Technical Assistance Manual. Washington, D.C. 20507, U.S. Equal Employment Opportunity Commission; January 1992.

Adaptable Housing. Washington, D.C.: US Department of Housing and Urban Development.

Adult basic life support. *Journal of the American Medical Association* 268(16):2184–2198, 1992.

The Agency for Health Care Policy and Research: *Clinical Practice Guideline: Treatment of Pressure Ulcers.* Silver Springs, MD; December, 1994.

The Agency for Health Care Policy and Research: *Quick Reference Guide.* Silver Springs, MD; December, 1994.

American Red Cross: *Community First Aid and Safety.* St. Louis, MO: Mosby-Year Book, 1993.

Americans With Disabilities Act Accessibility Requirements: U.S. Architectural and Transportation Barriers Compliance Board. December, 1991.

Amundsen LR: Assessing exercise tolerance: A review. *Physical Therapy* 59(5):534–537, 1979.

Apts D, Blankenship K: *The American Back School Manual.* Ashland, KY: American Back School, 1980.

Atlas of Orthotics, American Academy of Orthopedic Surgeons. St. Louis, MO: C. V. Mosby, 1975.

Back Owner's Manual. Daly City, CA: Physicians Art Service, 1991.

Back Pain. San Bruno, CA: Krames Communications, 1986.

Back Tips for Health Care Providers. San Bruno, CA: Krames Communications, 1987.

Barrier-Free House Plans. Des Plaines, IL; Professional Builder, 1350 East Touhy Ave, 1995.

Bergen A, Colongelo C: *Evaluating the Environment: Problem Solving Worksheet.* Camarillo, CA: Everest and Jennings, 1984.

Birdsall C: How accurate are your blood pressures? *American Journal of Nursing* 84(11):1414, 1984.

Blessey RL, et al: *Clinical Decision Making in Physical Therapy.* Philadelphia, PA: F.A. Davis, 1985.

Blood Borne Infections: A Practical Guide to OSHA Compliance. Arlington, TX: Johnson and Johnson Medical, 1992.

Body Substance Precautions in Schools: Recommendations. Columbus, OH: The Ohio Department of Health, 1991.

Bonewit K: *Clinical Procedures for Medical Assistants.* 3rd edition. Philadelphia, PA: W. B. Saunders, 1990.

Brown V, Graf S: Lecture notes and handouts. Columbus, OH: Physical Therapy Division, School of Allied Medical Professions, The Ohio State University, 1985.

Cardiopulmonary Resuscitation. Dallas, TX: American Heart Association, 1987.

Care and Service. Wheelchair Prescriptions: Booklet No. 4. Camarillo, CA: Everest and Jennings, 1983.

Carr J, Shepherd R: *A Motor Relearning Program for Stroke.* 2nd edition. Rockville, MD: Aspen, 1987.

Case-Smith J: *Practical Aspects of Using Outcomes Measures.* Model Program for Linking Allied Health Education, Research and Practice: Columbus, OH: pp. 82–93: November 1996.

Choosing a wheelchair system. *Journal of Rehabilitation Research and Development.* Clinical Supplement. Washington, D.C.: Department of Veterans Affairs. March (suppl 2): 1990.

Clarkson HM, Gilewich GB: *Musculoskeletal Assessment.* Baltimore, MD: Williams and Wilkins, 1989.

Code of Federal Regulations 28CFR Part 36: Nondiscrimination on the Basis of Disability by Public Accommodations and in Commercial Facilities. Washington, D.C.: July 1994.

Connolly JB: A new breed of consultant. *Clin Mgmt* 12:72–80, 1992.

Connolly JB: Understanding the ADA. *Clin Mgmt* 12:40–45, 1992.

Coruth F, Thompson F: *Transfer and Lifting Techniques for Extended Care.* Vancouver, BC: Evergreen Press, 1983.

Danger Signs and Symptoms: Clinical Skillbuilders. Springhouse, PA: Springhouse Corporation, 1990.

Daniels L, Worthingham C: *Muscle Testing: Techniques of Manual Examination.* 5th edition. Philadelphia, PA: W. B. Saunders, 1986.

Domenico RL, Ziegler WZ: *Practical Rehabilitation Techniques for Geriatric Aides.* Rockville, MD: Aspen Publishing, 1989.

Duff JF: *Youth Sports Injuries.* New York, NY: Macmillan, 1992.

Emergencies. Springhouse, PA: Springhouse Corporation, 1985.

Emergency Procedures: Clinical Skillbuilders. Springhouse, PA: Springhouse Corporation, 1991.

Erdos EE, Jared M, Steinheiser: *Basic intravenous therapy.* Seminar proceedings, NCS Health Care, 1992.

Fahland B, Grendahl BA: *Wheelchair Selection: More Than Choosing a Chair with Wheels.* Minneapolis, MN: American Rehabilitation Foundation, 1967.

First Aid for Choking. Dallas, TX: American Heart Association, 1988.

Fit Back Workout. San Bruno, CA: Krames Communications, 1990.

Freed M, Hofkosh J, Kaplan L, Neuhauser C: Choosing ambulatory aids. *Patient Care* October 15:20–35, 1987.

Freed M, Hofkosh J, Kaplan L, Neuhauser C: Using ambulatory aids. *Patient Care* 21(16):36–46, 1987.

Garritan S, Jones P, Kornberg T, Parkin C: Laboratory values in the intensive care unit. *Acute Care Persp* Winter 1995.

Ghasemi Z, Martin T: The role of the physical therapist in the intensive care unit. *Acute Care Persp* Winter 1995.

Gomella LG (ed.): *Clinician's Pocket Reference.* 6th edition. Norwalk, CT: Appleton and Lange, 1989.

Guidelines for Documentation. Presented to nursing personnel at Rosegate Convalescent Center, Columbus, OH, 1991.

Guidelines for Exposure Determination and Prevention. Cincinnati-Dayton, OH: Association for Practitioners in Infection Control, 1992.

Guidelines for prevention of transmission of human immunodeficiency virus and hepatitis B virus to health care and public safety workers. Atlanta, GA: Centers for Disease Control, *MMWR* 38(5–6):3–37, 1989.

Hamilton HK (ed.): *Nursing Procedures.* Springhouse, PA: Intermed Communications, 1983, pp. 249–262.

High Blood Pressure. New York, NY: American Heart Association, 1969.

Hill PH, et al. *Making Decisions.* Reading, MA: Addison-Wesley, 1979.

Hollis M: *Safe Lifting for Patient Care.* 2nd edition. Oxford, England: Blackwell Scientific Publications, 1985.

Hoppenfeld S: *Physical Examination of the Spine and Extremities.* New York, NY: Appleton-Century-Crofts, 1976.

Hospital infection control. In *Employee Orientation Notebook.* Columbus, OH: Riverside Methodist Hospital, 1992.

Jobst-Custom Graduated Compression Supports Measuring and Fitting Manual. Charlotte, NC: Jobst.

Kendall FP, McCreary EK: *Muscle Testing and Function.* 3rd edition. Baltimore, MD: Williams and Wilkins, 1983.

Kendall K: Evolution of Sacred Heart Hospital's Wound Assessment Sheet. *Acute Care Perspectives* (Newsletter of the Acute Care/Hospital Clinical Practice Section, American Physical Therapy Association), Pompton Plains, NJ, Summer, pp. 6–8, 1995.

Kennedy KL: *Wound Caring.* Eau Claire, WI: Professional Education Systems, Inc, January 1997.

Kennedy KL: Wound caring. Seminar, Columbus, OH; March 17, 1997.

Kenney WL: *ASCM's Guidelines for Exercise Testing and Prescription.* 5th edition. Baltimore, MD: Williams & Wilkins, 1995.

Kettenbach G: *Writing S.O.A.P. Notes.* Philadelphia, PA: F. A. Davis, 1990.

Kisner C, Colby LA: *Therapeutic Exercise: Foundations and Techniques.* 3rd edition. Philadelphia, PA: F. A. Davis, 1996.

Koblenzer L, Gyuricza B: *Nursing Concepts and Procedures Relevant to Physical Therapy.* Cleveland, OH: Physical Therapy Department, Department of Health Sciences, Cleveland State University, 1982.

Kumar V, Cotran RS, Robbin SL: *Basic Pathology.* 5th edition. Philadelphia: W. B. Saunders, 1992.

Lehmkuhl LD, Smith LK: *Brunnstrom's Clinical Kinesiology.* 4th edition. Philadelphia, PA: F. A. Davis, 1983.

Lewis C: Wheelchair use for the older patient. *Physical Therapy Forum* 11(23):4–7, 1992.

Lewis LV: *Fundamental Skills in Patient Care.* Philadelphia, PA: J. B. Lippincott, 1976.

Magee DJ: *Orthopedic Physical Assessment.* 2nd edition. Philadelphia: W. B. Saunders, 1992.

McArdle WD, Katch FI, Katch VL: *Essentials of Exercise Physiology.* 4th edition. Philadelphia: Lea & Febiger, 1994.

McCash T: *Procedures for the ADA.* Dublin, OH: Meacham and Apel Architects Inc., October 1991.

McCulloch JM, Kloth LC: Decision point: Wound dressings. *PT Magazine* 4:52–62, 1996.

Meyer K: *Ten Commandments for Communicating With Persons With Disabilities.* Axis Center for Public Awareness of People with Disabilities: Columbus, OH.

McCulloch JM, Kloth LC, Feddar JA: *Wound Healing Alternatives in Management.* 2nd edition. Philadelphia: F. A. Davis, 1995.

Measuring Blood Pressure: A Guide for Paramedical Personnel. West Point, PA: Merck, Sharp and Dohme.

Measuring the Patient. Wheelchair Prescriptions: Booklet No. 1. Camarillo, CA: Everest and Jennings, 1983.

Minor SD, Minor MA: *Patient Care Skills.* 2nd edition. Norwalk, CT: Appleton and Lange, 1990.

Mirone JA: Understanding the Americans with Disabilities Act. *Healthcare Trends Trans* 4:36–38, 1993.

Morey S: Pressure Ulcer Wound Care. Presented at Ohio Physical Therapy Association, April 17, 1997, Columbus, OH.

Murdock KR: ICU paraphernalia: Physical therapy implications. *Acute Care Persp* Winter 1995.

Najdeski P: Crutch measurement from the sitting position. *Physical Therapy* 57(7):826–827, 1977.

National Pressure Ulcer Advisory Panel: *A Selected Bibliography: Pressure Ulcer Assessment, Prevention and Treatment.* 3435 Main Street, Buffalo, NY; April 1995.

Norkin C, Levangie P: *Joint Structure and Function: A Comprehensive Analysis.* 2nd edition. Philadelphia, PA: F. A. Davis, 1990.

Nursing Photobook Annual. Springhouse, PA: Springhouse Corporation, 1987.

Occupational Safety and Health Administration, Department of Labor: Occupational exposure to bloodborne pathogens; Final rule. *Federal Register.* December 6, 1991.

Ohio Hospital Association: Occupational exposure to bloodborne pathogens; OSHA's final rule. *OHA Bulletin,* December 20, 1991.

Okamoto GA, Phillips TJ (eds.): *Physical Medicine and Rehabilitation.* Philadelphia, PA: W. B. Saunders, 1984.

O'Sullivan SB, Schmitz TJ: *Physical Rehabilitation: Assessment and Treatment.* 3rd edition. Philadelphia, PA: F. A. Davis, 1994.

O'Toole M (ed.): *Encyclopedia and Dictionary of Medicine, Nursing and Allied Health.* Philadelphia, PA: W. B. Saunders, 1992.

O'Toole M (ed.): *Miller-Keane Encyclopedia and Dictionary of Medicine, Nursing, and Allied Health.* 5th edition. Philadelphia: W. B. Saunders, 1992.

Palmer ML: Gross muscle testing. *Clinical Management* 5(4):18–24, 1985.

Palmer ML, Toms J: *Manual for Functional Training.* 3rd edition. Philadelphia, PA: F. A. Davis, 1992.

Perry AG, Potter PA: *Clinical Nursing Skills and Techniques.* 2nd edition. St. Louis, MO: C. V. Mosby, 1990, pp. 315–335, 403–405, 691–693, 733–756.

Person First. AXIS Center for Public Awareness of People with Disabilities: Columbus, OH: April 1995.

Polich S, Faynoor SM: Interpreting lab test values. *PT Magazine* 4:76–88, 1996.

Poor Posture Hurts. San Bruno, CA: Kramer Communications, 1986.

President's Committee on Employment of People with Disabilities: Washington, D.C. 20004–1107.

Procedures. Springhouse, PA: Intermed Communications, 1983, pp. 502–508, 568–572, 665–669.

Product Report: Wheelchair. Washington, DC: American Association of Retired Persons, 1990.

Project Action. Washington, D.C.; National Easter Seal Society.

Project ADA. Chicago, IL; National Easter Seal Society.

Purtilo R: *Health Professional and Patient Interaction.* 4th edition. Philadelphia, PA: W. B. Saunders, 1990.

Rantz MF, Courtial D: *Lifting, Moving and Transferring Patients.* 2nd edition. St. Louis, MO: C. V. Mosby, 1981.

Recommendations for Human Blood Pressure Determination by Sphygmomanometers. Dallas, TX: American Heart Association, 1984.

Recommendations for prevention of HIV transmission in health care settings. Atlanta, GA: Centers for Disease Control *MMWR,* 36(2S):377–382, 387–388, 1987.

Rules and Regulations Occupational Safety and Health Act. *Federal Register.* December, 1991; 56(235):64, 175, 182.

Safety and Handling. Wheelchair Prescriptions: Booklet No. 3. Camarillo, CA: Everest and Jennings, 1983.

Saunders HD: *For Your Back, A Self-Help Manual.* Minneapolis, MN: Viking Press, 1985.

Scott R, Cooperman J: Legal and ethical practice issues in physical therapy. Presented at Ohio Physical Therapy Association, April 16, 1997, Columbus, OH.

Scully RM, Barnes MR (eds.): *Physical Therapy.* Philadelphia, PA: J. B. Lippincott, 1989.

Swanson MA: *Crutches on the Go.* Bellevue, WA: Medic Publications, 1974.

Taylor PM, Taylor DK (eds.): *Conquering Athletic Injuries.* Champaign, IL: Leisure Press, 1988.

Techniques for Moving Patients. Deerfield, MA: Dray Publications.

Umiker W: *Management Skills for the New Health Care Supervisor.* Rockville, MD: Aspen, 1988.

Umphred DA (ed.): *Neurological Rehabilitation.* 2nd edition. St. Louis, MO: C. V. Mosby, 1990.

Update: Universal precautions for prevention of transmission of human immunodeficiency virus, hepatitis B virus and other bloodborne pathogens in health-care settings. Atlanta, GA: Centers for Disease Control *MMWR,* 37(24):377–382, 1988.

Voss DE, Ionta MK, Myers BJ: *Proprioceptive Neuromuscular Facilitation.* 3rd edition. Philadelphia, PA: Harper and Row, 1985.

Weiss M: Class notes and handouts. Columbus, OH: Physical Therapy Division, School of Allied Medical Professions, The Ohio State University, 1975.

Weiss M: Class notes and handouts. Canton, OH: Stark Technical College, 1982.

What Everyone Should Know About Diabetes. Greenfield, MA: Channing L. Bete Company.

Wheelchair Selection. Wheelchair Prescriptions: Booklet No. 2. Camarillo, CA: Everest and Jennings, 1983.

Wilson AB Jr: *Wheelchairs, A Prescription Guide.* Charlottesville, VA: Rehabilitation Press, 1986.

Wood EC, Becker PD: *Beard's Massage.* 4th edition. Philadelphia, PA: W. B. Saunders, 1990.

Wood LA (ed.): *Nursing Skills for Allied Health Services.* 3 vols. Philadelphia, PA: W. B. Saunders, 1975.

Index

Page numbers in *italics* refer to figures; page numbers followed by t refer to tabular material.